Praise for *Kill Switch*

Kill Switch by Richard K. Burt, MD, is a thoroughly researched, scholarly history of the relationship between humans and viruses beginning with smallpox, several centuries ago, and ending with COVID-19. It is written for the general public, with scientific concepts explained in layman's terms and copious historical background that is not typically available in routine sources. This book details the efforts of humanity to do battle with viruses over centuries, revealing the mistakes and subsequent corrections in the process of understanding viral etiology and the production of vaccines and antiviral drugs. Dr. Burt is an alumnus of the NIH, a leading physician-scientist in the field of bone-marrow transplantation, and a scholar of the highest integrity. This stunning book reveals the complexities of vaccine and drug production, as well as the good and poor decisions made by healthcare leadership up to the present day. It is truly a gift to the American people and should be read by everyone.

—Miriam C. Poirier, PhD, Scientist Emeritus, National Institutes of Health, National Cancer Institute, Laboratory of Cancer Biology and Genetics

Professor Burt has been a national, award-winning leader in the development of new treatment of autoimmune disease using stem cell transplantation for decades. His inventive treatment paradigms have advanced an entire field to the great benefit of many patients. As such, he understands innovation from the physician-scientist's point of view. This vantage allows Dr. Burt to guide your remarkable journey down a wandering path of insight, innovation, and discovery that leads to amazing and important breakthroughs in vaccines. His writing style is crisp and witty and engaging. Enjoy your journey!

—Charles Link, MD, FACP, Executive Chairman of Syncromune, Inc. USA

For me, *Kill Switch* was fascinating and hard to put down. Loaded with information on science, medicine, history, and politics, it is easy to read and well suited both for the medical professional and layperson alike. Well referenced and well written, Dr. Richard Burt presents the facts and allows you to draw your own conclusions as to whether the COVID-19 pandemic was indeed created in a Chinese lab with US taxpayer dollars.

—United States Congressman Dave Weldon, MD

This book is written by a physician-scientist who pioneered novel advances using stem cells for autoimmune diseases. Using his honed bench to bedside skills, Dr. Burt transports us into the world of viruses. Remarkably close to us and even together with us, there is a unique and constantly changing microworld of viruses that has a dramatic impact on population health and influences economics, politics, and public policy. In his extraordinary monograph, Professor Burt performed sophisticated and comprehensive insight into interaction of viruses and human beings. It is a thought-provoking analysis about the benefits and harms of this interaction. *Kill Switch* is incredibly unique as it may be used both as an encyclopedia about biology of viruses, their evolution, and development of vaccines, as well the thoughtful story about the challenges of the past and present world. With no doubt, this monograph will be of interest to all those who are concerned about the future of mankind.

—Professor Denis A. Fedorenko, MD, PhD, Pirogov's
National Medical Surgical Center, Moscow, Russia

Kill Switch conceptualizes viruses and global pandemics with a renewed vigor and perspective. It transports the audience into the interplay between viruses and the immune system and how that affects us individually and as a worldwide community. Dr. Burt's book offers a timely reminder of the devastating impact of past viral epidemics and underscores the importance of applying new insights—immunologic and otherwise—to mitigate future public health crises. Dr. Burt's thoughtful examination of these events, as presented in this multifaceted book, has many aspects and depths to be grasped by different readers and with each new reading. It provides a valuable and accessible synthesis of lesions learned—and those yet to be fully understood.

—Professor Shimon Slavin, MD, Scientific & Medical Director,
Biotherapy International The Center for Innovative Cancer
Immunotherapy & Cellular Medicine, Tel Aviv, Israel

Richard K. Burt's *Kill Switch* exemplifies a passionate commitment to free speech, independent thought, and intellectual courage—qualities crucial in today's scientific discourse. Dr. Burt challenges orthodox narratives, weaving detailed scientific explanations with significant historical events to enrich readers' understanding. Although some conclusions are controversial and merit careful consideration, *Kill Switch* serves as an important conversation starter, inviting further inquiry and debate. As a complement to conventional scientific literature, this book offers a valuable dissenting voice that highlights the necessity of open intellectual dialogue.

—Professor Joachim Burman, MD, PhD,
Uppsala University, Uppsala, Sweden

Dr. Richard Burt's pioneering work for over three decades has propelled science forward in the treatment of multiple diseases. I should know. Dr. Burt's work on hematopoietic stem cell transplant in treating multiple sclerosis patients saved my own life in 2018. In *Kill Switch*, a doctor and world-famous researcher provides a factual, dispassionate, and illuminating telling of the history of disease discovery, research, and treatment, from COVID-19, to AIDS, to HPV, to yellow fever. Dr. Burt speaks from deep inside the medical and scientific world to the reader outside the medical and scientific world about both the most beneficial and most controversial historical moments of disease discovery and treatment—ones many magazines have been too afraid to cover. Dr. Burt never shields the reader from controversial facts, such as the FDA continues to allow the use of animal cells for vaccine production or that some study participants for disease have been intentionally left untreated to observe them and advance the interests of science. Dr. Burt doesn't tell the reader how to interpret this information. He doesn't think for the reader. He only gives the reader the knowledge, *all* the knowledge, so that we can think for ourselves. Here is a doctor who treats both the patient and the reader as his intellectual equal, one whom he believes has a right to know the truth about how disease treatments were discovered. All the truth.

—Professor Sandra Didi, MA; University of Texas,
Fellow for the Association for the Study of Middle East
and Africa; Analyst for the US Military

Dr. Burt is a pioneering researcher and doctor. At the beginning of the COVID pandemic, I was fortunate to meet him on a plane flight. He informed me of NIH funding virus gain of function research in Wuhan, China. The fear to say anything other than that of the White House and lay media narrative was so palpable that within my own department when I mentioned Dr. Burt's information, I was warned not to repeat it. What went wrong in our society that even a chief of police would be made to fear asking honest questions? Over time, more information trickled out confirming what Dr. Burt had told me. In this book, only Dr. Burt can explain the history of science behind COVID and vaccines that leaves the reader with a logical and realistic understanding of what happened. There are many lifesaving lessons gained in this outstanding read. For people to have confidence in our institutions, we need people with integrity and courage to report the good and the bad. Enjoy your read, you will learn a lot that was not said.

—Richard Smith, Chief of Police (retired), Kansas City, Missouri

Dr. Richard Burt's *Kill Switch* makes insightful and thought-provoking reading for anyone interested in learning about the role of viruses in shaping history throughout the ages, how governments have responded to their threats, and how scientists have managed to harness their power to the benefit of humanity. By wrapping history around science, it makes both topics interesting. A refreshingly honest book you cannot set down—worthy of a Pulitzer.

—Professor Basil Sharrack, PhD,
University of Sheffield, United Kingdom

Kill Switch provides a highly readable history of viruses in human history. The book takes complicated scientific and medical ideas and translates them for the average reader. In telling this history, Dr. Burt makes unexpected cultural connections in the discovery of and treatment for different viruses, and when the book examines the origin of COVID-19, the story transforms into a medical thriller.

—Associate Professor Tod Chambers, PhD, Feinberg School of Medicine, Northwestern University, Chicago, Illinois

This book should be read by all medical students and health professionals, but also by laypeople and politicians to capture "*How Viruses Shaped Humanity*" and why life on our planet is more complex than wishful thinking. *Kill Switch* is a token of the vast knowledge of the author, Dr. Richard Burt, that will guide the readers through the looking glass into a deeper world. A splendid tribute based on facts, science, history, and compassion to human inquisitiveness when entering an invisible realm that alters our world. The question may be asked: Which side of the looking glass is real, and which is an emergent phenomenon?

—Professor Domique Farge, MD, PhD, Hospital St-Louis, Paris, France

Proviso: There is a submicroscopic world of viruses and smaller world of atoms that exists next to and within us. They affect and alter our life, society, and destiny. Scientists who enter that realm are daring greatly to benefit humanity. They are human with human fragilities and fears. If they stumble, become fixed in a single mind frame, or lost in their rabbit hole, they should still be respected for their courage to seek answers, but neither should the lessons learned be ignored. As such, this book should not be twisted to imply or conclude that any person mentioned herein set out on their trek to do intentional harm. On the contrary, the motivation behind this book is to show how good intentions may break bad, to provide a historical perspective for how we arrived at this junction, to stimulate independent thinking, and to empower our children as they and their children face the unknown without us.

KILL SWITCH

The History of How Viruses Shaped Humanity and Led to COVID-19

Richard K. Burt, MD

Forefront
BOOKS

Kill Switch: The History of How Viruses Shaped Humanity and Led to COVID-19

Published by Forefront Books, Nashville, Tennessee.
Distributed by Simon & Schuster.

Library of Congress Control Number: 2025909696

Print ISBN: 978-1-63763-467-7
E-book ISBN: 978-1-63763-468-4

Cover Design by Michelle Manley
Interior Design by PerfecType, Nashville, TN

Printed in the United States of America
25 26 27 28 29 30 [RR4] 10 9 8 7 6 5 4 3 2 1

FOREWORD ECCLESIASTICAL:

By Monsignor Tomasz Trafny, Former Head of Science and Faith Department at the Pontifical Council for Culture, Vatican, Italy

Medical research has reached levels of sophistication that within the same medical knowledge multiple ramifications have arisen of such complexity that doctors themselves are unable to follow anything but a few particular specializations. Often, people without medical training not only fail to understand the language, but do not even grasp the general concepts that frame the health conditions of themselves or their loved ones. On the one hand, therefore, one has the impression that medicine is turning more and more into a hermetic knowledge, far from nonexperts and, consequently, inaccessible to the majority of people. However, it would be difficult to find even a single human person who has never felt the need for this "special" knowledge in his or her life. We all feel that our lives are marked or even pervaded by the ever-changing diseases that require the intervention of the "possessors" of that hermetic knowledge we commonly call "doctors."

Dr. Richard K. Burt's book is a rare example of an extraordinary ability to communicate difficult concepts in an engaging, captivating, and understandable way, making them accessible to "laymen."

A comprehensible image of the efforts undertaken to eradicate certain diseases is outlined through the historical background, the presentation of the scientists and institutions behind complex medical research, the tracing of socio-economic contexts, and the ethical questions that arise every time scientific experimentations are done. At the same time, at the front of the reader, an important horizon of reflection opens up on progress and its price, understood not only in terms of the sacrifice (commitment) of thousands of researchers, but the actual sacrifice of human lives for a variety of reasons, unfortunately sometimes simply economic.

Scientific research, in fact, is an arduous endeavour often marked by multiple failures and errors that are not silenced in this book. On the contrary, pointing out some of them helps in addressing important ethical questions about how to prevent possible tragedies. In a more general context, it is a question that concerns each of us. How many times, in fact, have we made a wrong choice or taken a misstep with irreparable consequences? How many times have we thought if I could stop everything to avoid a disaster? Science found a possible solution, which is called the kill switch. The ultimate reflection of this book is precisely about this kind of switch that can prevent irreparable damage. Moreover, we should rather talk about a set of kill switches because there are many: the supervisory and control bodies or organizations, the evaluation processes of the results by the scientific community, the involvement of patients (informed consent), the ethical-legal codifications, the procedures to avoid conflict of interest, freedom from the censorship of truth, and so forth.

In addition, the reader will find many stimulating reflections on and explanations of scientific research, as well as multiple ethical questions such as the following: Is research truly driven by principles of altruism and empathy for those who suffer or rather by mere profit? Are we still free individuals who "own" ourselves or has a part of us already been acquired and perhaps patented by some pharmaceutical company or a research institute, after having signed a few disclaimers in preparation for a medical exam? Are we consciously participating in the advancement of human knowledge, or we are simply used as a mere resource of the biological material to be acquired?

Dr. Burt's *Kill Switch* raises both our personal and collective awareness. Without similar stimuli for broad societal and cultural discussion and, more importantly, without instruments such as kill switches, it could be that one day the only trace of our existence will be "the immortal drive"—"a record of our digital DNA floating alone in the vast emptiness and silence of space."

FOREWORD SECULAR: SEPARATION OF POWERS

By The Honorable Mark Kirk, Former United States Senator from Illinois, Former Member of the United States House of Representatives (IL-10)

During my tenure serving in the United States House of Representatives and Senate, I upheld fundamental principles that should guide both science and public policy: Trust must be earned, and transparency must be maintained. Dr. Richard Burt's *Kill Switch* is a thoughtful and unflinching exploration of how viruses and vaccines have shaped the course of human history and how modern medicine and our systems of checks and balances, though well-intentioned, have sometimes struggled to keep pace with the ethical challenges that come with scientific progress.

In *Kill Switch*, Dr. Burt takes us on an enlightening and relatable journey to understand the omnipotent viruses and how their vaccine counterparts have shaped public health, policy, and opinion. History reminds us that this viral force of nature has brought about the decline of empires and fueled diseases such as yellow fever, which caused more deaths than combat during the Spanish–American War and compelled a US military response, which led to significant public health advancements. Franklin D. Roosevelt's personal experience with polio led him to advocate for research and funding for polio treatment and vaccine development. The book *Kill Switch* details how viruses can arise naturally or from unintentional and intentional human action.

Through storytelling and anecdotal evidence, *Kill Switch* explores science's highest standards and greatest achievements while reminding us of the unintentional consequences of good intentions and that even in times of fear and uncertainty, democratic values should never be cast aside. I have always believed in the power of American science, and I worked alongside colleagues from both parties to support it. But science, like the government, must remain accountable to the people it serves. That means asking hard questions, allowing honest debate, admitting failures, and doing a root cause search when our institutions fall short. This emphasis on accountability is needed to reassure the public and instill confidence in the scientific community.

This book also explains how passage of the Bayh-Dole Act in 1980 inadvertently created an inherent conflict of interest. Today, this well-meaning law, designed to accelerate taxpayer-funded medical research, has led to a situation where the NIH, universities, and drug companies share profits, while icing out the taxpayers who paid for it and limiting reward to research scientists whose intellectual prowess invented it, while simultaneously pocketing billions of dollars in profit with little to no oversight or accountability. This situation begs the question: With no ombudsman or independent review body, what could possibly go wrong? A thorough reassessment is needed to understand how taxpayer-funded research has tied together corporate and academic interests and corrupted the bedrock principles of transparency, accountability, and noncoerced consent in medical practices.

Kill Switch is a wake-up call. We are all familiar with the saying about the road to hell being paved with good intentions. It is the role of a “kill switch” to prevent good intentions from straying off course. The Bayh-Dole Act unintentionally violated the separation of powers (monies) between government bureaucracies, universities, and Big Pharma corporations. Separation of power is an important kill switch that empowers individuals and keeps institutions accountable, preventing conflicts of interest that undermine public trust. We should hopefully all agree that in politics and virology, the separation of powers allows sunlight and public accountability. Separation of powers is a potent antiseptic.

I commend Dr. Burt, a valued son of Illinois, himself a product of the National Institutes of Health (NIH) and university life, for offering this work in the spirit of inquiry, not condemnation. He challenges us to examine the past with humility to shape the future with wisdom. As biotechnology creates new carbon-based life forms and as electrical impulses are used to create new metal-based artificial intelligence (AI), the importance of kill switches gains a new urgency. Dr. Burt has reminded us that respecting historical kill switches such as free speech, transparent unforced consent, independent outside accountability, and separation of powers, while incorporating new technologically appropriate kill switches for the unforeseeable complications of the technology that we are creating, is an important conversation. It’s a conversation worth having before it is too late.

CONTENTS

Time is the distance that makes us lose sight of the past.—RKB

INTRODUCTION

People do not understand science, because it is presented without the historical scaffolding that built it.—RKB

A kill switch is any check and balance that prevents good intentions from going wrong. During the 1990s, humanity started creating new viruses that never previously existed on earth. This harrowing reality poses a number of serious questions. Have we judiciously thought through what could go wrong? Should a genetic kill switch be engineered into these new viruses?

Traditional kill switches include outside investigation, noncoerced consent, separation of powers, and free speech. While most of us are not allowed to self-investigate, government institutions are routinely charged with investigating themselves. Career government institutionalists thus experience a conflict of interests, because by looking the other way, they can ensure their own reputation, promotion, and job security. A review process located outside of the institution would be the appropriate kill switch against institutional misbehavior, one that would avoid such conflicts of interest. A fundamental kill switch that checks risky or deceitful behavior is transparent, noncoerced consent. Free speech is so sacred a kill switch that it is enshrined in the First Amendment to the US Constitution. Has our system lost respect for these commonsense, operational restraints?

This book is a story of how we ended up where we are when it comes to our relationship with viruses and vaccines. It tells a story of human courage, ingenuity, and success as well as the fear, mistakes, denial, and losses that we've experienced on the way. It is an attempt to open peaceful and thoughtful discussion, to provide some peace for the millions who have died during the recent pandemic. It is an attempt to seek some resolution for the many who have lost loved ones, whose families were broken apart, whose spirits were broken, and who still suffer from COVID-19 pandemic post-traumatic stress disorder. Loss and grief progress through stages of denial, anger, depression, acceptance, and finally resolution to help others, even when we cannot help ourselves. May this book facilitate that process.

Viral research and vaccines are surrounded by controversy. The goal is not to say who is right or wrong but rather to present the controversies and to examine how we arrived at this place. The goal is not to blame any one person but to look at the underlying system.

In an attempt to explain viruses and molecular biology (biology at the level of atoms) to the lay person, this book reconstructs the historical scaffolding that got us to where we are today. In doing so, this book demonstrates how viruses are an integral character in the human story.

CHAPTER 1

COVID-19: The Foreboding First Report

Words are a violence to protect some by destroying others.—RKB

Dr. Zhang Jixian in Wuhan, China, was the first to notice what subsequently became known as the COVID-19 pandemic. On December 26, 2019, when evaluating images of the lungs from an elderly couple with cough and fever, Dr. Zhang recognized clinical and imaging similarities to the viral SARS pneumonia pandemic that occurred in 2003. (SARS is an abbreviation for severe acute respiratory distress syndrome.)

Dr. Zhang ordered an X-ray of the lung of the couple's son. It showed the same smoky, ground-glass appearance present in the parents' lungs, an appearance distinct from the dense consolidation that normally occurs with bacterial infections. Zhang knew that for all family members of different ages to have the same acute lung disease at the same time meant that it was infectious. This pneumonia was later named COVID-19, an abbreviation for coronavirus disease 2019.

Throughout this book, it is important to remember the similarity between the COVID-19 pandemic that started in 2019 and SARS outbreak that occurred in 2003. Both COVID-19 and SARS are caused by coronaviruses (abbreviated CoV). The proper name of SARS is SARS-CoV-1. The proper name for COVID-19 is SARS-CoV-2. SARS-CoV-1 caused the first human coronavirus infection and localized epidemic in 2003 that lasted about six months. SARS-CoV-2 caused a worldwide pandemic that began sixteen years later in 2019 and continues to this day.

On December 27, 2019, Dr. Zhang's observation of a virus lung infection that mimicked the 2003 SARS-CoV-1 virus was reported to the Wuhan Center for Disease Control. On December 30 the Wuhan Municipal Health Commission released an emergency notice of "pneumonia of unknown cause."[1] In order to control the narrative, the Chinese government substituted the euphemism "unknown cause" for SARS-like pneumonia.

The First Public Report of SARS

On that same day as the official release referring to a "pneumonia of unknown cause," Dr. Li Wenliang saw a report from a patient in the Wuhan Central Hospital emergency department, in which the words SARS coronavirus was circled.[2] Dr. Li informed his medical school colleagues on a private WeChat social media account stating: "7 confirmed cases of SARS were reported from Wuhan Seafood market." Later Dr. Li posted on WeChat "the latest news is, it has been confirmed to be coronavirus infections, but the exact virus strain is being subtyped." This information spread on social media like wildfire because the Chinese people knew how lethal the 2003 Chinese SARS epidemic had been.

Four days after his WeChat, Dr. Li was interrogated by the Wuhan Public Security Bureau. The Security Bureau issued a public warning and censured him for the crime of publishing untrue statements about SARS. Dr. Li was forced to sign a letter recanting his statements and was threatened with incarceration for any further "false" information. China Central Television (the Chinese equivalent to CNN) then publicly humiliated and shamed Dr. Li for "rumor mongering," a "character assassination" technique and misdirection also utilized by our own Western media.

On January 8, five days after his interrogation and humiliation by Chinese police and Chinese Central Television, Dr. Li caught COVID-19 from an infected patient whom he was seeing in Wuhan Central Hospital. To protect his family and avoid their exposure to COVID-19, he did not return home. Dr. Li never saw his family again.

Dr. Li was admitted on January 12 to the medical intensive care unit. On February 6 his blood oxygen levels dropped dangerously low. Because his lungs were unable to oxygenate his blood, he was placed on a heart-lung machine for extracorporeal (outside of the body) oxygenation. Later that evening he died.[3] Social media posts using his name were being monitored by the Chinese government to prevent "rumor mongering," and reports of his death from that day were deleted. In the afternoon of the following day, the hospital announced his death. His wife was pregnant at the time of his death. Four months after his death, his widow gave birth to their son.

The Chinese people demanded a response from the Chinese government.[4] The social media posting #WeWantFreedomofSpeech gained two million followers in only five hours before it was taken down by government monitors. Two months after Dr. Li's death, the Chinese central government reversed itself and declared Dr. Li to be a state martyr who gave his life for the Chinese people.[5]

Summary

COVID-19 went on to become a worldwide pandemic, killing to date approximately eight million people. To prevent another outbreak, we need to know where SARS-CoV-2 came from. But how does one begin to answer this question? We need to start by first learning about viruses—what they are, when we discovered them, and how human beings have addressed them in the past. As Carl Sagan said, "You have to know the past to understand the present."[6]

CHAPTER 2

Viruses: A Transition Between the "Living" and the "Dead"

A virus was the original inhabitant of this planet.—The X-Files *(1998 film)*

Blessed is the meek virus, for it inherited the earth.—RKB

Our modern term *virus* is derived from the Latin word *virus*, meaning "poison." This same word is also the root for our word *virulent*. Viruses have killed hundreds of millions of people throughout human history. The strongest human is nothing compared to a minuscule and seemingly meek virus that cannot be seen even with the most powerful light microscope.

While the word *virus* has an ominous inference, 8 to 10 percent of our own cell's genetic structure is composed of embedded viral genes.[7] Another 40 percent of our genetic structure is composed of noninfectious virus-like, and perhaps virus-derived, segments, including retrotransposons that can jump or transpose to another region of DNA within the same cell.[8] Viruses are invisible ghosts that fluctuate between the dead and the living, lurking in our environment and in our genetic code, and we are only just beginning to unravel their many functions. Is it possible that life started as a virus and that we are the evolutionary descendants of viruses?

Viruses compose the largest biomass on this planet—larger than all bacteria, animals, and humans combined. Case in point, the human gut is full of viruses. It is estimated that one gram (0.03 ounces) of human stool contains one billion viruses.[9] Wow! Viruses are a conundrum. They have the propensity to harm and kill us, but we would not exist without them. Because humans and viruses are intertwined, altering viruses has unexpected consequences.

Is a Virus Alive or Dead?

Outside of its host cell, a virus is inert with no metabolic activity and is no more alive than a rock. Inside the host cell, a virus is metabolically active. Depending on the virus and cell infected, it can make its host cell produce and release more than ten thousand copies of itself.

It is debatable whether viruses are alive or dead, because their "life cycle" continuously transitions back and forth between their dead or inert state when they are outside a cell, and their living or metabolically active state when they are inside a cell.[10] Viruses may be the evolutionary step or the missing link that bridges the gap between the dead and the living. What came first, the chicken or the egg? The answer may be a virus.

The Size of a Virus

An average human is 1.7 meters (5 foot 6 inches) tall. A human is made up of more than fifty to seventy trillion cells. Our word *cell* is from the Latin *cella*, which means "storeroom" (like the English word "cellar"). Cells have a surrounding fatty (lipid) wall behind which everything that makes us is stored and manufactured. The length of a human cell is 0.025 centimeters (25 micrometers). Bacteria are 1 micrometer in size, which is twenty-five times smaller than a cell. In comparison, most viruses are between 10 to 50 nanometers, which is about fifty to one hundred times smaller than bacteria.[11]

Cells and bacteria were first made visible to the human eye by the light microscope. The single-lens light microscope was discovered in the early 1700s by Antonie van Leeuwenhoek, a Dutch merchant who got the idea after using a magnifying lens to inspect threads of cloth.[12] Modern compound microscopes—the contemporary descendants of van Leeuwenhoek's invention—use two or more lenses and have a magnification a thousandfold greater than the human eye.[13]

The emergence of the light microscope allowed for the initial formulations of germ and cell theory. Germ theory states that infections are caused by organisms like bacteria and viruses too small to be seen by the human eye.[14] The German physician Rudolf Virchow (1821–1902) was one of the educators to promote the use of microscopes. Virchow correctly proposed that new cells arise by the division of preexisting cells.[15] It was because of the light microscope that Virchow and many other scientists could make strides in our understanding of bacteria and cells.[16] Because of the light microscope, like the "Show-Me" state of Missouri, seeing is believing.

Viruses were too small to be detected by these instruments, which kept them imperceptible to the human eye. However, this does not mean that scientists were unaware of their existence. The field of virology started when Charles Edouard Chamberland (1851–1908) and Louis Pasteur (1822–1895) at the Pasteur Institute in Paris invented a porcelain water filter, now known as the Pasteur-Chamberland filter.[17] While bacteria and other larger microscopic particles would be caught in the filter, viruses could still pass through with the water and cause an infection when ingested. This prompted Pasteur and Chamberland to theorize the existence of something smaller than bacteria, leading to the emergence of the field of virology.

The invention of the electron microscope by the German electrical engineer Ernst Ruska in the 1930s confirmed the theories of Pasteur and others concerning viruses. Ruska was awarded the 1986

Nobel Prize in Physics because of his discovery (see Box 2.1).[18] Instead of using a lens to bend visible light that has a wavelength of 400 to 700 nanometers (one nanometer equals one billionth of a meter), an electron microscope shoots a beam of electrons that permits one

Name	**Virus genetic material** (Chapter 8)	**Electron Microscopy Morphology**	**Structure** (Schematic)
Smallpox	DNA	Brick shaped (football like) with dumbbell core	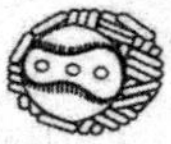
Rabies	RNA	Bullet shaped	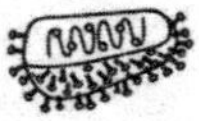
Yellow Fever	RNA	Spherical with cauliflower buds	
Poliomyelitis	RNA	Spherical	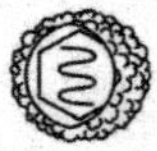
HIV	RNA	Spherical with cone or bullseye shaped core	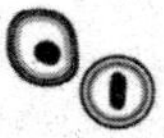
HPV	DNA	Icosahedral	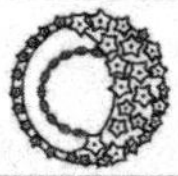
Ebola	RNA	Filaments (worm like)	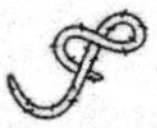
H5N1	RNA	Sphere with club shaped spikes like a crown	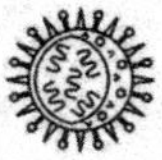
Covid	RNA	Sphere with club shaped spikes like a crown	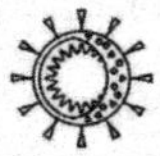

TABLE 2.1: The morphology or structure and characteristics of viruses covered in the chapters of this book. COVID = coronavirus disease (2019), DNA = deoxyribonucleic acid, H5N1 = a bird flu that can infect humans, HIV = human immunodeficiency virus, HPV = human papilloma virus, RNA = ribonucleic acid.

million times magnification. The higher magnification is due to an electron's wavelength of approximately one nanometer, a hundredfold smaller than the wavelength of visible light. The electron microscope allowed previously invisible viruses to become visible, a boon for the growing field of virology.[19] (The three-dimensional structure of the particular viruses discussed in this book are shown in table 2.1.)

Box 2.1: The Nobel Prize

Alfred Nobel invented dynamite. His brother Ludwig founded Branobel, the family oil company. Branobel is Russian for "Brothers Nobel." The Nobel family were called the "Russian Rockefellers."[20] However, they were not Russian. They were Swedish.

A Paris newspaper mistook Ludwig to be the inventor of dynamite, and upon Ludwig's death, the obituary read: "The merchant of death is dead."[21] According to one account, Alfred, the brother who invented dynamite, was so affected by the newspaper's headline that upon his own death, he willed his estate to establish the Nobel prize.

Alfred Nobel left one quarter of a billion dollars in today's money for an annual prize in literature and peace to be awarded in Oslo, and in chemistry, physics, and medicine to be awarded in Stockholm. It is rumored that Alfred excluded mathematics, because the woman he loved married a mathematician.[22] In 1895, Alfred Nobel in his last will and testament donated a fortune to Sweden to establish the Nobel prize, not to Russia from where the oil wealth originated.

In April 1920, the Red Army confiscated (nationalized) the Branobel oil fields. One month later, in May 1920, Standard Oil (the Rockefellers) bought most shares of Branobel. Standard Oil incorrectly gambled that the Bolsheviks could not remain in power. A chill traveled down the spine of the wealthy in America for fear that "nationalization" could happen to them.[23] Like Branobel had done, the desire by multi-national corporations to monopolize Russia's natural resources that cover eleven time zones and Russia's opposition to their desires linger until today.

Virology

Virology is the study of the viruses, including their types, structure, methods of infection, and the diseases they cause. In the early twentieth century, it was discovered that viruses could be made less virulent (attenuated) after multiple passages through an animal host or through animal cells cultured (grown) in the laboratory. From the beginning of the twentieth century until the present day, the field of virology has focused on developing animal hosts and cells to culture and study viruses. The advent of molecular biology during the last half of the twentieth century (see section two) enabled viruses to be further studied and modified at a molecular level, allowing for genetic manipulation.

Compared to a human cell's genetic structure that contains deoxyribonucleic acid (DNA) (chapter 8), a virus's genetic structure may consist of either DNA or ribonucleic acid (RNA) (chapter 9). Compared to the human cell that has about twenty-five thousand DNA genes, a RNA virus usually has from one to fifteen genes, while a DNA virus (depending on the virus) usually has from two to two hundred genes.

Vaccines

A vaccine delivers a virus (or part of a virus) into one's body with the intended goal of prompting the body to establish an immunity to the disease caused by the virus. To start this process, vaccines may contain an alive but less virulent form of the virus, a killed and thus permanently non-replicating and noninfectious virus, or the outer shell protein of a virus (called a virus-like particle), or some of the genetic material of the virus. Vaccines are injected (or swallowed in the case of polio vaccine) to give you immunity against a future viral infection.

Vaccine development markedly accelerated after the introduction of molecular biology techniques in 1960 (see the timeline in Figure

2.1).[24] Mandatory vaccinations markedly accelerated after the 1980 Bayh Dole Act gave universities, government bureaucracies, and pharmaceutical companies shared profits in drug and vaccine sales (see chapter 16). The 1986 Vaccine Injury Compensation Program likewise gave pharmaceutical companies immunity from being sued for vaccine-related injuries (see chapter 11).

In 1970, children were typically immunized with only three vaccines (DPT [diphtheria, tetanus, and pertussis], polio, and smallpox).

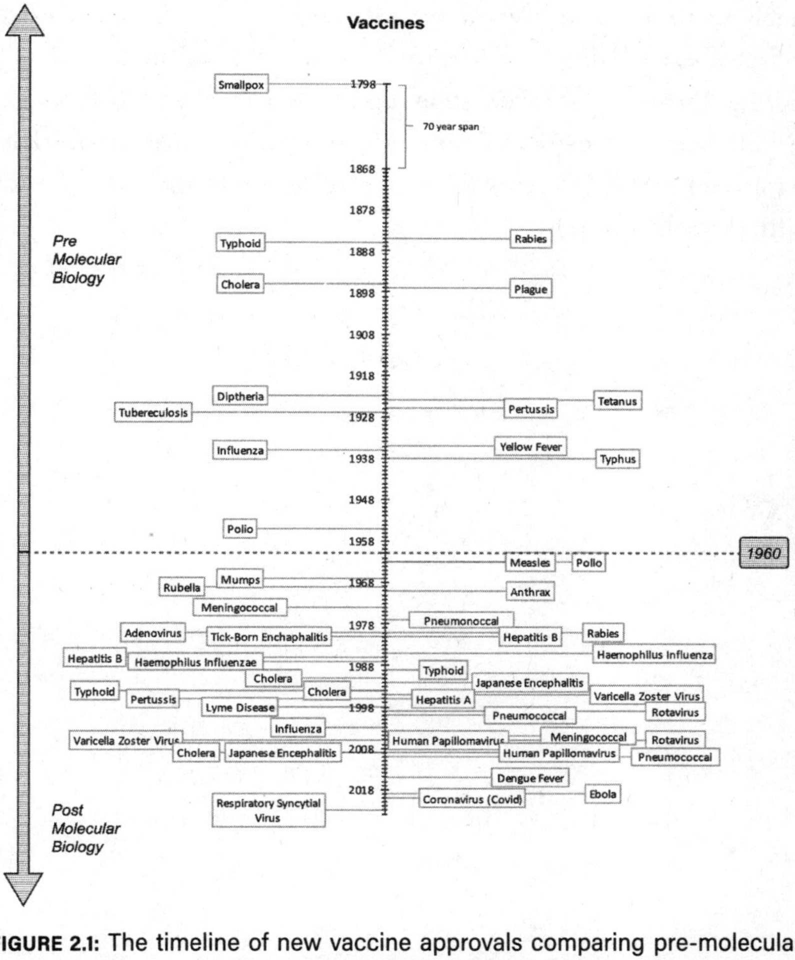

FIGURE 2.1: The timeline of new vaccine approvals comparing pre-molecular biology era before 1960 and the post-molecular biology era after 1960.

As of 2020, children in America typically receive more than twenty-five vaccinations within the first twenty-four months of life. Babies are now repeatedly vaccinated at one, two, four, six, twelve to fifteen, and eighteen to twenty-three months after birth.[25]

Summary

Is this rapid increase of infant vaccination saving lives, or have we gone too far and too fast and thereby overestimated our abilities to safely control viruses? What sort of safeguards might allow us to escape from treading into trepidatious inroads? To understand the full significance of these questions and answer them with appropriate circumspection, we need to start with our earliest human interactions with these invisible agents and examine how our antecedents dealt with their ill effects.

SECTION ONE

Pre-Molecular Biology Era of Intact Live or Dead Viral Vaccines

CHAPTER 3

Smallpox: The Death of Empires

The world's first vaccine was pus from an infected person's lesion. The second vaccine was pus from a cow's lesion.—RKB

The smallpox virus normally enters a person by inhalation through the lungs. The initial indicators are the usual, nonspecific symptoms of most viral infections: a high fever (102 to 104 degrees Fahrenheit), headache, backache, abdominal pain, nausea, and vomiting.

For smallpox, a few days after the fever subsides, lesions begin to appear in the mouth, throat, and tongue, which are followed by flat skin lesions over the entire body that evolve into raised vesicles (small blisters), which then morph into pustules (pus-filled blisters). Smallpox pustules are round, elevated, and tense to touch. Each pustule is the size of a pencil top eraser or pea. The skin lesions may evolve more quickly (modified smallpox), may rarely be flat (flat-type smallpox), or may be associated with diffuse mucosal bleeding (hemorrhagic smallpox).[26] Lesions crust over and start to scar after two to three weeks, with those that occur over the cornea (eye) causing blindness due to scarring.[27]

The most common form of smallpox, which is called usual smallpox, has a mortality rate of 30 percent. The number of pustules in usual smallpox ranges from a few to several thousand. Modified smallpox occurs in reinfected patients or those infected after vaccination. Due to prior immunity, its course is relatively benign. Flat-type and hemorrhagic smallpox have very high mortality rates. Smallpox-related death usually occurs during the second or third week of infection with injury to the lungs, liver, and kidneys.[28] There are no effective antiviral drugs for smallpox. Bacterial antibiotics have no benefit in preventing or delaying death.

The name "smallpox" was used in medieval Europe to differentiate it from "large pox," which is now known as syphilis. A recent book on the devastation caused by smallpox during this period has characterized its lesions as the "speckled monster."[29] Smallpox was so common and feared in Renaissance Europe that it was mentioned in Shakespeare's *Romeo and Juliet*. In this play, the dying Mercutio's last utterance is: "A pox on both your houses," a double entendre used today to mean that warring factions will bring death to each other and to innocent bystanders.

The Death of Empires

The period of 96–180 AD is often referred to by historians as the era of the five good emperors. Characterized as an epoch of general peace and prosperity, this golden age of Roman history ended under the reign of Marcus Aurelius Antoninus (r. 161–180), the so-called philosopher king of Rome. Even today, Marcus Aurelius's *Meditations* are still studied in philosophy classes, including his famous maxim: "The best revenge is to be unlike him who performed the injury."[30]

Besides his philosophical prowess, Marcus Aurelius is also the namesake of the Antonine plague (c. 165–180 AD), a devastating epidemic that marred the entire Roman Empire during his reign. In fact, some historians even attribute Marcus Aurelius's death to this plague.[31] Roman legions warring in Mesopotamia likely contracted the Antonine plague during their military skirmishes with the Parthians during the winter of 165 AD. These soldiers suffered from headache, fever, diarrhea, pustular and scarring skin lesions, and trouble breathing. These symptoms may now, in retrospect, be attributed to a virus, most likely the smallpox virus.[32] When these Roman soldiers returned to their homes or were relocated to other military campaigns, they brought the Antonine plague with them.

Accustomed to cramped quarters, Roman legions suffered high mortality rates from the plague. So many legionaries died that the northern frontier was left indefensible. In desperation, greater numbers of Germanic tribes were recruited into the army and paid by the Romans to fight against other invading Germanic tribes. The invincible Roman legions faltered, and news of this weakness hastened barbarian tribal migration from their harsh northern latitudes toward the warm Mediterranean climate. The influx was greater than Roman society could assimilate. The golden age of Rome and nearly two hundred years of empire-wide peace (*Pax Romana*) ended. Smallpox marked the beginning of Rome's decline.[33]

The Roman Empire was not the only political superpower affected by smallpox. Smallpox also caused the collapse of Aztec and Inca empires. The smallpox plague that Europeans accidentally brought with them brutalized the indigenous peoples of Central and South America.[34] It killed roughly twenty million Native Americans[35]—far more than any conquistador's sword. In New England, the British used smallpox as a form of germ warfare.[36] During Pontiac's Rebellion (1763–1764)—a military conflict that arose out of the ashes of the French and Indian War—Lord Jeffrey Amherst, a commander of the English Army in North America, distributed smallpox-laden blankets as a gift to local Indian tribes that were allied with the French.[37] The town of Amherst and Amherst College, both in Massachusetts, are today named in his honor.

Variolation: The First Vaccine

At some point, human beings began to recognize that those who survived an initial bout with smallpox were immune from future infection. To improve their odds for survival, medieval Europeans began practicing *variolation*, a term that derives from the Latin *variola*, which means "cutting the skin."[38] (The smallpox virus was thus named the variola virus because of this.) Variolation involved cutting the skin of a person who had never contracted smallpox with a knife deliberately contaminated with the pus from a smallpox pustule. In doing so, variolation afforded lifelong immunity from smallpox. Variolation was also called *inoculation*, which derives from the Latin verb *inoculo*, meaning "to engraft" (that is, to engraft the smallpox virus).

The use of inoculation as a way of combatting smallpox was not restricted to Western Europe. Such practices also were used in the luxury slave trade occurring in the Balkans, Middle East, and North Africa from the Renaissance into the early twentieth century. Sultans and other elites living in the Ottoman Empire had a preference for young and fair-skinned Circassian concubines from the Caucasus Mountains.[39] To preserve their value, captured Circassian slavegirls were inoculated by their captors with smallpox in parts of their bodies where the scar would not be visible.[40]

The variolation method was a successful early means of preemptively combating smallpox. Today, we know that route of entry of a virus affects its toxicity.[41] By exposing individuals to smallpox through the skin, variolation provides the immune system more time to develop the necessary antibodies for immunity before onset of systemic disease and organ failure. As a result, the mortality of variolation is significantly less (3 percent) compared to the mortality from a natural aerosolized smallpox infection inhaled through the lungs (15 to 30 percent).[42]

Cowpox Inoculation: The Second Vaccine

In 1796 a British physician, Dr. Edward Jenner, noticed that farm girls milking cows developed mild cowpox skin lesions but never suffered from smallpox.[43] He reasoned that cowpox protected them from smallpox and began performing inoculation from cowpox lesions. After inoculating (injecting or vaccinating) people with cowpox virus, he injected them with live smallpox virus. Nobody developed smallpox. The cowpox virus caused immunity to smallpox. Derived from the Latin word for cow (*vacca*), the cowpox virus used in the inoculation process was called a *vaccine*. Likewise, the injection of cowpox into the skin was referred to as *vaccination*.

Dr. Jenner was a visionary who started the field of vaccines.[44] We also owe to him the term "cuckoo," meaning deranged behavior. He documented the cuckoo bird as a squatter that laid its egg in another bird's nest. Upon hatching, the cuckoo hatchling evicts the parents' fledgling newborn chicks from the nest so the foster parents of the murdered chicks will raise it.[45]

Box 3.1: What Does It Mean to "Passage a Virus"?

Viruses were originally passaged *in vivo,* that is, inside a live animal. Today, the passage of a virus is usually done outside the body (*ex vivo*) in a laboratory culture of animal cells or in living bird embryos. Like selectively breeding wild animals to be domesticated for certain traits, passaging "domesticates" the virus by selecting strains that are less aggressive when reinjected into a susceptible host.

Passage *ex vivo* is done in a laboratory dish or vial containing nutrient media, and controlled temperature, acidity, and carbon dioxide and oxygen concentration necessary to keep the cell alive. If the cell type and conditions are appropriate, the virus seeded in the media will infect the cells and start reproducing and shedding new viruses into the media supernatant above the cells. Each passage is done by collecting the supernatant and infecting a fresh dish or vial of cells. This is done sequentially in serial passages.

Serial passage of a virus may attenuate the virus (i.e., make it less toxic). This allows it to be used in a vaccine. Attenuation is caused by the natural evolution of spontaneous genetic mutations in the virus. Although not generally recognized as a potential or serious complication until the late 1960s, passage of viruses in animals or in animal cells may cause contamination of the vaccine with another virus that may introduce a previously nonhuman virus into the human population.

In the early 1900s cowpox (and horsepox, which worked equally well) were initially passaged (Box 3.1) in the skin of infected animals. To maintain a routine supply of vaccine, smallpox was later passaged in cells in a laboratory dish (Box 3.2).[46] To differentiate the smallpox vaccine virus from wild-type cowpox, it was termed *vaccinia*. A vaccinia sample still available from 1902 was sequenced in 2017 and found to be genetically more like horsepox than cowpox.[47]

Box 3.2: Vaccine Strains Against the Human Smallpox Virus

The cowpox virus used in smallpox vaccines are divided into first-, second-, and third-generation variations.[48] First-generation vaccines, as developed by Edward Jenner, were from the pus of a live animal pox virus pustule.

The second-generation vaccines came from virus cultured *ex vivo* in animal cells in the laboratory. In 1967 the World Health Organization approved four second-generation vaccine strains.[49] Serious acute complications of vaccination with first- and second-generation vaccines were fever and rare cases of inflammation of the heart (pericarditis) or brain (encephalitis).

In the late 1970s, third-generation vaccines were attenuated further by performing more passages in different animals or in cell culture.[50] Two third-generation vaccine strains were Modified Vaccinia Ankara (MVA) and LC16m8.

The MVA strain was developed in Germany in 1977 and was derived from a first-generation vaccinia virus. It was passaged in cows, donkeys, chicken fibroblasts, and finally in the vascular membrane of embryonated chick eggs.[51] The LC16m8 strain was developed in Japan in 1975 from a first-generation strain. It was repeatedly passaged in a laboratory culture of rabbit kidney cells.[52] Unlike first- and second-generation vaccines, MVA and LC16m8 vaccinia strains caused minimal fever or other acute side effects. In 1980 the World Health Organization declared the world free of smallpox, and vaccinations against smallpox stopped.[53]

Summary

The last documented case of smallpox occurred in 1977 in Somalia following a worldwide vaccination program initiated by the World Health Organization.[54] Over the duration of human history, innumerable people have suffered and died from smallpox. The scourge of this virus that had decimated families and armies, ended empires, and forever changed human history was eliminated from earth by vaccination with domesticated live cowpox and horsepox viruses. A few vials of the original wild type of smallpox virus have been frozen and are in storage.[55]

Smallpox is the only virus that has been driven to extinction by human activity. Is it possible that this good news may have a delayed downside? Humans have already caused the extinction of innumerable animal species with detrimental impact to our ecosystem. As Linda Krueger, director of the Nature Conservancy, writes, "The rapid loss of biodiversity that we are witnessing is about much more than nature. The collapse of ecosystems will threaten the wellbeing and livelihoods of everyone on the planet."[56] Will limiting or changing the biodiversity of natural viruses have unforeseen ramifications as well? As we will see in coming chapters, human actions do have unexpected consequences.

CHAPTER 4

The Rabies Virus: The First "Dead" Vaccine

Whether you like it or not, everything is connected. A connection exists between vaccines, inflammatory reactions, and autoimmunity.—RKB

Rabies has been present since the beginning of written history. Symptoms are frenzy, rage, excessive salivation, trembling at noise, and an agonizing thirst accompanied (paradoxically) by a fear of water (hydrophobia). These symptoms are followed by convulsion, seizures, and death. In some cases, instead of rage (furious rabies) the person or animal becomes paralyzed (paralytic rabies).

The association of rabies with rage or frenzy can be traced back to its name. The word "rabies" is derived from the Latin verb *rabere*, meaning "to rage," which is related to the ancient Sanskrit *rabhas*, meaning "to do violence." The rabies virus belongs to the lyssavirus category of viruses, which are named after Lyssa, the Greek goddess of frenzy and fury.

To this day, rabies has no effective antiviral treatment. Once symptoms present in humans, rabies is nearly 100 percent fatal, resulting in the highest case fatality ratio of any known infection.

After onset of symptoms, approximately eleven people have been documented to survive.[57]

Virtually any mammal, including domestic cats and wild foxes, raccoons, and skunks, may transmit rabies. The domestic dog bite is the most common worldwide cause of rabies.[58] After dog bites, bat bites are the second most common cause. The most common reason for rabies occurring without a known cause (cryptogenic) is from a bat bite.[59]

Symptoms usually begin one to three months after an animal bite but may present as early as ten days to as long as six years following initial contact.[60] After onset of symptoms, death occurs within one to two weeks.[61] Saliva with a heavy viral load, multiple bites, or bites on the face that have less distance to travel before reaching the brain manifest a shorter time interval before onset of symptoms. Because clinical signs may not occur for months or occasionally years after an animal bite, rabies has rarely occurred in the recipient of an organ transplant from an infected but presymptomatic donor.[62]

Infection is transmitted through a bite, lick, or scratch. Once the virus-infected saliva of a rabid animal enters a wound, it travels backward (i.e., retrograde) up nerves to the spinal cord and brain. Nerve cells have arms (known as axons) that may be several feet long. Material is moved within a nerve cell along a microtubule "highway," on which a group of proteins called the dynein motor complex act as a bus to transport material. Rabies makes a protein that allows the virus to hitchhike onto dynein motor proteins that travel backward along the microtubule highway to the nerve's center or body, which is where the rabies virus replicates.[63]

After replicating, the virus travels down neurons, enters saliva, and after a bite from the rabid animal repeats this cycle in another victim. The rabies virus consists of only five genes that allow it to infect nerves, travel up the nerve, replicate, travel back down nerves, enter saliva, and cause spasm of throat muscles that synchronize swallowing.[64] Rabid individuals drool saliva from the mouth and fear water despite their great thirst, because swallowing induces throat spasms.

Rabies Vaccine

Nearly a century after the English physician Edward Jenner injected a cowpox virus into people as a vaccine to prevent smallpox (see chapter 3), the French physician Louis Pasteur developed the world's next viral vaccine. Pasteur is considered the father of the field of immunology (the study of the immune system).[65] He developed this vaccine by injecting the dried spinal cord of rabies-infected rabbits into various animals. The animals did not develop rabies if the spinal cord had been desiccated (dried) for more than six days before it was injected.[66] In 1885 Pasteur used this treatment to inoculate a nine-year-old boy who was bitten multiple times by a rabid dog.[67] The boy, Joseph Meister, never developed rabies. He spent his adult life as a Pasteur Institute employee.

Despite experiencing success, Pasteur was criticized for injecting people with an air-dried virus that, at times, was still alive. By 1908 the rabies vaccine was produced more reliably and with greater sterility through the use of formalin, which "killed" (i.e., inactivated) the virus (Box 4.1).[68] Whether air dried or chemically inactivated, as more people were vaccinated, some patients developed inflammation of the brain that caused neurologic deficits including paralysis.[69] This vaccine-related complication is called experimental allergic encephalomyelitis (EAE).[70]

Box 4.1: Formalin Fixing

Killing a virus but keeping it physically intact so your body's immune cells recognize it and make an immune response is the art of fixing or "embalming" a virus.[71] Virus embalming is done with formalin, which is aqueous formaldehyde created when the gas is bubbled through water until it ceases to dissolve, resulting in a liquid solution that contains 37 percent formaldehyde.[72]

The embalming capabilities of formalin were first discovered by the German doctor Ferdinand Blum.[73]

Formalin crosslinks proteins that prevent them from decomposing. This is called "fixing tissue."[74] Tissue fixing revolutionized the fields of anatomy and histology (studying tissue under a microscope) and allowed production of dead viral vaccines. By crosslinking proteins, formalin kills viruses but preserves their three-dimensional structure, to which a recipient's immune system develops immunity. Today, either formalin or beta-propiolactone may be used to inactivate (kill) the viruses used in vaccines.

Rabies Vaccine and Autoimmune Allergic Encephalomyelitis

The first rabies vaccines were complicated by encephalomyelitis (inflammation of the brain) due to contamination of the vaccine with spinal cord tissue. To decrease the risk of allergic encephalitis, rabbit spinal cords ceased being used. Instead, newborn (suckling) mouse brains or embryonated eggs were infected with rabies and used as a vaccine source. Autoimmune inflammation of the brain, spinal cord, nerve roots coming off the spinal cord, or peripheral nerves was less common, but still occurred.[75] *Ex vivo* cell culture techniques allowed production of rabies vaccine in non-neurologic cells that eliminated vaccine-related neurologic autoimmune complications.

Spinal cord contaminated rabies vaccine caused neurologic deficits. Unlike rabies, the patients did not develop hydrophobia (fear of water), excessive salivation, or rage, and they cannot transfer their symptoms to another person.[76] Over time, it was realized that myelin proteins in brain and spinal cord tissue contaminating the vaccine caused these symptoms referred to as experimental allergic encephalomyelitis (EAE).[77]

To minimize EAE, the rabies virus is now produced in non-nervous cells that do not contain myelin.[78] As rabies-induced EAE was eliminated, it morphed into a tool to study animal models for multiple sclerosis, a human neurologic autoimmune disease. As a result, EAE is now called experimental *autoimmune* (not allergic) encephalitis, an animal equivalent of multiple sclerosis.[79] The original rabies vaccine contaminated with myelin from the central nervous system opened the door to understanding how a virus or a viral vaccine could initiate an autoimmune disease.

Myelin is a fatty, proteinaceous material that wraps around neurons to increase electrical conduction velocity.[80] If myelin is co-injected with an adjuvant that stimulates the immune system, such as the dead rabies virus (or other vaccine such as measles), the immune system responds against both the virus and the injected myelin. The response is both immunity to rabies and an autoimmune neurologic disease.

Rabies Vaccination

Rabies vaccine guidelines recommend vaccination of high-risk individuals before exposure and treatment of all people after exposure.[81] Pre-exposure prophylaxis is recommended for animal workers such as veterinarians and travelers to rabies endemic areas of the world. Post-exposure prophylaxis is given to every person exposed to rabies or suspected of exposure. Provided post-exposure prophylaxis is given before onset of symptoms, rabies can be almost always prevented. Treatment of a rabid bite involves the cleaning and sterilization of the wound, infusion of anti-rabies antibodies (immunoglobulins), and vaccination against rabies using the dead rabies virus. The rabies vaccine is given on day zero, three, fourteen, and twenty-eight after the bite, if the victim was never previously vaccinated, and on days zero and three if they were previously vaccinated.

Rabies virus from dog bites has been virtually eliminated in North America not by the preemptive vaccination of unexposed people but by the vaccination of pets, especially dogs.[82] It is the only domestic pet vaccine required by law in most states. Currently in America, only one to three cases of rabies are reported annually.[83] In Europe, the immunization of wild carnivores such as foxes that infected domestic dogs also helped decrease the incidence of human rabies.[84] This was done through the use of an appetizing bait containing the killed rabies virus. Certain initial baits such as eggs did not work, as the foxes would store the eggs to be eaten later, during which time the vaccine would degrade. The first successful oral vaccine trial of wild foxes was performed in Switzerland through the use of chicken heads.[85] In a macabre and grotesque picture, one hundred fifty thousand chicken heads containing dead rabies virus were air dropped by helicopter onto the countryside.

Summary

Currently, tens of thousands of people, mostly in Asia and Africa, die each year from rabies. Nearly half of those deaths are children.[86] The high death rates in these areas derive largely from the lack of effective policies to vaccinate animals and lack of universal access to vaccination once bitten.

Like the smallpox vaccine, the rabies vaccine is a miracle, a virus kill switch that has saved countless lives. Rabies vaccination also inadvertently taught us that a vaccine contaminated with pieces of an organ's tissue can cause your body to attack that organ and cause autoimmune disease. Using that knowledge, scientists vaccinate animals to cause autoimmune diseases as a tool to study autoimmunity in the laboratory. We might say that errors and problems are our teachers. But it is better to prevent such errors before they occur than to deal with them afterward, and this is what vaccines are designed to do. Yet, as we saw in this chapter, problems may also arise from vaccines.

CHAPTER 5

Yellow Fever: Humanity's Martyrs and Opportunists

If you think you are too small to make a difference, you haven't spent the night with a mosquito.—The Dalai Lama

How do we approach questions? Scientists routinely submit to being questioned. To protect patient privacy, medical doctors decline third-party patient questions. Journalists insist on questioning others but do not submit themselves to questioning.—RKB

The symptoms of yellow fever are the usual viral symptoms of muscle aches, loss of appetite, fever, headache, photophobia (i.e., sensitivity to light), backache, lassitude (i.e., fatigue), nausea, and vomiting. These symptoms resolve within three to five days.[87] Twenty-four to forty-eight hours after recovery, about 15 percent of patients redevelop new symptoms of high fever and prostration (i.e., mental and physical exhaustion). From there, multiple organs will start to fail, including the liver, kidneys, heart, and brain. Patients vomit blood, the whites of their eyes and their skin yellow from jaundice, and their stools become especially foul smelling. Next, their urination decreases or stops, confusion and delirium occur, and their blood pressure drops. Diffuse bleeding from the mouth and rectum, seizures, and coma ensue before death.

Yellow fever is so named because the patient turns yellow with fever. The yellow color is due to the liver's inability to excrete bile or, more specifically, a component of bile called bilirubin. Other names for yellow fever are the American plague, yellow jacket, and *vomito negro*.[88] The latter Spanish name derives from the black vomit that occurs. As the patient's liver fails, it stops making blood-clotting proteins, and blood starts to ooze into the patient's gut.[89] The acidity in the stomach degrades red blood, resulting in vomit with the appearance of black ground coffee.

The American Plague

Yellow fever is called the American plague due to its presence in the United States from its very founding.[90] America's first well-documented epidemic of yellow fever occurred in Philadelphia in 1793.[91] At that time, Philadelphia was a bustling port city of fifty thousand people and the (temporary) capital of the United States. As the seat of the federal government, Philadelphia was where George Washington resided during most of his two terms as president.

In the summer of 1793 Caribbean immigrants and slaves crowded the port of Philadelphia, including some who arrived on the *Hankey*, a British merchant ship that previously anchored in West Africa before reaching the Caribbean. Later referred to as "the ship of death," the *Hankey* would proceed to leave a trail of yellow fever at every port of call, most notably Philadelphia.[92] When the deaths from yellow fever started rising, around 40 percent of Philadelphia's inhabitants (mostly federal government employees and wealthy private citizens) hurriedly abandoned the city. During this time, George Washington escaped to his country estate at Mount Vernon. Alexander Hamilton, whose picture is on the ten-dollar bill, similarly fled to New York but was denied entry.[93] Hamilton developed yellow fever and survived. Approximately five thousand of the thirty-thousand residents trapped in Philadelphia died from yellow fever. The epidemic finally stopped in the autumn of 1793 when the temperature dropped.

Yellow fever was also called "yellow jacket" during this time, as ships under quarantine flew a yellow flag.[94] To this day, ships hoist a yellow flag to warn that a contagious disease is onboard, informing other ships to stay away. The term "quarantine" derives from the Latin word *quadraginta*, meaning "forty." This is because such quarantines often lasted around forty days. Why forty days was chosen as the standard quarantine interval for infections is not known. One speculation is that this number was drawn from the biblical time of Jesus's fasting in the desert during which he withstood the devil's temptations.[95]

Ships bearing the yellow flag could not enter port and were required to stay offshore until completing quarantine. Such experiences may have inspired various tales about ghost ships like the *Flying Dutchman*, which legends stated was never allowed to make port, forever cursed to sail the seven seas. As one author from 1790 summarized the legend, "The Dutchman . . . wanted to get into harbour but could not . . . and was lost and that ever since in very bad weather her vision appears."[96] Although we have no early account explicitly linking the *Flying Dutchman* with yellow fever, as historian Billy Smith claims, "the tale of the *Flying Dutchman* was part of the lore that the [yellow fever] plague generated."[97]

A forty-day quarantine would have been an economic disaster. Inflationary pressure would cause prices to skyrocket on the mainland, as anything perishable on a merchant ship, such as fruits, vegetables, or meats, would rot. Businesses financially backing these ships would sometimes go bankrupt. Jobs would be lost. Like the effects of the disease itself, the economic effects of a yellow fever quarantine would have been hardest on the poor. Since nobody knew the exact incubation interval before onset of yellow fever symptoms (now known to be three to five days),[98] the arbitrary quarantine interval of forty days would have been unnecessarily long and caused significant hardship for working-class individuals.

In some states, the quarantine duration was instead left to local discretion. However, this was also not without problems. For example, in 1878 the steamship *Emily D. Souder* sailing from Havana was quarantined for only a few hours before being allowed to berth in New Orleans. The inspectors found that the ship's purser, John Cark, was a little under the weather. This was attributed to a hangover from the crew drinking rum the night before. The day after disembarking, Clark developed yellow fever, and a few days later he died. The ship's engineer, Thomas Elliot, also developed yellow fever and died.[99] Before long, New Orleans was in the midst of a yellow fever epidemic, resulting in the death of nearly 10 percent of the city's population.

This 1878 yellow fever epidemic sailed from New Orleans up the Mississippi River on steamboats and into the river harbor of Memphis, Tennessee. Over half of Memphis's forty-five thousand residents (mostly those with financial means) stampeded over each other to escape the city. Fear of the invisible grim reaper was so palpable that some did not even bother to gather personal belongings or lock their homes. Of the remaining twenty thousand inhabitants of Memphis, approximately seventeen thousand were infected with yellow fever, and about five thousand of those infected died.[100]

The Sinking of the USS *Maine*

Two decades after the 1878 epidemic, yellow fever played a lethal role in the Spanish-America War.[101] The battleship USS *Maine* arrived in the harbor of Havana, Cuba, in January of 1898 in order to protect American interests in the ongoing Cuban War of Independence. On the evening of February 15, 1898, the USS *Maine* suddenly heaved out of the water with a deafening explosion followed by the screaming of men lost in smoke and flames.[102] The ship's captain and officers frantically worked to rescue crew trapped in the lower decks before being completely submerged. Spanish sailors and officers on shore jumped into boats and rowed into the flaming USS *Maine* to help pull out maimed and burned American sailors. Spanish doctors and nurses worked around the clock to save as many injured sailors as they could. Of 355 enlisted men and officers on the USS *Maine*, 261 died. The captain of the battleship, Charles D. Sigsbee, telegrammed the secretary of the Navy in Washington, DC, reporting on the Spanish help, goodwill, and sympathy for his crew. Captain Sigsbee concluded his cable with this message: "Many Spanish Officers including representative of General Blanco now with me to express Sympathy."[103]

Word of the USS *Maine* spread like wildfire thanks to the newspaper magnates of the era. Two of these media barons included the Harvard-educated William Randolph Hearst—who was immortalized in the movie *Citizen Kane*[104]—and his rival, the Hungarian immigrant Joseph Pulitzer, the namesake of the Pulitzer Prize for journalism. Both Hearst's *New York Journal* and Pulitzer's *New York World* sensationalized the sinking of the USS *Maine* within their respective publications, emotionally manipulating the tragedy to increase sales revenue. Coincidentally nicknamed "yellow journalism," such emotionally charged, opportunistic, and profit-seeking reporting has maintained its deep roots in mainstream American corporate media ever since.[105]

To boost circulation, these newspapers spun the USS *Maine* catastrophe as an act of Spanish aggression. The newspaper headlines read "Destruction of the Warship Maine Was the Work of an Enemy."[106] The catchy phrase, "Remember the Maine. To hell with Spain," swept across America and prompted public outcry for war.[107] The resulting Spanish-American War began on April 21, 1898. It was over in less than four months. When the war started, Spain was a hollowed-out, bankrupt shell of its former self. It did not have the military power or finances to fight the much stronger American military. What allowed Spain to hang on for as long as they did was an unexpected and stealthy ally: yellow fever. During the Spanish-American War many more soldiers died from diseases like typhoid, malaria, and yellow fever than from battle wounds.

In the end, Spain as the losing party of the war surrendered Cuba, Puerto Rico, Guam, and the Philippines to America. This secured America as a maritime military power and ingloriously ended the Spanish Empire, which at its height was the fifth largest empire in world history. To this day Guam and Puerto Rico remain US territories.

Eighty years after the war had passed, a 1976 forensic examination headed by Admiral Hyman G. Rickover, the father of America's "Nuclear Navy," determined that the USS *Maine* explosion resulted from an unintentional error in ship design. The fatal flaw was that the battleship's coal bunker was located next to the ammunition's magazine. An accidental fire in the former likely spread to the latter, causing an explosion that changed the course of history.[108]

The Yellow Fever Commission

Since more American soldiers died during the Spanish-American War from infection than from the horrors of battle, the United States organized the Yellow Fever Commission, headed by physician and Army Major Walter Reed, to determine its cause.[109] Walter Reed grew up the son of a poor, rural Methodist minister. He was well educated in medicine, history, and classical Greek and Latin. Because he did not have the proper upper-class background, money, or credentials to start his own private medical practice, he became a military surgeon.[110]

The Yellow Fever Commission consisted of Walter Reed, Jesse Lazear, James Carroll, and Aristides Agramonte.[111] They traveled to the newly acquired American territory of Cuba to study yellow fever. They were met by a Cuban native Carlos Juan Finlay, an epidemiologist who noticed a correlation between the annual number of mosquitos and the number of yellow fever cases.[112] In 1881, twenty years before the Yellow Fever Commission was established, he presented a paper to the Havana Academy of Sciences called "The Mosquito Hypothetically Considered as the Agent of Transmission of Yellow Fever."[113] Except for being mocked with the nickname "Mosquito Man," he was ignored.

Reed decided to test Finlay's mosquito hypothesis, resulting in James Carroll and Jesse Lazear subjecting themselves to the bite of mosquitos that had fed on the blood of yellow fever patients.[114] A few days later, both developed high fever, intense pain, and fatigue. Lazear would die twelve days later from the virus, while Carroll recovered but suffered permanent cardiac damage. Despite his heart problems, after his initial recovery Carroll completed the last official duty of the Yellow Fever Commission. He demonstrated that yellow fever could be transmitted by an infectious patient's blood even after being passed through a filter capable of removing bacteria. This established yellow fever as an infectious agent smaller than a bacterium—that is, a virus.[115]

In a presentation to the American Public Health Association in Indianapolis, Reed reported on mosquito-transmitted yellow fever.[116] His data was considered speculative and insufficient proof for a mosquito vector. The *Washington Post* summarized Walter Reed's mosquito hypothesis as: "Of all, the silly and nonsensical rigmarole about yellow fever that has yet found its way into print—and there has been enough of it to load a fleet—the silliest beyond compare is to be found in the arguments and theories engendered by the mosquito hypothesis."[117] In response, Reed set up Camp Lazear, named after his recently deceased colleague, six miles from Havana. Camp Lazear was designed to prove or disprove whether mosquitos could transmit yellow fever.[118]

At Camp Lazear, US military and Spanish immigrant volunteers who signed a consent form were recruited to sleep in one building containing the soiled linen and bodily fluids from yellow fever–infected patients. This was to determine if poor hygiene and body fluids (vomit, urine, sweat, stool) passed yellow fever along to other subjects, as was typical for bacteria like cholera. The other building contained clean linens, but those subjects were bitten by mosquitos that had fed on the blood from people with yellow fever. On Christmas Day, 1900, the first volunteer in the mosquito room developed yellow fever. As time went by, only subjects in the mosquito room developed yellow fever.

The volunteers were paid $200 in gold to participate and $500 in gold if they contracted yellow fever. By today's standards, these payments are approximately $8,000 and $20,000, respectively. Even though the patients were consenting volunteers, this study may be viewed as unethical by current norms. In truth, however, the true involuntary aspect was the US government forcing military personnel to remain posted in a yellow fever–infested Cuba in the first place. The soldiers stationed in Cuba became infected with yellow fever regardless of the conclusion of the Yellow Fever Commission study. Those soldiers had three options: (1) hope for the small possibility of running out the gauntlet of time and escape yellow fever infection; (2) get infected outside of the study without compensation or payment; or (3) volunteer to get paid and offered the best military care if infected.

The identification of mosquitos as the reservoir for yellow fever explained why yellow fever occurred in America as intermittent epidemics and then disappeared. The yellow fever virus is zoonotic, meaning it is spread by mosquitos drinking the blood of an infected subject and then transmitting it after feeding upon another human. During the winter season, the insects carrying the fever would die out, causing the spread of the fever to cease as well. Despite the innumerable epidemics, yellow fever has never mutated or learned how to jump from one human to another without a mosquito intermediary.

The identification of the mosquito as the cause of yellow fever stopped epidemics in America. Pesticides were developed to kill adult mosquitos. Standing water was drained to prevent breeding, and stagnant water was covered with oil to suffocate larvae. For discovering its secrets, the members of the Yellow Fever Commission were received as heroes. As noted, Jesse Lazear died after contracting yellow fever. A dormitory at Johns Hopkins University, his alma mater, and a stained-glass window at the Washington National Cathedral are now dedicated to him.

Walter Reed died in 1902, two years after formation of the commission. The United States' flagship military medical hospital, the Walter Reed National Military Medical Center, was named in his honor in 1905.

James Carroll died in 1907. He was interred with full military honors in the Washington National Cemetery. In 1915 the last surviving member of the Yellow Fever Commission, Aristides Agramonte, published the inside story of his comrades' sacrifices in *Science Monthly*, the prestigious journal of the American Society of Science.[119]

Although neither an American nor a formal commission member, Carlos Finlay, who first proposed and informed the commission of his belief that mosquitos caused yellow fever, died in 1915. Before his death, he was nominated for a Nobel Prize. The statue *El Obelisco* (The Obelisk) stands in his memory in Havana, Cuba. The United Nations Educational, Scientific, and Cultural Organization (UNESCO) established the Carlos J. Finlay Prize for microbiology in 1980 in his honor.

The West African Commission

In 1925, ten years after the death of the last member of the Yellow Fever Commission, the West African Commission was organized by the Rockefeller Foundation.[120] Once again, a US Army physician, this time Colonel Henry Beeuwkes, led the commission. The primary goal of this commission was to discover the source of and find a treatment for yellow fever. They set up a base camp in Yaba, Nigeria.

An African man named Asibi, who was living in nearby Ghana and afflicted with yellow fever, donated a blood sample to the West African Commission. Using Asibi's blood, yellow fever was transmitted to monkeys imported from India. The Indian subcontinent was free (and to this day remains free) of yellow fever. Unlike African monkeys that had been exposed and were resistant to reinfection, Indian monkeys acquired yellow fever with a course identical to humans.[121] They died or recovered with immunity. The yellow fever virus could now be transmitted between and studied in laboratory monkeys. The West African Commission discovered that serum from monkeys that survived infection protected other susceptible monkeys. Although not understood at the time, this protective effect was due to passive immunity from the transfer of antibodies against the virus. The transfer of a previously infected patients' serum to stop a new virus infection was most recently used in China in 2019 to successfully treat COVID-19.

Like James Lazear of the Cuban Yellow Fever Commission, three West African Commission members died at the yellow fever altar. Shortly after reporting on successful transmission of yellow fever to monkeys, Adrian Stokes died in 1927 from yellow fever.[122] While injecting monkeys to better identify the infectious agent involved, Hideyo Noguchi, a second investigator, also succumbed to yellow fever.[123] A third member of the commission, William Young, who performed Noguchi's autopsy, died shortly afterward from yellow fever.[124]

The West African Commission helped establish tropical Africa, with its hot and humid climate, as the endemic site and reservoir for yellow fever. The initial transportation of yellow fever to the Americas accompanied the African slave trade during the sixteenth and seventeenth centuries. During this interval, intermittent epidemics occurred in Latin America, the Caribbean, and tropical South America.

Max Theiler and the Only Nobel Prize for a Vaccine

To develop a vaccine for yellow fever, an animal model was needed. The West African Commission provided it with the passage of the Asibi strain in Indian monkeys. Dr. Max Theiler with the Rockefeller Foundation discovered that passage of the Asibi strain could be done by direct inoculation into the brains of mice. However, passage in a mouse brain caused the vaccine to develop excessive fatal neurologic toxicity when reinjected into monkeys. So too passage of the virus in a monkey liver resulted in a vaccine that caused excessive fatal liver disease. To develop a vaccine safe for humans, a production source other than mice or monkeys was needed.

A breakthrough finally occurred in 1937. In three sequential publications in the *Journal of Experimental Medicine* that year, Theiler and other members of the Rockefeller Foundation recounted how they used the Asibi strain to develop a safe vaccine for yellow fever.[125] By culturing the Asibi strain in mouse embryonic tissue with serum isolated from monkey blood and then shifting it into minced whole chick embryos and finally chick embryos that had their head and spinal cord tissue removed, Theiler and his team were able to diminish vaccine-related neurotoxicity. After 176 passages, this strain of yellow fever virus, now called 17D, had lost neurologic and liver toxicity but still could elicit an immune response.[126]

The 17D yellow fever virus strain was "alive" but attenuated with few serious clinical adverse symptoms. Theiler's 17D variant became the universal yellow fever strain used in vaccines worldwide. The basic technique for yellow fever vaccine production from the 17D strain is: (1) inoculate the 17D virus with a syringe into seven-day-old embryonated chicken eggs (i.e., eggs with a live embryo inside); (2) incubate the inoculated eggs for four days; (3) crack the egg open and remove the eleven-day-old embryo; (4) mince the embryo in a blender (in early vaccine lots human serum was added to this step); (5) centrifuge (i.e., spin) the minced embryo organs to separate them from the fluid (called supernatant) that is rich in virus; and (6) freeze the supernatant (the vaccine) on dry ice. Later advances in freeze-drying technology have led to the lyophilization (sublimation of ice to a water vapor under vacuum) of the vaccine to form a dry powder. Before vaccination, the freeze-dried vaccine is rehydrated with salt water and injected under the skin much like a mosquito bite.

Max Theiler received the 1951 Nobel Prize in Physiology or Medicine for his work on developing the 17D yellow fever vaccine. It remains the only Nobel Prize ever awarded for a vaccine. During his Nobel committee address, Theiler addressed the sacrifices of the Yellow Fever and West African Commissions: "I like to feel that in honoring me . . . you are honoring all those workers in the laboratory, field, and jungle who have contributed so much under conditions of hardship and danger . . . those who gave their lives in gaining knowledge. . . . They were truly martyrs of science."[127]

Hepatitis B and Avian Leukosis Virus Contamination of the 17D Yellow Fever Vaccine

Following the initial development of the 17D yellow fever vaccine, Brazil was chosen as the first site for a large trial. This was because of the coexistence of monkey and human hosts in Brazil along with its tropical weather with no seasonal elimination of the mosquito reservoir, which led to recurrent yellow fever epidemics. Another reason for this decision was that the Rockefeller Foundation from New York had set up a yellow fever laboratory within the Brazilian Oswaldo Cruz Institute in Rio de Janeiro.[128]

Between 1937 and 1941 a number of Brazilians who received the vaccine developed liver damage and jaundice weeks to months after vaccination. The Brazilians recognized this complication through follow-up visits conducted with vaccine recipients months after their vaccination. In contrast, American physicians generally did not engage in intermediate- or long-term follow-up with vaccinated patients. The Oswaldo Cruz Institute determined that these effects were caused by human serum being added to the minced chick embryos in the production of the vaccine.[129] Brazil's "kill switch" is that they stopped using human serum for vaccine production. Because they had followed America's vaccine recipe, Angelo Moreira da Costa Lima, an investigator at the Oswaldo Cruz Institute, accused the Americans who provided the vaccine technology of using Brazilians as guinea pigs.[130]

Investigators in Rio de Janeiro informed the Rockefeller Institute in New York City of this complication. For unclear reasons, the Americans did not heed Brazil's warning and continued to produce the vaccine using human serum. They ignored Brazil's "kill switch" communication. The contaminated vaccine was even given to US soldiers during World War II. Later, it was realized that the yellow fever vaccine was contaminated with hepatitis B virus.

Once a human is infected, hepatitis B lives forever within the human host. It kills a minority from acute inflammation of the liver. For most people, hepatitis B becomes a chronic liver infection. After several years or decades, the chronic form of hepatitis B kills the infected person from slow liver fibrosis, cirrhosis, and either liver failure and/or liver cancer. More than fifty thousand US soldiers sent to fight in World War II developed hepatitis B infection after yellow fever vaccination.[131] Due to the sensitivities of World War II and troop morale, the press, even to this day, has remained silent about this. The veterans who suffered these complications were never notified, nor were their families compensated.

Two decades later in 1962, the avian (bird) leukosis virus was found to contaminate most yellow fever vaccines.[132] Avian leukosis virus is transmitted vertically from infected hen to embryonated egg and then to the vaccine recipient. It causes cancer in chickens.[133] In the only apparent study performed in 2,659 veterans with relatively short follow-up, there was no epidemiologic correlation found between cancer and the yellow fever vaccination.[134] Beginning in 1967, only chicken eggs from chickens free of avian leukosis virus would be used for vaccine production.[135] Long-term effects from introducing avian leukosis virus into humans are unknown.

Vaccine-Associated Brain (Neurotropic) and Liver (Viscerotrophic) Damage

Yellow fever vaccine complications have not completely disappeared. It is a live vaccine that was extensively passaged to avoid viral-induced liver or brain damage. Yet rare cases of yellow fever vaccine associated neurologic (brain) disease (YFAND)[136] and yellow fever vaccine associated viscerotrophic (liver) disease (YFAVD)[137] continue to be rarely documented after vaccination. YFAND is defined as the occurrence of fever, seizures, and brain dysfunction within thirty days of vaccination when other causes of brain inflammation are ruled out and the yellow fever virus is isolated from the fluid around the brain. YFAVD is characterized by fever and a failing liver with yellow fever virus isolated from the blood, liver, or kidney following yellow fever vaccination.

In 2001, YFAND and YFAVD were reported in ten patients.[138] Two weeks later, six of the ten vaccinated patients had died. The unsatisfactory explanation reported for the cause was "idiosyncratic" or "peculiar" host susceptibility.[139] In plain words, the attenuated virus retained lethal toxicity for subgroups of people.

Susceptible people have weak immune systems that cannot clear this weakened live vaccine virus before it causes liver or brain damage. This includes people over sixty years old, children less than nine months old, and patients on immune suppressive drugs. Brain or liver deaths may occur in a patient being immune suppressed from an organ transplant if the organ donor was recently vaccinated.[140] Neither blood nor organs should be donated for at least three weeks after the donor has received the yellow fever vaccine.

Summary

Several toxicity lessons have been learned from the development and deployment of the yellow fever vaccination. First, growing a virus with a human serum may spread another lethal human virus (in this case, hepatitis B). Second, the hubris of America's elite institutions to neglect follow-up treatment of yellow fever vaccine recipients led them to reject an accurate "kill switch" warning about producing the vaccine in human serum. Third, growing a virus in animal cells—even cells as sterile as embryonated chick eggs—may result in the transmission of a cancer-causing virus (in this case, avian leukosis virus) into the human population. Finally, a live attenuated (i.e., weakened) vaccine virus may still be lethal if injected into an immune compromised person.

The yellow fever vaccine continues to use the original Asibi-derived Theiler 17D strain and sub strains (17D204 and 17DD) grown in embryonated chick eggs. This is because natural infection is worse than vaccine complications. Unvaccinated populations suffer 15 percent mortality when naturally infected. Approximately two hundred thousand unvaccinated people get yellow fever each year, of which thirty thousand die predominately in endemic regions of Africa. Deaths from the vaccine occur but are rare (1 to 2.5 cases per million vaccinations).[141] Like natural infection, vaccination affords lifelong immunity.[142] However, vaccination is officially recommended every ten years for people traveling to endemic tropical and subtropical areas.[143]

The yellow fever vaccine has taught us that how we prepare a vaccine, be it with human serum or with animal cells, may transmit other injurious human or animal viruses to the vaccine recipient. Unless thoughtful cautions and safeguards are put into place, such tragic consequences can (and will) continue to happen in the development of future vaccines, as we'll see in the chapters to follow.

CHAPTER 6

Poliomyelitis: A Live or Dead Vaccine Grown in Monkey Kidney Cells

The polio pandemic paradoxically arose from cleanliness, i.e., removing sewage from drinking water.—RKB

Poliomyelitis (often abbreviation as polio) derives from two Greek words: *polios* "gray" and *myelos* "matter." The poliomyelitis virus infects the gray-matter nerve cells (neurons) of the spine and brain. It is classified as an enterovirus, which means it is a virus of the intestine (from the Greek *enteron* "entrails, bowel"). Its portal of entry into the body is via the digestive tract following oral ingestion. Poliomyelitis is transmitted between people by ingestion of water or food contaminated with human feces or from poor handwashing.

After oral transmission, poliovirus replicates in a type of immune cell called B cells in lymphoid (i.e., immune cell) aggregates known as Peyer's patches within the wall of the distal small bowel.[144] From there, the virus enters the bloodstream and reenters the lumen of the bowel to be transmitted through excreted feces to another person. The virus is cleared from the blood within seven days by antibodies generated by the immune system. During the interval required to generate antibodies to stop viral circulation, a break in the blood-brain barrier may allow poliovirus to enter the brain or spinal cord and cause paralysis.

The majority (80 to 90 percent) of poliomyelitis infections are asymptomatic. About 10 to 20 percent of infected subjects develop headache, neck stiffness, or a transient sensation of pins and needles or tingling. Approximately 1 percent of infected patients develop flaccid paralysis with residual deformed limbs, which requires the use of leg braces, crutches, or wheelchairs. In cases with respiratory paralysis, the patient is confined within a mechanical breathing device. For some, the infection results in death.

Since poliomyelitis is contracted from soiled water or food, it would be natural to think, as most people did and perhaps still do, that the populations most at risk would be those living under squalid and unsanitary conditions. The opposite is true. Polio is a disease associated with developed nations and a middle- or upper-income economic status.[145]

Before the twentieth century almost all people were exposed to polio during infancy. This resulted in asymptomatic infections and lifelong immunity, because infants are protected if infected while breastfeeding. Passive transfer of antibodies against poliovirus occurred via their mother's milk.[146] When exposed to live poliovirus, the infant immune system, under the protection of their mother's immunity, has time to develop its own immune cells to generate its own permanent supply of antibodies that prevent future infections.

The industrial revolution and broad acceptance of the germ theory as a cause for infections brought about sanitary improvements, like the separation of drinking water from sewage and fastidious handwashing before meals. There is a saying that "cleanliness is next to godliness," but ironically these hygienic advances resulted in reduced exposure to poliovirus in infants starting in the late nineteenth century in the United States and Europe, leading to a paralytic polio epidemic. As an unexpected late complication of good intentions to sterilize the water supply, polio-naïve children and adults became sitting targets.

Sister Elizabeth Kenny

One of the significant figures in the history of the treatment of poliomyelitis is Sister Elizabeth Kenny (1880–1952), an Australian nurse of Irish ancestry who grew up poor.[147] During the 1930s and 1940s, Kenny started using physical therapy as a means of rehabilitating paralyzed polio victims. While Kenny was not privileged with elite social status or the opportunity for a proper medical education, she did have the compassion, common sense, and courage to start muscle massage, joint movement, and warm compress therapy at onset of poliomyelitis weakness. Kenny realized that human touch, if started early on, was beneficial both psychologically and medically for infected individuals. Many of her patients and their families who witnessed the results reported regaining the ability to move and/or walk.

Sister Kenny's treatment flew in the face of the medical dogma of her day, which held that at the time of paralysis onset the affected limb or body should undergo strict immobilization. This was also a much cheaper treatment option, as one detached attendant could care for many immobilized patients. Several physicians viewed Sister Kenny's success with jealous disdain. One medical journal at the time even said her idea was "not original" and, "It is not certain whether Sister Kenny gets good results because of the meticulous application of good."[148] She was criticized by those with credentials and titles, yet her early physical therapy saved more children from wheelchairs than anyone else until the advent of the polio vaccine.

To this day, there are no effective antiviral drugs for poliomyelitis. Sister Kenny's approach is now universally accepted as the patient's best chance for full or partial recovery, if initiated early after onset of symptoms. Sister Kenny's inner fortitude and love for her patients kept her going despite painful and (in retrospect) completely inappropriate criticism. Her autobiography, *And They Shall Walk*, was published in 1943.[149] She died in 1952 before start of the first vaccine trial. Her last book, *My Battle and Victory*, was published posthumously in 1955.[150]

The Man in the Iron Lung

The story of polio also cannot be told without mentioning the iron lung and Frederick Snite (1910–1954). The iron lung was invented by the engineer Philip Drinker in 1928. It is an airtight hollow iron tube that surrounds the patient's body with only their head sticking outside of it. By alternating air pressure on the body inside the iron lung, it provides a push-pull motion on the chest to move air out of and into the lungs. Out of the many thousands of poliovirus-infected patients who were confined to this apparatus, Frederick Snite became the symbolic "man in the iron lung."[151]

Snite was born into a wealthy Chicago family. In 1936 while on a trip to Beijing, China, twenty-five-year-old Snite contracted polio with respiratory weakness and distress. After being paralyzed from the neck down, Snite's life was saved by putting him inside the only iron lung available in China. To return home, he traveled over seven hundred miles in an ambulance from Beijing to the port of Shanghai while remaining in his iron lung. Along the way, crowds gathered to see the novelty of a person's head sticking outside of a nine-hundred-pound capsule. If at any time the generators attached to the iron lung failed, emergency blacksmith-like bellows would be used to hand pump air pressure changes into and out of his iron casket.

In Shanghai, Snite was loaded onto the luxury ocean liner *President Coolidge* and along with numerous medical personnel sailed back to America. Snite lay lifeless on his back, unable to move or roll to his side, unable to comb his hair, feed himself, shave, cough, wipe his nose, or wipe after a bowel movement. He had to be intermittently suction with a thin tube placed down his throat to clear airway secretions. A portable respirator strapped on his chest would allow short intervals outside of the iron lung for aids to wash and clean his body and attend to any pressure ulcers.

For most people, Frederick's fate would be worse than death, but he had an indomitable spirit. He got married, fathered children, and would attend football games at his alma mater, Notre Dame. A place was allocated in the stands to accommodate his iron lung. During the games, he would lie on his back face up staring at the sky with a mirror tilted over his head so he could watch the game. Fans would cheer the home team, but whenever Snite entered the stadium, a wild mayhem of pandemonium would rock the entire arena. A sportswriter nicknamed the players in the backfield of Notre Dame "The Four Horsemen." Snite's nickname was the Fifth Horseman. After eighteen years in an iron lung, Snite's withered, motionless, and fragile body gave out. His funeral service, attended by 1,500 people, was held at Saint Luke's Catholic Church in River Forest, Illinois (a Chicago suburb).

Franklin D. Roosevelt and the National Foundation for Infantile Paralysis

Franklin D. Roosevelt was the thirty-second president of the United States. He was born in 1882 into one of New York's wealthiest families in a mansion on the Roosevelt estate overlooking the Hudson River. In 1921, at age thirty-nine, he developed polio, which at that time was called infantile paralysis because it usually affected children. Polio left him paralyzed from the waist down and in a wheelchair. In 1926, Roosevelt bought the Warm Springs Resort in Georgia and transformed it into a mineral water hydrotherapy and rehabilitation center for polio patients, including himself.[152]

In 1932, Roosevelt was elected US president and subsequently was reelected for a total of four terms. In a wheelchair, he led America through the Great Depression (1929–1938) and through World War II (1941–1945). Roosevelt threw the weight of the Office of the President behind developing a vaccine for polio. In 1938, Roosevelt established the National Foundation for Infantile Paralysis (often abbreviated as the National Foundation). Due to powerful mental images of children in crutches and Frederick Snite in an iron lung, and due to the support from figures like Roosevelt, the National Foundation was very successful in raising money to help patients with polio and to discover a vaccine.

The National Foundation for Infantile Paralysis was headed by Basil O'Conner, a friend of President Roosevelt. It was later renamed the March of Dimes.[153] The name March of Dimes came from a National Foundation marketing slogan used to raise money. With the collapse of the economy and loss of wealth during the Great Depression, the National Foundation solicited movie theaters to run a teaser on polio that aired just before the main film started, asking for people to donate their spare dimes. By collecting pocket change from large numbers of people, the National Foundation generated tremendous revenue.

The National Foundation donated the money it raised to help patients suffering from polio. Anyone with polio who requested help had their expenses paid. People did not have to prove or justify their debt or financial condition. Their word of needing help was good enough for the charity to provide financial aid. From 1938 until 1955 when the Salk vaccine was approved, the March of Dimes spent $233 million paying patient bills, which is roughly equivalent to $2.5 trillion in today's economy.[154]

Today tax-exempt charities will almost never pay for a patient's medical expenses. There still exist a few rare and unique organizations, such as St. Jude's Children's Research Hospital in Memphis,

Tennessee, that adhere to the principle of helping anyone who needs help. Most current medical organizations or societies arrange extravagant self-promotional advertising events hosted by "famous" people, and their executive staff are not infrequently flown around the world and paid a six- or seven-figure income, yet nothing is given by these organizations to help pay the bills of financially strapped patients in need.

When not paying the medical bills of polio patients, the National Foundation spent most of the rest of its income on funding polio research and a vaccine trial. In fact, they funded the largest vaccine trial ever performed in America. Under the visionary leadership of Basil O'Conner, the National Foundation recognized that the first step in development of a vaccine was to fund basic research. It provided a grant to Drs. Howard Howe and David Bodian at Johns Hopkins School of Medicine in Baltimore, Maryland, to study the neuropathology of poliovirus. After receiving a report in 1939 that two chimpanzees at the zoo in Cologne, Germany, developed paralytic paralysis, Howe and Bodian discovered that poliovirus from a patient's stool could infect chimpanzees and monkeys.[155] Cynomolgus monkeys from the Philippines and especially the more prevalent and easier to obtain Rhesus monkeys from India thus became animal models for poliovirus research and, later, for vaccine production.

To determine if there were different types of polioviruses that caused paralysis, cross-protection studies were performed on these monkeys. After injection into the brain of one strain of virus, monkeys that survived infection were re-exposed by the injection of a different viral strain into the brain. If the monkeys remained healthy, they were immune, meaning that the second virus injected into them was of the same strain as the first. If the monkeys again developed paralysis, then the second injected virus was from a different strain. By doing this with many different strains of poliovirus, they found three distinct viral subtypes that caused paralysis. All three distinct paralytic poliovirus subtypes (types 1, 2, and 3) would have to be included into any vaccine.[156]

Hundreds of thousands of rhesus and cynomolgus monkeys were used for polio research and vaccine production during this period. In just 1955 alone, two hundred thousand monkeys were imported for vaccine production.[157] Monkeys were bought in New Delhi and shipped to New York via London. In that year, 394 monkeys died from suffocation in an unvented truck while transiting through London. The Indian population was in an uproar, as in the Hindu religion animals, like humans, have souls and thus should not be mistreated.[158] After the institution of safeguards, the shipments continued.

To make a vaccine, large quantities of virus would be needed. Beginning in 1941, the National Foundation funded John Enders at Harvard to determine the best conditions to grow poliovirus in laboratory cells. Instead of using a stationary flask, tubes were laid horizontally into holes in a wood block that slowly rotated so the cells inside the flask contiguously encountered both air and media.[159] Enders was able to grow polio in different cell types, including in monkey kidney cells.[160] (The history of using cells to grow poliomyelitis virus for vaccines is described in Box 6.1.) Growing virus in cells incubated in a laboratory facilitated access to an abundant supply of virus for polio vaccine trials. Enders also demonstrated successful *ex vivo* (outside of the body) cell culture of other viruses including measles. In 1954, he was awarded the Nobel Prize in Medicine or Physiology for growing poliovirus in laboratory cells.[161]

Box 6.1: Cells Used to Produce Poliovirus Vaccines

Poliomyelitis virus was first produced in freshly harvested monkey kidney cells that have a limited life span in culture, resulting in the death of untold numbers of monkeys. In 1962, Leonard Hayflick at the Wistar Institute established a human cell line called WI-38 (an abbreviation for Wistar Institute Fetus 38).[162]

It was collected from the three-month-old fetus of a patient undergoing an elective legal abortion in Sweden. Like all nonembryonic cells, WI-38 is not immortal and is exhausted or undergoes senescence at approximately fifty passages (called the Hayflick Limit). WI-38 was the first *human* cell line used for vaccine production and is still used to manufacture the rubella (also known as German measles) vaccine.

Poliovirus vaccine is currently grown in Vero cells (an Esperanto abbreviation for *verda reno*, meaning "green kidney") that are an immortalized African green monkey kidney cell line generated in Japan.[163] The Vero cell line can grow indefinitely in culture. It provides an unlimited renewable and well-characterized single cell line that is negative for "known" adventitious (i.e., harmful) infectious agents.

Enders's work not only changed the landscape of virus research but altered the landscape of medical research funding as well. The National Foundation ran into a problem when trying to fund Enders's research, as Harvard would not allow Enders to accept the money unless an additional 28 percent of the total research budget was added to support Harvard's bureaucracy ("facility and administration," also known as "indirect costs"). The National Foundation relented. The university's argument was that the more research money an investigator attracted, the more facilities and administration were needed.[164]

Over time, facility and administration costs on medical research grants have become standard practice, and the percent taken by universities has gradually escalated. Facility and administration payment to the institution for most grants is now often greater than 50 percent and, in some institutions, as high as 80 to 90 percent. (A February 2025 law that limits indirect costs to 15 percent has been temporarily blocked following a district court injunction.) It is a medieval labor relationship, one that renders untenured and, in some cases, tenured university researchers as temporary employees expected to acquire grants to pay not only for their own salary and research but also for their employer's salary and office space.

Polio Vaccines

Enders's breakthrough in growing poliovirus in cells provided an ample supply of poliovirus for vaccines. During the 1950s, three investigators (Koprowski, Salk, and Sabin) took the lead in developing poliovirus vaccines.

The Koprowski Live Polio Vaccine

From his prior experience working on the live yellow fever vaccine trial in Brazil, Hilary Koprowski at Lederle Laboratories in New York believed that a live but weakened (i.e., attenuated) virus would give the best immune response against polio.[165] He attenuated poliovirus by orally feeding it to cotton rats. After oral ingestion by rats, the virus was collected from rat feces to vaccinate infants. Koprowski developed two strains used for vaccines, called SM and TN. In 1950, nineteen New York children were vaccinated with rat-attenuated live oral polio vaccine. They developed antibodies (an immune response) to polio with no reported ill effects.[166]

Due to these initial reports of safety and development of immunity, in 1955 the Koprowski oral vaccine was given to infants in Northern Ireland. In this trial, the virus was collected from stool of vaccinated infants and injected into the brains of healthy monkeys as a safety check to ensure that the vaccine was safe. Several of the injected monkeys developed paralysis.[167] After oral ingestion by humans, the attenuated Koprowski polio vaccine, weakened by passage in rats, had reverted into its natural paralytic form. Vaccination of humans with the Koprowski live rat-attenuated vaccine was immediately stopped.

As a result, the first polio vaccine trial was a failure. That being said, it was wisely stopped early due to the kill switch used in the study. It was a safeguard that likely saved countless lives.

In 1957, Koprowski moved to the Wistar Institute in Philadelphia. To further attenuate the virus, the SM strain was fed to and then collected from the stool of severely disabled and institutionalized infants in Sonoma, California.[168] As infants, they could not provide consent for participation in the study. The children developed immunity, and some unvaccinated playmates also got infected and became immune following exposure to their infected playmates' feces.[169] They called this new strain CHAT after Charlton, the name of a six-month-old infant that was among those fed the SM strain.[170]

Vaccination using the Koprowski strain of live CHAT virus restarted in 1957 in the Congo.[171] Needless to say, bad luck continued to follow the Koprowski vaccine trials. These outstanding issues—a failed UK trial due to reversion to pathogenic virus, further attenuation by infecting a mentally disabled infant who could not give consent, and a controversial African trial—will be discussed in further detail in chapter 10.

Salk's Dead Poliovirus Vaccine

The second vaccine trail was undertaken by Jonas Salk at the University of Pittsburgh and the National Foundation. Due to safety concerns about using a live virus—like the one used in the Koprowski vaccine—the National Foundation focused on developing a dead, formalin-fixed virus for its vaccine trial, similar to the Pasteur Institute's use of a formalin-killed rabies vaccine (see chapter 4, especially Box 4.1).[172]

Salk chose to passage poliovirus from infected monkey kidney cells through a coarse filter and then through a finer porcelain filter to remove any cellular tissue or bacteria that could contaminate the vaccine. This filtrate containing poliovirus was adjusted for multiple variables, including exposure to formalin concentration, temperature, acidity, and virus concentration. The treated filtrate of dead virus was injected into monkeys to confirm that the virus was dead. This was followed by the injection of live poliovirus into the vaccinated monkey to confirm that the monkey had developed immunity and would not become paralyzed.

Using Salk's vaccine, the National Foundation undertook America's largest vaccine trial up to that point in history.[173] An army of teachers, physicians, and nurses were required to treat 1,400,000 children. Each of these children needed three intramuscular injections to develop immunity.

The Salk vaccine trial had an "observed" group consisting of children who either received the vaccine or were just observed and not injected. In this group, 330 of 725,173 (0.045 percent) untreated "observed" children contracted polio, while 38 of 221,988 (.017 percent) vaccinated children got polio. The Salk trials also had another, more scientifically rigorous group in which treatment was randomized and blinded for both the child and the medical staff. Children received either injections of the vaccine or injections of a placebo without medical staff or participants knowing who received the vaccine and who received the placebo. In this group, 115 of 201,229 (0.057 percent) children injected with placebo got polio, while 33 of 200,745 (0.016 percent) injected with the vaccine got polio. The Salk vaccine was successful.

In just six years, the National Foundation did the impossible. From 1949 to 1955, Howard Howe discovered the three different paralytic strains needed for a vaccine; Enders discovered how to mass produce poliovirus in monkey kidney cells in the laboratory; and Salk perfected the use of monkey kidney cells to mass produce poliovirus that was then formalin killed to produce the Salk vaccine, and a successful clinical trial was completed.[174]

The Salk polio vaccine was the most important and politically recognized health priority in America at that time. The Salk vaccine was not without checks and balances. One of these checks was Bernice Eddy, who at the time worked at the US government's largest medical research facility: the National Institutes of Health (NIH). Bernice discovered that the Salk vaccine, which was produced by a company called Cutter Laboratories, contained a disease-causing live pathogenic virus that caused paralysis in monkeys.[175] Her superiors at the NIH squashed her findings. The NIH did not investigate Cutter vaccine production process, and the vaccine produced by Cutter Laboratories was approved for license. The NIH ignored the results of this safeguard.

Vaccination with the Salk-Cutter vaccine would end up infecting 120,000 children with live poliovirus. Around forty thousand of these children developed polio symptoms, fifty-one of them were permanently paralyzed, and five died.[176] The overarching issues causing live virus contamination stemmed from the fact that the Cutter Laboratories manufacturing facility placed the tanks containing live virus in the same room as tanks containing virus undergoing formalin inactivation, allowing for easy cross-contamination. The viruses in the formalin tank had also clumped, allowing some of them to resist chemical (formalin) inactivation.

Despite rejection of her results by the NIH, Eddy continued to work on polio vaccine safety.[177] In 1959, she tested rhesus monkey kidney-derived polio vaccine samples by injecting it into 154 newborn hamsters, after which 109 hamsters developed cancers.[178] For a second time, her results threatened the world's largest health initiative. Instead of activating a stop or kill switch, the NIH banned Eddy from doing any further polio vaccine safety testing.

The virus in the Salk polio vaccine causing the cancer in hamsters was a monkey virus called SV40, an abbreviation for simian vacuolating virus 40.[179] Between 1955 and 1963, hundreds of millions of people who received the Salk vaccine (or Sabin vaccine, see below) were unknowingly co-infected with the SV40 monkey virus.[180] This occurred because the poliovirus used for vaccine production was grown in live monkey kidney cells harvested from monkeys infected with SV40 virus. Through these vaccines, SV40 was able to cross species and enter the human population. Today, it is thought that SV40 persists among humans through respiratory spread (i.e., coughing).[181]

For more than fifty years, the academic explanation and medical dogma concerning Eddy's experiment was that SV40 caused cancers in hamsters but not in people.[182] This opinion was bolstered in part by an epidemiological study on lack of SV40's association with cancer.[183] It is important to note, however, that while epidemiology checks for gross association between two events, it does not prove a cause and effect relationship. Moreover, a negative epidemiology study does not necessarily disprove a cause and effect correlation either. The cancer caused by SV40 occurs in only a few rare types of cancer that were probably not adequately represented in the epidemiological study. Additionally, while SV40 is a component in the development of certain rare cancers, it is only one of several genetic changes on that ladder.

In 1992, more than forty years after Eddy's work, SV40-specific DNA was found in children with certain types of brain cancers (ependymomas and choroid plexus).[184] In 1994 and 1996, SV40 DNA was also found in human lung mesothelioma cancers and bone cancers (sarcomas).[185] In 1997, Dr. Michele Carbone discovered that the SV40 virus contributes to some cancers by interfering with the function of an anti-cancer suppressor gene called p53. Several human cancers are characterized by functional loss of the anti-cancer p53 gene.[186]

We now know that SV40 persists throughout the host's life either in a hibernating (latent) form or in a replicating form that contributes to human cancers in the brain (astroctyomas, glioblastomas, meningiomas), bone (sarcomas), lymphocyte immune cells (lymphomas), and membranes lining the lungs (mesotheliomas). When compared to controls, a significant percentage of these cancers are positive for SV40.[187] Moreover, the annual incidence of human bone tumors,[188] brain cancer,[189] and lymphomas[190] is increasing. More than half a century after Eddy's original test results, SV40 is now viewed as a cofactor contributing to these cancers.

The story of Bernice Eddy offers a lucid example of how public confidence and trust in the ability of the medical industry (Cutter Laboratories) and the government (NIH) to be honest brokers in ensuring safe vaccine creation and production were undermined. Can government agencies and institutions be trusted to impartially self-investigate? We will return to this topic in chapters 15 and 16.

Notwithstanding the issues identified by Eddy, the Salk vaccine succeeded in ending the poliovirus pandemic in the United States. Before the Salk vaccine, the incidence of polio in America was 58,000 cases a year. After release of the Salk vaccine in 1955, the incidence of polio dropped in 1957 to 5,600 cases, and in 1961 to only 161 cases.[191]

Sabin's Live Oral Polio Vaccine

Albert Sabin was at Cincinnati Children's Hospital and eventually served as president of the Weisman Institute in Israel. He nominated Maxwell Theiler for the 1951 Nobel Prize in Physiology or Medicine for developing a live yellow fever vaccine (see chapter 5). Sabin was skeptical of Salk's use of a dead virus and instead advocated for a live, attenuated polio virus vaccine trial like Maxwell Theiler did for yellow fever.[192] At that point, the National Foundation had spent a fortune on a successful dead vaccine trial but had been stung by the Cutter Laboratories fiasco. They had no appetite for another polio vaccine trial, especially one using a live vaccine.

Sabin was born in Russia and turned his attention to Russia to initiate an attenuated polio vaccine trial.[193] By moving his trials to another country, Sabin was following the precedence set by the yellow fever vaccine. Yellow fever vaccination had been successfully undertaken with a live vaccine trial provided by the Rockefeller Foundation in Brazil (chapter 5). Just like the Salk vaccine, poliovirus in the Sabin vaccine was cultured in and purified from monkey kidney cells. Long-term passage of poliovirus outside of the body in monkey kidney cells allowed for selection of attenuated strains that did not cause paralysis when reinjected into monkeys.

In contrast to the Salk vaccine, which contained dead poliovirus that had to be injected into muscle on three separate occasions, the Sabin live attenuated vaccine only needed to be taken once by swallowing a liquid formulation.[194] Once ingested, the live Sabin virus replicated in the gut and was excreted in the stool. Through poor hand washing and drinking water fecal-oral transmission, the vaccinated person's stool spread live polioviris infection and thus immunity to unvaccinated family, friends, and neighbors.

Despite the Cold War between Russia (at that time called the USSR) and the United States, Sabin was allowed on a humanitarian basis to collaborate with the Soviets.[195] He provided viral seed stocks from which Soviet scientists at the Polio Research Institute in Moscow prepared millions of vaccine doses. In 1959, Russia began vaccinating children with a live poliovirus.

The USSR trial was even larger than the American Salk trial and included approximately ten million children.[196] There was no unvaccinated control group, because it was reasoned that fecal spread of the live vaccine virus would contaminate the control group. In vaccinated Soviet republics, the annual incidence of polio markedly dropped. The Sabin vaccine was deemed safe and effective. It gave a greater spread of herd immunity and, due to its one-time oral delivery and less prohibitive cost, became the preferred polio vaccine worldwide, including in America. The catchy 1964 song "A Spoonful of Sugar" from the Walt Disney film *Mary Poppins* was a subliminal reference to the Sabin vaccine: "A spoonful of sugar helps the medicine go down; the medicine go down . . . in a most delightful way."

Vaccine-Induced Paralysis

One unexpected long-term complication of the Sabin vaccine was that some injected patients became "long term excretors" of the virus.[197] The longest known time interval that a non-immunocompromised patient has excreted vaccine-derived poliomyelitis in their stool following vaccination is eighteen years.[198] A second rare complication was that the virus could cause paralysis in individuals by mutating and reverting to its virulent form. Vaccine-induced paralysis associated with polio is officially called the slightly less accusatory term "vaccine-associated paralytic poliomyelitis."[199] Several decades after the Sabin trials, it was learned that a single nucleotide mutation can revert the Sabin poliovirus back to its neurotoxic paralytic form.[200]

The last documented wild-type poliovirus infection in America occurred in 1979. Since 1979, all cases of paralytic poliomyelitis have been vaccine induced. Between 1990 and 1999, sixty-one cases of paralytic poliomyelitis were documented; 97 percent of these were vaccine-induced paralytic poliomyelitis (one was imported from outside America, and one was of unknown origin).[201] Upon emerging as the predominate cause for paralytic poliomyelitis in America, the live Sabin vaccine has been gradually phased out. By 2000, America returned from where it started—that is, to using the dead Salk vaccine exclusively.[202] The Salk vaccine is the primary vaccine used in the United States today.

Switching to a nonreplicative (dead) Salk vaccine decreased the cases of vaccine-induced paralysis in America, but to date it has not eliminated cases from prior live oral poliovirus vaccination. In 2005, a stool sample on an immune-deficient infant in Minnesota tested positive for the vaccine-associated poliomyelitis virus.[203] Samples of the stool of twenty-three neighboring children demonstrated that eight of them (38 percent) tested positive for the Sabin vaccine poliomyelitis virus. None of the children suffered paralysis.

In 2011, a case of vaccine-induced paralysis was isolated in the stool of a forty-four-year-old Minnesota woman with immune deficiency.[204] She became paralyzed from her neck down and died after being unable to breathe. It was determined that she was infected twelve years earlier when her child received the live oral Sabin polio vaccine. Both Minnesota cases were in immune-deficient patients.

In 2022, an otherwise healthy adult male in New York developed sudden, flaccid lower-leg paralysis from vaccine-induced paralysis.[205] Live Sabin vaccine that reverted to its paralytic form was recovered from his stool. It was also identified in the wastewater from two neighboring counties.

The abovementioned cases are not solitary outliers. Over the past couple decades there has been a worldwide uptick of vaccine-induced paralytic poliomyelitis. In 2020 alone, there were 1,081 cases of vaccine-induced paralysis across the globe. Due to the prevalent use of the live Sabin polio vaccine in the past, vaccine-associated paralysis is now ten times more common than paralysis from natural poliovirus infection.[206]

Vaccine-induced paralysis is predominantly caused by poliomyelitis type 2. The last natural paralysis caused by poliovirus type 2 occurred in India in 1999. The World Health Organization has since developed a new oral vaccine using live polio virus type 2 that is genetically mutated to be more resistant to reverse mutation into a paralytic strain.[207] In less-developed countries, the Sabin polio vaccine is still used due to the expense and logistics surrounding the use of the dead polio vaccine.

Summary

The polio vaccine story is a heroic narrative of an entire country contributing to stop the most feared virus of its time. It is also a story of altruism; Salk, the National Foundation for Infantile Paralysis (i.e., the March of Dimes), and Sabin refused to personally profit from the vaccine. They did not patent their vaccines and refused royalties on its sale.[208]

The story of the polio vaccine also weaves into more harrowing territory. It speaks of how human technology and sanitary advancements paradoxically caused a global pandemic. It raises ethical concerns regarding massive primate experimentation,[209] the exploitation of institutionalized and developmentally disabled children who lacked consent,[210] and the double standard of Africans and Indians being treated with the riskier but more cost-effective Sabin vaccine while Americans are being treated with the safer Salk vaccine.[211] It is also a story of unforeseen complications, such as the introduction of the cancer-causing SV40 virus to the human population,[212] the Cutter vaccine virus fiasco,[213] long-term Sabin poliovirus excretors infecting their neighbors' water supply,[214] and the spontaneous reversion of live poliovirus vaccine into its paralytic form to cause vaccine-induced paralysis that is now the most common cause of polio in America.[215] Finally, it is a story about how the National Institutes of Health suppressed and denied mistakes that resulted in vaccine-related deaths.[216]

The story of the polio vaccine is a revealing account of success and unexpected harmful short- and long-term consequences that come from vaccine development and usage. It is an example of the immense risks we face in developing vaccines. It demonstrates the importance of having kill switches and safeguards in place.

Determining whether poliomyelitic paralysis is from a naturally acquired wild-type infection or is vaccine-induced requires advances in molecular biology (e.g., total genetic sequencing). By the 1960s, the tools to study life at a molecular level (i.e., molecular biology) were being discovered. Molecular biology is now used to study and manipulate viruses as well as to design new viral vaccines. This has created a whole new set of problems for us, as we'll see in the third section of this book. To prepare for that road ahead, the next three chapters will review the basics of molecular biology. Stay with me (don't worry, there will be no math equations).

SECTION TWO

Molecular Biology

CHAPTER 7

Atoms: Self-Contained Packages of Electrical Charge

Empty space is an electromagnetic field, and atoms are packages of electricity that communicate by emitting light.—RKB

Atoms make up the basic building blocks of everything in the universe. An atom is one tenth of a billionth of a meter in diameter. There are approximately one hundred different types of naturally occurring atoms. In 1869, the Russian chemist Dmitri Mendeleev organized atoms into the periodic table, placing atoms with similar properties in the same column.[217] The periodic table (see Table 7.1) has survived the test of time, insofar as the empty spaces in his original table predicted the discovery of future atoms. The periodic table separates atoms into metals, metalloids, and non-metals.

Atoms are composed of a center or nucleus with positively charged protons around which a cloud of electrons with a negative charge circulate.[218] Hydrogen, the smallest atom, has one proton and one electron. Carbon, the backbone of life, has six protons and six electrons. Since they are electrically neutral, neutrons will not be discussed. Electromagnetic charge causes an attraction between opposite charges and repulsion between similar charges. It is this force

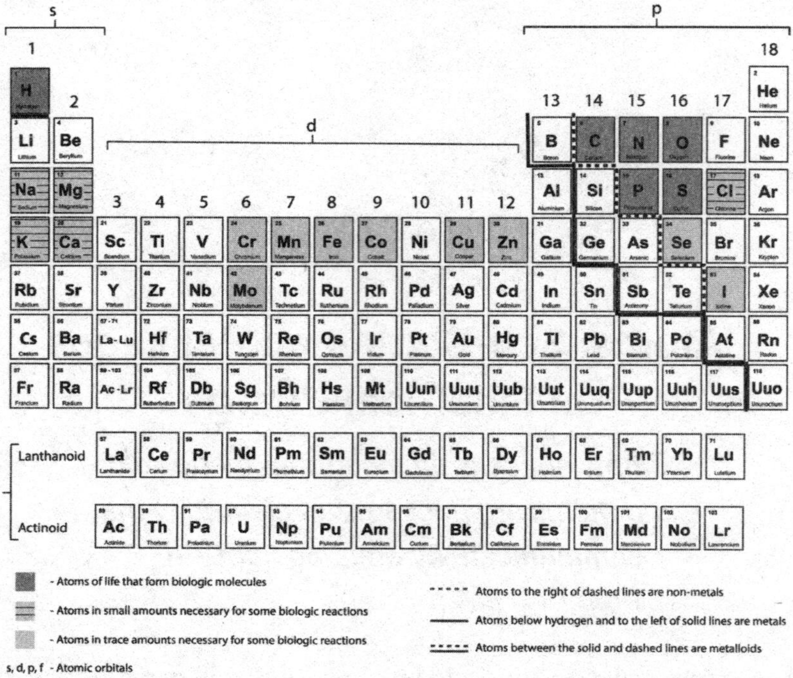

TABLE 7.1: The periodic table. The atomic number (number of protons) in each atom is in the top left of each entry above the atom's name (atomic mass is omitted). *Metals* are below hydrogen and to the left of the solid dark line. *Metalloids* with properties between metals and non-metals are between the solid and dashed lines. *Non-metals* are to the right of the dashed line. Metals in the far left of the table with *s* orbitals like to give up electrons to become charged atoms (ions). Transition metals like to communally share their *d* orbital outer electron with all other metal atoms. Non-metals that have *p* orbitals like to accept an electron from other atoms. The final right-hand column of atoms (column 18) is composed of the noble elements (atoms) with filled *s*, *d*, and *p* orbitals. They are chemically inert as electrically neutral atoms.

that holds matter together and makes chemical and biologic reactions possible. Each type of atom (in its resting, nonionized state) has a unique number of electrically charged protons (i.e., atomic number) with the same number of electrically charged electrons. Each atom has a unique name and abbreviation.

Electromagnetic Force

The ancient Greeks first recognized electricity in the form of static electricity. When they rubbed amber (tree resin) with animal fur, the amber would move or attract light objects, like one's own hair. Today, children often encounter static electricity by rubbing their bare feet on thick carpets before touching a metal doorknob causing an electric spark. Not coincidentally, our word "electricity" derives from the Greek word for amber (*electron*).

We do not usually sense electricity, because it is in all atoms everywhere, and within atoms positive and negative charges are usually balanced with a net charge of zero. Electricity exerts no external force when the net charge is zero. But it is there. Electricity is what holds atoms together and connects atoms to each other to form molecules that form us.

Electricity and magnetism constitute a single force—put differently, they are two sides of the same coin—that herein will be referred to as electromagnetism or simply electricity. A force is something that causes an object to move. There are only four known forces in the universe.[219] The force of gravity is experienced as an attraction between objects. It holds us to this earth and extends over cosmic distances. The two other forces, the strong force and the weak force, are quantum forces that are only experienced within the very minute distance inside an atom's nucleus.

Electromagnetism governs everything from the world between atoms and molecules to everyday life around us. The electric force may be either positive or negative. Like electric charges repel and opposite charges attract. Positive protons in the nucleus of an atom should push away from each other and fly apart. It is the presence of the strong force (which is a stronger force than electromagnetism) within the nucleus that explains why positively charged protons do not repel and fly apart.

Negatively charged electrons are attracted to and circulate around the positively charged protons in the nucleus. Because of that attraction, electrons should spiral into the center of the nucleus. The Nobel Laureate and Danish physicist Niels Bohr (1885–1962) was the first to use quantum mechanics to explain why electrons do not collapse into the nucleus.[220] Electron orbitals are quantized, which means that their orbitals and energy levels are finite or discrete and not infinite or continuous. Electrons cannot exist in between orbitals and cannot fall into the proton when in the closest orbital to the nucleus. In the quantum world of atoms, electrons can only jump between specific orbitals. When energy is provided or taken out, electrons perform orbital jumps without existing within the space between orbitals.

Life is an emergent property of atomic and molecular electromagnetic forces. Everything in biology depends on electromagnetic attraction or repulsion. That being said, however, where does the electromagnetic force come from? According to Richard Feynman, who won the 1965 Nobel Prize in Physics for a theory called quantum electrodynamics,[221] magnetic and electric attraction or repulsion arises from exchange of very short-lived light particles called virtual photons. Quantum electrodynamics is just a theory, but it would be ironic if science was moving full circle to rediscover Genesis 1:3, where God decrees on the first day of creation "Let there be light."

The Difference Between Metals and Non-Metals

A metal likes to give up the electron in its outermost orbital. As a result, metals have strong bonds because each atom circulates its outermost electron among all the other atoms that make up a piece of metal. Metals are generally good conductors of electricity. They are defined by their degree of ductability (i.e., their ability to deform under pressure without breaking) and by their malleability (i.e., their ability to be hammered into different shapes). The best metal conductors of electricity are copper, silver, and gold. In contrast, a non-metal likes to accept an electron into its outermost orbital. Non-metals develop a localized strong bond between two or more neighboring atoms called covalent bonds that often allow organic molecules to rotate, bend, or twist. Non-metals are generally not good conductors of electricity. They are insulators.[222]

Natural rubber that is composed of the non-metals carbon and hydrogen is a poor conductor of electricity. It is a good insulator. Glass and dry sand are composed predominantly of the non-metals silicon and oxygen and are also an insulator. Air is composed of non-metals like nitrogen and oxygen and is an insulator. Water (H_2O) is an exception to this pattern. Even though it is composed of two non-metals (hydrogen and oxygen), water has an asymmetrical or polar distribution of electrons, making it a good conductor of electricity. When water vapor condenses in the air, the air becomes a conductor of electricity and lightning may occur.

Moving electrons form electricity. They are everywhere, whizzing around each atom, causing chemical reactions in our cells and in the wires that power our appliances, electric cars, cell phones, and computers. A lightning bolt is composed on average of 150 quintillion moving electrons. A lightning rod that stands high in the air and is buried in the ground will transfer lightning into the ground, because the earth is a good conductor of electricity. The earth conducts electricity because it is a giant ball of metals and water. Lightning going into or out of the earth is like a teardrop going into or out of the ocean. Due to moving molten metals within the earth's core, the earth projects a giant electromagnetic field into space to form an unseen protective bubble around us.

Metals

Sixty-six of the ninety-nine natural elements are metals. The formal names of metals are derived by adding the suffix -ium or -um to their Latin name (e.g., Aurium [Au] from the Latin *aurum* is gold).

Metals compose 2.5 percent of the human body. This is mostly due to calcium, which makes up 1.5 percent of the body through the formation of bones and teeth that is deposited outside of living cells. Within a living cell, a few metals, while not common, are important for a cell's function and life. The metals sodium (Na) and potassium (K) normally give up a single electron and develop a single positive ionic (electric) charge. The metals calcium (Ca) and magnesium (Mg) usually give up two electrons. Positively charged sodium, potassium, calcium, and magnesium pair (i.e., form ions) with chlorine (Cl), a non-metal that accepts electrons from metals to become a negatively charged chloride. These charged metals are a cell's electrical circuit. They contribute to electrical charge differences between the inside and outside of a cell, resulting in nerve impulses, the release of hormones, muscle contraction, the transmission of messages, and movement.

A few other metals are present in trace amounts in carbon-based life. They contribute to specialized functions by how their charge helps biological reactions. For example, iron helps carry oxygen in red blood cells. Cobalt, chromium, copper, zinc, manganese, molybdenum, and selenium also impart unique functions to a few proteins.[223] Metals are often toxic to carbon-based life when they are present in excess, occur in a different form, or are charged. Excessive iron, for instance, causes liver damage (cirrhosis). Pure or elemental sodium is explosive when exposed to water.

The body uses certain routes like the kidney (urine), liver (stool), hair, and skin to excrete unwanted metals. What the body cannot excrete, it hides by burying the metal within certain organs or in bone. Human bone is the graveyard used by the body to bury many trace metals, or at least until the graveyard is full. In such cases, like zombies arising from the dead, bones will leak out such metals. As a result, lead, mercury, and aluminum may show up on the list of trace elements in the body, but they are unwanted hitchhikers and have no useful purpose or "good" intentions once inside a living cell.

Metals in their charged or ionic form may alter a protein's function or denature (i.e., destroy) the normal shape of a biologic molecule. Because the DNA of genes is negatively charged, positively charged metals may bind to and disrupt genes. Charged metals interrupt or destroy the electromagnetic interactions that generate the vitality and symphony of life. Yet, despite this, modern medicine indiscriminately injects metals into people with little afterthought. Case in point, medical imaging is performed by injecting the metals technetium, gadolinium, indium, gallium, or zirconium in the body.[224] Total joint replacements are made of cobalt, chromium, molybdenum, titanium, aluminum, and vanadium.[225] Heart valves are also made of titanium.[226] The long-term ability of these metals to revert to a toxic charged state inside a carbon-based life is still unknown.

Non-Metals: The Six Atoms That Form the Molecules of Life

Biology is derived from the two Greek words *bios* meaning "life" and *logos* meaning "study." The biology of life is the study of carbon (C) and five other atoms: hydrogen (H), oxygen (O), nitrogen (N), phosphorus (P), and sulfur (S). These six elements are bonded or grouped together into molecules that compose 99 percent of every cell. The branch of chemistry that studies how these six atoms combine to form life is called organic chemistry.

The glue or force that binds together the six atoms of life to form molecules with a carbon backbone comes from the covalent bonds that bind those atoms together. Covalent binding is not easily destroyed by motion or heat. But in organic molecules, it allows twisting and rotation of atoms, facilitating a large variation in three-dimensional molecular structure between covalently bonded atoms.

Ionic, polar, and van der Waals forces are weak electric bonds that allow for reversible or repeated chemical reactions that occur in living organisms. These bonds are three hundred times weaker than metallic bonds or non-metal covalent bonds that hold atoms together. Ionic bonding occurs when a metal gives up an electron to become positively charged, while a non-metal accepts the electron to become negatively charged. An example is sodium chloride ($Na^+ Cl^-$), which is table salt. Organic molecules generate electromagnetic attraction or repulsion due to polar or van der Waals charge variation within biologic molecules that arises from unequal sharing of electrons by atoms in the molecule (see Box 7.1). Electric charge variation within biologic molecules causes biologic reactions. These electrical reactions are the source of life. Biological molecules are categorized by their structure as sugars, proteins, glycoproteins, lipids (fats), or nuclei acids such as deoxyribonucleic acid (DNA).[227]

Box 7.1: A Thumbnail Sketch of Non-Metal Covalent, Polar, and van der Waals Electrical Forces

Covalent bonds are the superglue that bind the atoms in organic molecules together. Covalent bonding between non-metal atoms was described by Linus Pauling's valence bond theory and Robert Mulliken's molecular orbital theory. Linus Pauling was awarded two Nobel Prizes (1952 and 1962).[228] Robert Mulliken received the Nobel Prize in 1966.[229] In valence bond theory, electrons are shared or distributed between two atoms to make a covalent bond. In molecular orbital theory, atomic orbitals are redistributed into new binding or anti-binding molecular orbitals that are shared across several neighboring atoms (not just two neighboring atoms) within the molecule.

Whether occurring between two or a limited number of neighboring atoms, covalent bonds generate secondary electromagnetic charges. Asymmetrical distribution of the electrons between two atoms results in a weak electromagnetic force called a polar bond that attracts or repels other molecules. When covalent binding occurs across several atoms, resonance of the electron wave will cause peaks and troughs that increase or decrease the probability of an electron being present in different regions of the molecule. This gives rise to electrical differences within a molecule that generate electromagnetic forces called van der Waals forces. The reversible chemical interactions of biological molecules depend on weak electromagnetic attraction and repulsion arising from polar and van der Waals forces that are three hundred times weaker than covalent bonds.

Non-metal atoms in the periodic table, if bonded together in a different order, do not form the flexible molecules that comprise living organisms. Carbon forms the backbone of biologic molecules, but when bonded only to itself, carbon is inorganic—that is, nonliving. Carbon-carbon binding may, depending on its structure, occur as diamond (tetrahedron), graphite (hexagonal), graphene (single-layer hexagonal honeycomb), nanotubes (hollow cylinder), or fullerenes (soccer balls of pentagons and hexagons).

The German chemist Fritz Haber was awarded the 1918 Nobel Prize for his work with non-metals. He invented nitrogen fertilizer.[230] His Nobel Prize was controversial because he also invented chlorine gas (two chlorine atoms bonded to each other) and an explosive called TNT composed of carbon, hydrogen, nitrogen, and oxygen (C7H5N3O6). Chlorine gas and TNT were first used in World War I as an effective means to kill soldiers. Haber's personal life is an example of what can go wrong when science is not anchored to a kill switch of checks and balances. Rumored to be distraught over her husband's inventions, Haber's wife killed herself with her husband's military pistol the same day that the first chlorine gas attack was executed on the Allied troops.[231] After World War I, the 1925 Geneva Protocol banned the use of chlorine gas in warfare.

Summary

Electromagnetism is the language by which atoms and molecules communicate and function. It is present everywhere. Atoms and molecules would not exist without strong electromagnetic bonds. Life and biologic reactions would not exist without weak electromagnetic ionic, polar, or van der Waals interactions. Our consciousness is an emergent product of nerve cell electromagnetic interactions. Much like computers, we as human beings also function using an electric binary code (i.e., positive or negative charge). Yet, for the most part, we are illiterate, blind, and deaf to the mysterious "hieroglyphics" of atomic and molecular electromagnetic communications. As Thomas Edison, the inventor of the light bulb, once said: "I have come to the conclusion that I never did know anything about electricity."

One constant that has appeared in mathematical equations used to study electromagnetism at an atomic level is called the fine-structure constant. That constant is roughly 1/137. In quantum (atomic) physics, some people give the number 137 an almost mystical reverence. If that number was just slightly weaker or stronger, electrons would be bound too loose or too tight to protons. In either case, atoms as we know them would not exist, matter would not exist, the universe would not exist, and we would not exist. The fine-structure constant is telling us something about the electromagnetic force that made atoms and the universe possible. We just do not understand what. As the Nobel Laureate Wolfgang Pauli said: "When I die my first question . . . will be: What is the meaning of the fine structure constant?" In an odd alignment of strange coincidences, Wolfgang Pauli died in room 137.

Mercury and aluminum are metals added to vaccines. Yet we have given scant consideration of how they or their electric charges interact with organic molecules. Mercury and aluminum will be discussed in chapters 12 and 13, respectively.

CHAPTER 8

DNA: The Evolutionary Memory of Who We Are

Watson and Mullis flew higher than Icarus but were burned just the same.—RKB

Deoxyribonucleic acid (DNA) is our genetic material. It is the embodied record of our ancestry and our offspring. It is nature's recorded memory of our past, present, and future. The discovery of DNA had an inauspicious and slow beginning. In 1869, the Swiss chemist Friedrich Miescher collected pus from patients' bandages to characterize the protein in white blood cells that fights infection. What he discovered instead was a substance that he called nuclein. It was very high in phosphorous atoms and resistant to things that degrade protein (see chapter 9). He realized that nuclein was a new type of organic molecule. He wrote: "It seems probable to me that a whole family of such slightly varying phosphorous-containing substances will appear." He was right; Miescher had discovered DNA. Dr. Miescher was almost one hundred years ahead of his time.[232]

Fifty years later, in 1919, the chemist Phoebus Levene identified these nucleins as deoxyribonucleic acid (DNA) and learned that DNA was composed of a phosphate, a sugar (deoxyribose), and four nucleoside bases: adenine (A), guanine (G), thymidine (T), and cytosine (C).[233] While Levene discovered the components of DNA, the order, structure, and function of the DNA molecule remained unknown.

In 1944, Oswald Avery at Rockefeller Hospital published a paper showing that inherited traits, which at that time were called transforming factors, were transmitted to offspring by DNA.[234] He did this by studying bacteria. As a single-cell organism, bacteria are a simpler model to study than multi-cellular organisms. It was known that when cultured together in a broth, dead bacteria could transform live bacteria by passing their characteristics on to them. This transforming factor would then be inherited by the live bacteria's progeny. Crude extracts from dead bacteria could also provide the transforming factor.

Avery washed or purified the crude transforming factor extract from cells by adding a lipid soap and salt to disrupt the cells' membrane, which was followed by adding rubbing alcohol (isopropyl alcohol) to precipitate or settle the invisible transforming factor out of solution. The transforming factor precipitated out of solution as a white, slimy, and sinewy material that would wrap around and suspend like strings hanging from your finger. The procedure Avery used is so simple that it can be done in your own kitchen on any living organism like a tomato or strawberry. You can separate out and hold the fruit's white gooey genes (DNA) in your own hand.

Purified transforming factor was resistant to things that degrade protein but, after exposure to something that degrades DNA, would lose its transforming activity. Avery concluded that the transforming factor that passed on inherited material was DNA. The term "transforming factor" was replaced by Avery with the word "gene," which derives from the Greek word *genea* meaning "procreation, offspring." The finding that genes are made of DNA was a fundamental discovery. Avery was nominated for but never received a Nobel Prize.[235]

The American biochemist Erwin Chargaff, who had previously read Avery's paper, advanced Avery's research by reporting in 1950 that DNA, regardless of species, had the same amount (or ratio) of adenine to thymidine and guanine to cytosine.[236] This meant that adenine was always paired with thymidine, and guanine was always paired with cytosine. What was still missing, however, was a complete understanding of the structure of DNA. For that, we must change the scene to Cambridge.

Watson, Crick, and the Magicians at Cambridge

Cambridge University in the United Kingdom is a collection of thirty-one colleges located fifty-five miles north of London in its namesake city. A few blocks from Cambridge University stands a British pub called the Eagle. It is a stone and wood building on a cobblestone sidewalk that was constructed in 1667. Next to the entrance of the Eagle is a small, modest, and easily overlooked plaque that commemorates this pub as the place where James Watson and Francis Crick announced the discovery of DNA's three-dimensional structure, a eureka moment that has been called discovering "the secret of life."

DNA is a chain of repeating units called nucleotides (see Figure 8.1).[237] In human beings, DNA consists of three billion nucleotides, which are divided into forty-six separate chains called chromosomes. The key to understanding DNA was determining the three-dimensional structure of the DNA chain. Watson and Crick achieved this by using X-ray diffraction (also known as X-ray crystallography). X-ray diffraction gives a picture that looks like a medical X-ray of dark and light colors but in a seemingly incomprehensible pattern.[238] X-ray diffraction is not magic, in that the images it produces require rigorous analysis and interpretation. It is hard work (see Box 8.1).

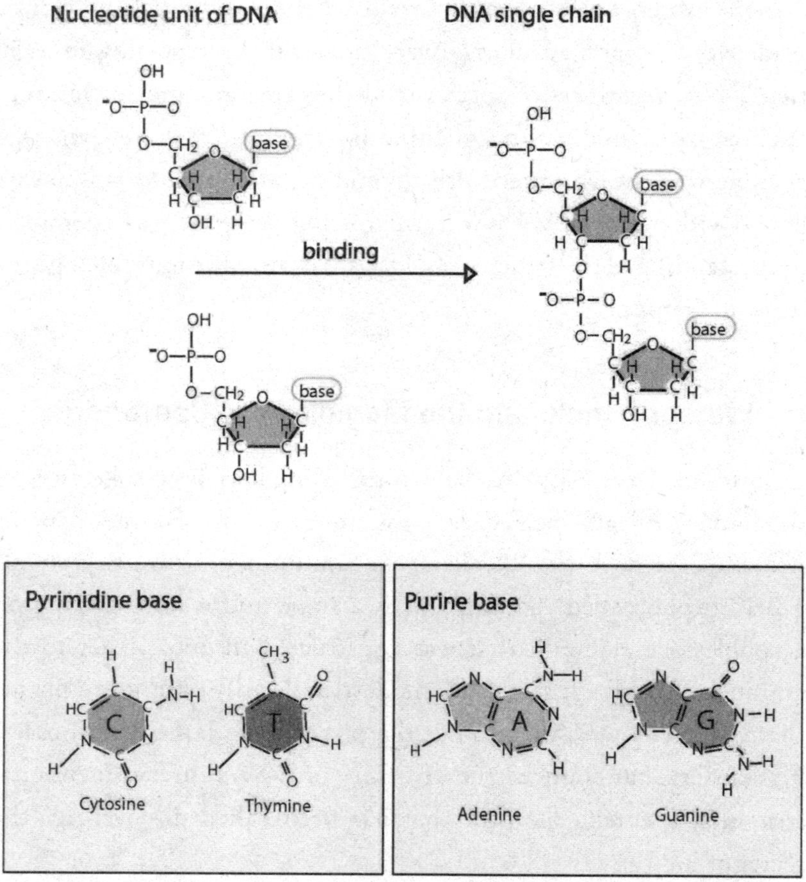

FIGURE 8.1: Nucleotide bases (cytosine, thymine, adenine, guanine) of deoxyribonucleic acid (DNA). Human DNA contains three billion base pairs of nucleotides linked together into forty-six separate chromosomes.

Box 8.1. A Thumbnail Sketch of X-Ray Diffraction

In medical X-rays, the skeleton can be easily visualized from soft tissue because of differences in X-ray penetration.[239] Instead of determining the amount of radiation passing directly through an object, the scatter of X-rays in a tangential or sideways direction after hitting an object is called X-ray diffraction. A father and son team, William and Lawrence Bragg, won the Nobel

Prize in 1915 for explaining the diffraction of X-rays on rows or planes of atoms within a crystal.[240]

More than two dozen Nobel prizes have been awarded for determining the structure of organic molecules by X-ray crystallography.[241] While this sounds like a simple way to win a Nobel prize, it is not. It may take years of work, experience, and luck.

The first problem is getting organic material to form crystals.[242] A large amount of very pure organic material and sterile conditions (bacteria eat organic molecules) is required. Conditions for precipitation out of solution (crystallization) include concentration of agents (salt, sugars, alcohol) in the water solution, temperature, cryoprotection if using low temperature, solvent evaporation rate, acidity (pH), and, if available, seeding with a microcrystal (called nucleation) to initiate crystallization. Organic crystals may be as soft as butter, making fishing the crystal out of solution difficult.

Once fished out of solution, the second problem is determining 3-dimensional structure from the X-ray scatter that is now done with computer based mathematical analysis. Once the crystal's structure is identified, it may not be a molecule's normal shape since the conditions used to precipitate a biologic molecule out of solution may not be physiologic conditions. For DNA, the low salt or more hydrated B form of DNA is the physiologic double-helix "staircase" structure of DNA.[243]

The X-ray diffraction pattern of DNA (Figure 8.2) looks like a Rorschach inkblot test. When the first images came out, nobody knew what it really meant. Watson and Crick built and studied numerous models from this data. Their "eureka" moment came when they realized that the X-ray diffraction pattern was from two DNA helical chains coiled around the same axis.[244] From there, Watson and Crick determined that the two chains were held together by weak polar binding (see chapter 7) of adenine-thymidine and guanine-cytosine pairs (Figure 8.3).

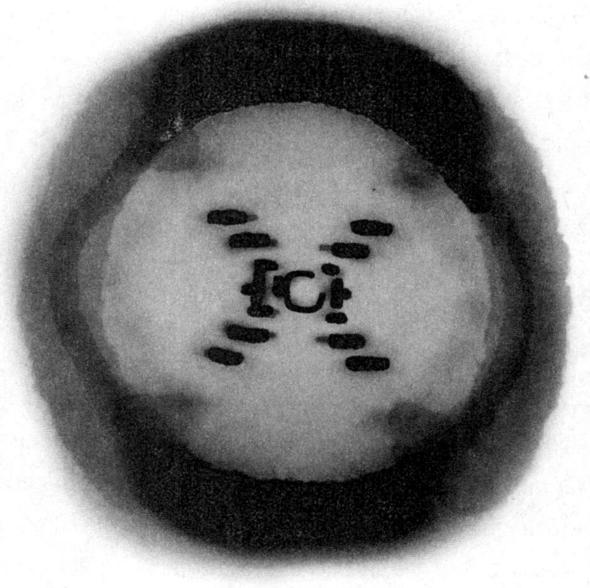

FIGURE 8.2: Schematic representation of X-ray diffraction picture of DNA.

Due to the predictable pattern of adenine and thymidine always binding to each other, and guanine and cytosine always binding to each other, it follows that one chain of DNA is always complementary to the other, such that each chain can serve as the template for the replication of the other chain. A newly synthesized daughter cell DNA thus possesses the same sequence of DNA bases as the original parental strand, ensuring that progeny will have the same genetic or inheritable information (see Figure 8.3).

In 1962, ninety-seven years after the initial finding of nuclein by Friedrich Miescher, the Nobel Prize was conferred to James Watson, Francis Crick, and Maurice Wilkins for their discovery of the double helix.[245] The X-ray diffraction of DNA was performed by Maurice Wilkins and Rosalind Franklin, and the interpretation of the diffraction pattern was done by Watson and Crick. Rosalind Franklin died in 1958 at age thirty-seven from ovarian cancer four years before the Nobel Prize was awarded. Franklin did not receive official recognition

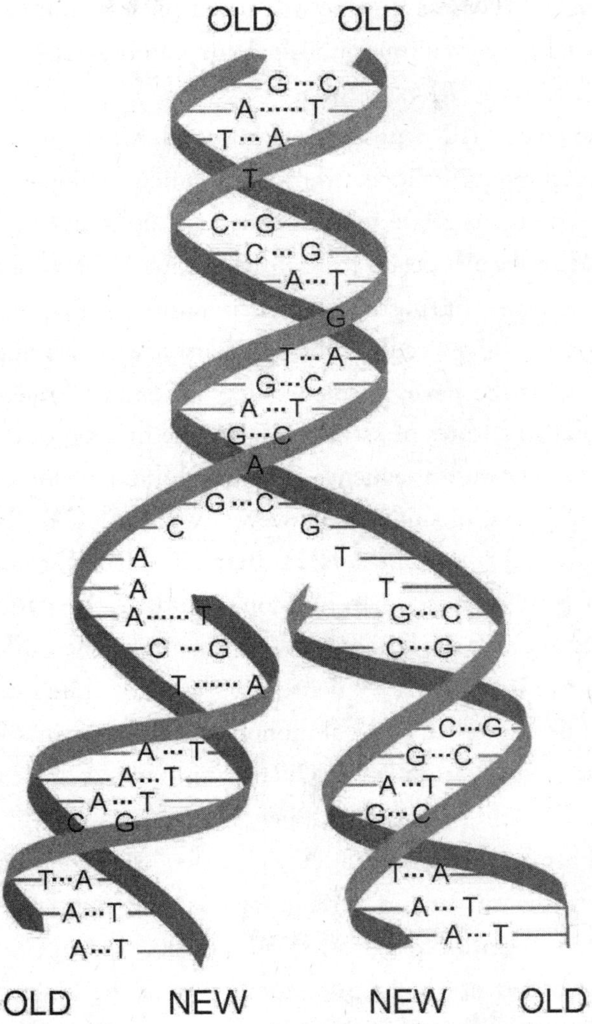

FIGURE 8.3: Double-stranded DNA undergoing replication to duplicate itself during the creation of new cells. A = adenine, C = cytosine, G = guanine, T = thymine. The ribbons are the sugar (deoxyribose) backbone of DNA.

from the Nobel Committee for her contribution, insofar as Nobel Prizes cannot be awarded posthumously.

Crick, Wilkins, and Watson never patented their discovery. It was done simply to help humanity. Francis Crick finished his career in La Jolla, California, as a member of the Salk Institute, which was named after Jonas Salk, whose vaccine was based on formalin-killed poliovirus (chapter 6). Wilkins published his autobiography, *The Third Man of the Double Helix*, in 2003.[246]

Watson accepted a position at Harvard, where he was instrumental in changing its focus from developmental biology and physiology (how organs relate to each other) to molecular biology (how atoms and molecules relate to each other). In 1962, he became the director of Cold Spring Harbor Laboratory, which became the world's mecca for molecular biology. Watson was also appointed to be the head of the newly formed Human Genome Project. Run by the National Institutes of Health (NIH), the mission of the Human Genome Project was to sequence the entire human genome (the complete set of genes and DNA). However, Watson left his position in 1992 after the director of the NIH, Bernadine Healy, recommended patenting gene sequences. In Watson's words: "The nations of the world must see that the human genome belongs to the world's people, as opposed to its nations."[247] Watson later stated, "Life's instructions ought not be controlled by legal monopolies at the whim of Congress or the courts."[248] Watson left the NIH within weeks of its announcement that it would patent human genes.

The Human Genome Project pitted the "common ownership of humanity's shared genetic heritage against the right to financially benefit from scientific progress."[249] The dispute over gene patenting eventually ended up in the Supreme Court of the United States in a case between the Association for Molecular Pathology versus a myriad of genetic companies. In 2013, the Supreme Court ruled that an entire gene could not be patented because nobody made it, but this decision still allowed one to patent the nucleotide coding sequence of a natural gene, provided that the intervening nonprotein coding DNA sequences were removed.[250] This compromise seems paradoxically inconsistent because noncoding DNA sequences are normally removed by nature when the cell translates the gene's nucleotide sequence into a protein (chapter 9).

Although ultimately unsuccessful, Watson fought to keep nature's secrets free for all humanity. Because of incendiary statements related to his beliefs on the role of genes in human behavior, he became, in his own words, an "unperson." To avoid bankruptcy, he had to sell his Nobel Award.[251] It was bought at auction in 2014 for $4.1 million US by Alisher Usmanov, a Russian billionaire who, out of respect, promptly returned the Nobel Prize medal to Watson.[252]

Due to the discovery of the double helix structure by the Cambridge magicians, the second half of the twentieth century revolutionized our understanding of DNA. Knowing the structure of DNA helped later biologists explain how DNA faithfully replicates. It opened the door to numerous biological techniques to manipulate DNA that could break and reform the weak electromagnetic polar bonds between DNA bases while not affecting the stronger covalent bonds of the DNA backbone. While there are many different techniques today that take advantage of differences in electromagnetic bond strength, for our immediate purposes we will focus only the polymerase chain reaction.

Kary Mullis and Polymerase Chain Reaction

The polymerase chain reaction (also known as PCR) is an automated technique used to copy and rapidly multiply a piece of DNA. PCR was invented in 1985 by Kary Mullis. During the late 1960s, Mullis was a student at the University of California at Berkeley. At that time, Berkeley was one of America's epicenters for drugs, rock and roll, and sex. Emulating the *Zeitgeist* of the age, Mullis was a free-spirited, free-thinking genius whose thoughts flowered in that environment. It was even reported that Mullis used to synthesize his own hallucinogens.

As Mullis titled one of the chapters in his 1998 autobiography: "A Lab Is Just Another Place to Play."[253]

For some, Mullis was an irresponsible and impetus-driven adolescent. But others recognized him as an eccentric genius. Case in point, in 1968, as a twenty-two-year-old college student, he published his article "The Cosmological Significance of Time Reversal" in *Nature*, the world's most prestigious science publication.[254] In that sense, one might say Mullis's genius left him misunderstood. In his own words: "Welcome to Earth. It's a little confusing at first. That is why you have to come back over and over again before you learn to really enjoy yourself."[255]

PCR is an automated thermocycling (temperature cycling) procedure involving three steps: DNA denaturation (using heat to pull DNA strands apart), annealing (matching small pieces of DNA together at a lower temperature), and extension (lengthening the growing strands of new DNA) (Figure 8.4).[256] In his development of PCR, Mullis used Taq polymerase isolated from a bacteria called *Thermus aquaticus* (which means "hot water" in Latin) that lives in near boiling volcanic hot springs. (Taq is an abbreviation for *Thermus aquaticus*.)

DNA polymerase is the cellular protein that duplicates a strand of DNA to make two DNA strands. Unlike human DNA polymerase, Taq DNA polymerase does not lose function (also known as denaturation) at high temperatures. The Taq DNA polymerase is larger than the human DNA polymerase and is held together by more electromagnetic polar bonds, which prevents it from degrading in heat.

To perform PCR, a solution is prepared that contains: (1) double-stranded DNA to be replicated; (2) single-strand DNA primers; (3) individual DNA nucleotides; and (4) Taq DNA polymerase. First, the solution is heated to near-boiling temperature to denature or break apart the polar "electromagnetic" attraction holding the two DNA chains together. The double-stranded DNA

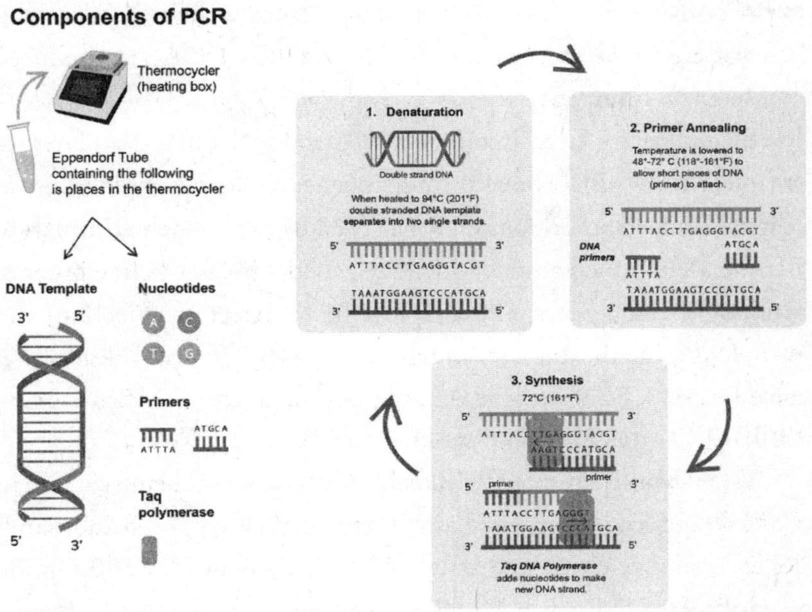

FIGURE 8.4: Scheme of polymerase chain reaction (PCR). There are three steps to PCR: denaturation, primer annealing, and synthesis. In the first round of amplification, two strands become four, then four become eight, with each amplification cycle doubling the amount of DNA.

then separates into single strands of DNA. However, the boiling does not break the strong covalent bonds holding together the single DNA chains. It is like when you're cooking a stew. The boiling may soften the root vegetables and meats in the stew, but the individual atoms comprising the ingredients do not fly apart and disappear in front of you.

Next, the temperature is lowered, allowing the nucleotide primers to anneal (i.e., bind) to the complementary nucleotide sequence on the parent DNA template. From there, the temperature is raised to allow Taq DNA polymerase to make new DNA strands by individually adding nucleotides that are complementary to the parental DNA nucleotide sequence. This cycle is then automatically repeated thirty to thirty-five times inside an instrument called a thermocycler. Millions of copies of the original double-stranded DNA are produced within a few minutes.

By replicating large amounts of identical DNA in a short amount of time, Mullis's PCR breakthrough opened up a new world of possibilities. Since its invention, PCR has been used to match criminals to a crime, determine paternity, identify genetic diseases before onset of symptoms, clone genes, allow rapid tests to detect an infection, and even determine the ancestry of ancient peoples from long-dead skeletons. In 2020, PCR became the standard rapid test used to diagnose COVID-19 virus infection (see chapter 15).

When Mullis invented PCR technology, he was a chemist at Cetus, a San Francisco–based company. Cetus gave Kary a ten-thousand-dollar severance check and then sold Kary's patent for $300 million to Hoffmann-LaRoche. Mullis walked away from science, having been burned by his creative passion, and turned instead to surfing the ocean waves in La Jolla, California. In 1993, he was awarded the Nobel Prize in Chemistry for discovering PCR.[257] He passed in 2019.

Due to PCR technology, the sequencing of the entire human genome—composed of three billion nucleotide base pairs and the genes encoded by these base pairs—was completed in 2003 following a worldwide effort. Surprisingly, only 1 to 2 percent of the human genome consists of genes used to make proteins (see chapter 9). Equally surprising is that the amount of DNA in a particular organism's cell does not necessarily correlate with intelligence. An onion has sixteen billion nucleotide base pairs, five times as much as a human.[258]

The amount of DNA that is *not* used to make proteins roughly increases with evolutionary complexity. Single-cell bacteria have roughly 50 percent nonprotein base pair nucleotides and 50 percent protein-coding base pair nucleotides. By comparison, in humans 98 to 99 percent of nucleotides are nonprotein coding base pairs. A multi-cellular organism with highly specialized cells must turn genes on and off based on what cell they are in and what environmental signals it receives. You do not want, for instance, a nerve cell expressing genes that make hair. It appears that these regions in DNA that do not make proteins are involved in epigenetics, meaning they are the administrators and regulators of gene expression. A massive and ongoing project involving many different scientific centers called ENCODE (an abbreviation for Encyclopedia of DNA Elements) is continuing to decipher exactly what all this nonprotein DNA is doing.

Summary

DNA is the template that holds the genetic code that we inherit from our ancestors. This makes our knowledge of our DNA invaluable. Case in point, in 2008 a digital record of the entire DNA nucleotide sequences of a select cohort of human beings—including the athlete Lance Armstrong and the Cambridge University physicist Stephen Hawking—were stored on a hard drive called "the immortal drive." This drive was then sent to the International Space Station orbiting earth.[259] The immortal drive serves as a human DNA time capsule designed to survive the extinction of our species. Rather than have the only memory of humanity being a record of our digital DNA floating alone in the vast emptiness and silence of space, we should exercise the foresight of a kill switch to prevent good intentions from going bad.

CHAPTER 9

Proteins: The Building Blocks of Life

While DNA is the artistic director, proteins are the corps de ballet in the dance of life.—RKB

In 1837, the Dutch chemist Gerardus Mulder correctly predicted that the "basic material" (German: *Grundstoff*) of all living forms consisted of a combination of six different types of atoms: carbon, hydrogen, oxygen, nitrogen, sulfur, and phosphorus. It seems Gerardus Mulder had better intuition than Fox Mulder on *The X-Files*. He correctly proposed that this *Grundstoff* is made by plants and then transferred to herbivores and then into carnivores.[260] A year later, Mulder replaced *Grundstoff* with the new term "protein," which was derived from the Greek word *prōtos*, meaning "first in rank" or "first position."[261]

The discovery of DNA in 1869 by Friedrich Miescher (chapter 8) was ignored for decades, because DNA was initially thought to be just another protein. We later learned that the building blocks of proteins do not contain the phosphorous present in DNA. Furthermore, the building blocks of DNA do not contain the sulfur present in some amino acids and proteins.

While the repeating building blocks of DNA are the four nucleotides (A, T, G, and C) (chapter 8), the building blocks that compose proteins are known as amino acids. Amino acids are named as such because they consist of an amino group (NH2) attached to a carboxylic acid (COOH) group via an intermediary carbon atom (Figure 9.1). The carbon atom between the amino group and carboxyl group is attached to a hydrogen atom and to a side chain, which is known as an R group. There are twenty different R groups, one for each of the twenty different amino acids used to make proteins (Figure 9.2).

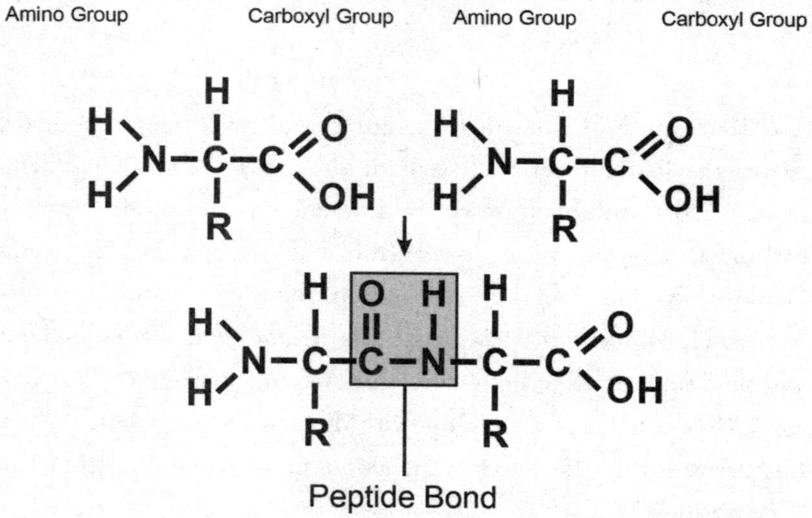

FIGURE 9.1: Bonding between two amino acids to form a dipeptide composed of two amino acids. C = carbon, H = hydrogen, N = nitrogen, R = side chain that is unique to each amino acid.

Peptides (defined as consisting of less than fifty amino acids) and proteins (defined as consisting of more than fifty amino acids) are made of a chain of amino acids covalently bonded to each other. Plants make more than three hundred different types of amino acids, but only twenty of these are used by herbivores, carnivores, and omnivores

Amino Acid R Groups

Name (abbreviation)	R-Group	Charge
Glycine (Gly) (G)	H	Nonpolar, aliphatic
Alanine (Ala) (A)	CH_3	Nonpolar, aliphatic
Valine (Val) (V)	$CH(CH_3)_2$	Nonpolar, aliphatic
Leucine (Leu) (L)	$CH_2-CH(CH_3)_2$	Nonpolar, aliphatic
Methionine (Met) (M)	$CH_2-CH_2-S-CH_3$	Nonpolar, aliphatic
Isoleucine (Ile) (I)	$CH(H_3C)-CH_2-CH_3$	Nonpolar, aliphatic
Serine (Ser) (S)	CH_2-OH	Polar, uncharged
Threonine (Thr) (T)	$H-C(CH_3)-OH$	Polar, uncharged
Cysteine (Cys) (C)	CH_2-SH	Polar, uncharged
Proline (Pro) (P)	H_2C / CH_2-CH_2	Polar, uncharged
Asparagine (Asn) (N)	$CH_2-C(=O)NH_2$	Polar, uncharged
Glutamine (Glu) (Q)	$CH_2-CH_2-C(=O)NH_2$	Polar, uncharged
Lysine (Lys) (K)	$CH_2-CH_2-CH_2-CH_2-NH_3^+$	Positively charged
Arginine (Arg) (R)	$CH_2-CH_2-CH_2-CH_2-C(=NH_2^+)-NH_2$	Positively charged
Histidine (His) (H)	CH_2-C (CH, NH^+, N, CH ring)	Positively charged
Asparate (Asp) (D)	CH_2-COO^-	Negatively charged
Glutamate (Gln) (E)	$CH_2-CH_2-COO^-$	Negatively charged
Phenylalanine (Phe) (F)	CH_2- (ring)	Nonpolar, aromatic
Tyrosine (Tyr) (Y)	CH_2- (ring) $-OH$	Nonpolar, aromatic
Tryptophan (Trp) (W)	CH_2- (ring, NH)	Nonpolar, aromatic

FIGURE 9.2: The twenty amino acids used to make peptides and proteins. Each amino acid has two abbreviations that may be used interchangeably. For example, alanine may be written as Ala or A.

to synthesize proteins.[262] These twenty are called proteinogenic amino acids, meaning they are used to create protein (Figure 9.2).[263]

The twenty amino acids used to make proteins have been highly conserved throughout billions of years of evolution. It is not clear why only a small percentage of the numerous types of amino acids made by plants are used to make proteins.[264] It is speculated that non-proteinogenic amino acids may be used by plants as a chemical defense to poison bacteria, fungi, or herbivores that eat them. Non-proteinogenic amino acids may also be used as a language to signal danger to other plants. In animals, a handful of non-proteinogenic amino acids that have no peptide bond to another amino acid are used for unique functions. Gamma-amino butyric acid (GABA), for instance, is a single amino acid used in human brains to modulate excitation between nerve cells.[265]

Meteorites on earth have been sliced open and found to contain amino acids such as alanine and glycine used to make proteins.[266] For years scientists wondered whether these amino acids were a contaminant or if they really did originate in space. In 2018, Japan launched the spaceship Hayabusa2 (meaning Falcon 2 in Japanese) that landed on the near-earth asteroid called Ryugu (meaning dragon place). Hayabusa2 captured a sample of the asteroid and returned it to earth. Analysis of the asteroid sample revealed twenty different amino acids, confirming that the building blocks of proteins exist in outer space.[267]

Of further note is the dwarf planet Farout (officially named 2018VG18), which was discovered in 2018 in the Kuiper belt, a donut-shaped ring of icy objects and asteroids about three times farther from the sun than Pluto.[268] Farout is a trans-Neptunian object composed of tholins, a word coined by Carl Sagan that refers to long chains (polymers) of carbon, oxygen, nitrogen, sulfur, and hydrogen.[269] Tholin atoms contain the molecular material used to make proteins. Is it possible that life on our planet was seeded by material from the Kuiper belt falling onto the surface of Earth, a predominately metal planet? The creation of the term *protein* from the Greek word meaning "first in rank" may have been more clairvoyant than first imagined when originally coined by Mulder in 1838.

The search for amino acids outside our planet is also being conducted on Mars. On February 18, 2021, NASA's Perseverance Rover landed in the Jezero Crater on Mars. It is equipped with a drill to sample and store Martian rocks and soil inside cylinders. Later, the cylinders will be returned to Earth for analysis of amino acids (among other things).[270]

Amino acids combine via peptide bonds to form proteins. Proteins have many functions. To list a few, proteins act as enzymes responsible for chemical reactions. They can send messages within cells in a process called signal transduction. Proteins signal other cells with hormones or other proteins such as insulin to control blood sugar, and they can form channels within cell membranes to move sodium, potassium, and other ions and material into and out of cells. Proteins also perform cellular synthesis and degradation, and they allow for the movement of cells and animals. Proteins make antibodies, toxins, and anti-toxins, and they produce the structural framework of cellulose for plants along with connective tissues such as tendons, hair, elastin, and collagen that hold animals together.

There are millions of proteins in human cells.[271] So how can only twenty different amino acids generate so many different proteins? A peptide containing only two amino acids covalently bonded together is called a dipeptide. A dipeptide has a potential of 20^2 (i.e., 400) different combinations of the twenty proteinogenic amino acids. A protein made of three hundred amino acids could consist of 20^{300} (over a septillion) different combinations of the same twenty amino acids. As you can see, the twenty proteinogenic amino acids that function as the backbone of all proteins can combine to make an innumerable number of different proteins with different functions.

These proteinogenic amino acids convey different charges and different bulk (steric) strain to different areas of the protein. Differences in amino acid electrical charge produce electrical attraction and repulsion in different locations in the protein. Electric charge variation from amino acids and from the solvent in the cell (salt water) folds each protein into a unique three-dimensional structure, which imparts to it a unique function.

To study a protein, it must first be purified. The techniques used to isolate and purify proteins take advantage of differences in protein size (or mass) and in protein electric charge. One such technique is known as gel electrophoresis.

Isolating Proteins by Gel Electrophoresis

Electrophoresis means migration in an electric field. Arne Tiselius, a Swedish biochemist at the University of Uppsala, was awarded the Nobel Prize in Chemistry in 1948 for his work on the electrophoresis of proteins. He constructed a five-feet-high and twenty-five-feet-long instrument that separated serum proteins based on electric charge migration through a liquid medium.[272] Tiselius's device was large, expensive, and impractical.

Tiselius's technique was perfected by the development of gel electrophoresis, which replaced the liquid medium with a gel and shrank the instrument to a portable desktop size. A gel is a more effective medium than a liquid due to its minute porous holes that retard protein migration by size.[273] Agarose gel electrophoresis was invented in 1975 by Oxford professor Edwin Southern. Commonly referred to as the Southern blot in his honor, Agarose gel electrophoresis is a common procedure used to separate fragments of DNA. In 1981, a polyacrylamide gel was developed that has since been used to separate proteins by size and charge; it is whimsically referred to as a western blot.

In polyacrylamide gel electrophoresis, proteins are loaded into a small well (hole) at the end of a clear polyacrylamide gel. When an electric current is turned on, the electrodes at the two ends of the gel acquire opposite charges (positive and negative), causing proteins in the well to migrate through the semi-solid gel. The rate of migration depends on the protein charge and size. Since its initial development, polyacrylamide gel electrophoresis has become an inexpensive and simple tabletop method to separate and purify proteins according to size and charge (Figure 9.3).

John Fenn and Isolating Proteins by Electrospray Ionization

Another method of isolating proteins for analysis is known as electrospray ionization. Electrospray ionization depends on turning a liquid

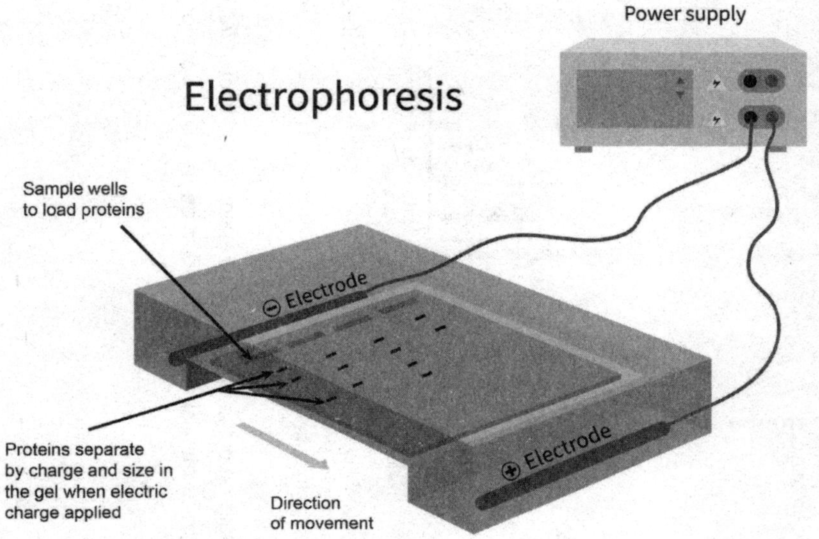

FIGURE 9.3: Portable electrophoresis gel device used to separate proteins by charge and size.

solution of proteins into a gas of ionized proteins. Proteins in a liquid solution are passed through a small caliber needle while a positive charge is applied to the needle wall. As a result, positive-charged proteins collect inside an ionized droplet at the open end of the needle.

When a charge is added to the end of the capillary, each droplet fragments into invisible ionized peptides that are deflected by a magnetic field before reaching the detector (see Figure 9.4). The droplet disappears so rapidly that the pop of air rushing to replace the sudden vacuum left behind is almost audible. The power of an invisible electromagnetic force to make a stationary piece of matter instantaneously vanish is humbling. This analytical tool is called mass spectroscopy because the detector identifies a spectrum (hence the name spectroscopy) of charged proteins separated in the magnetic field by the mass-to-charge ratio of each protein or peptide.[274]

Electrospray spectroscopy was invented by Professor John Fenn in the late 1980s.[275] Born in 1917, Fenn grew up during the Great Depression, with his family jumping between whatever odd jobs

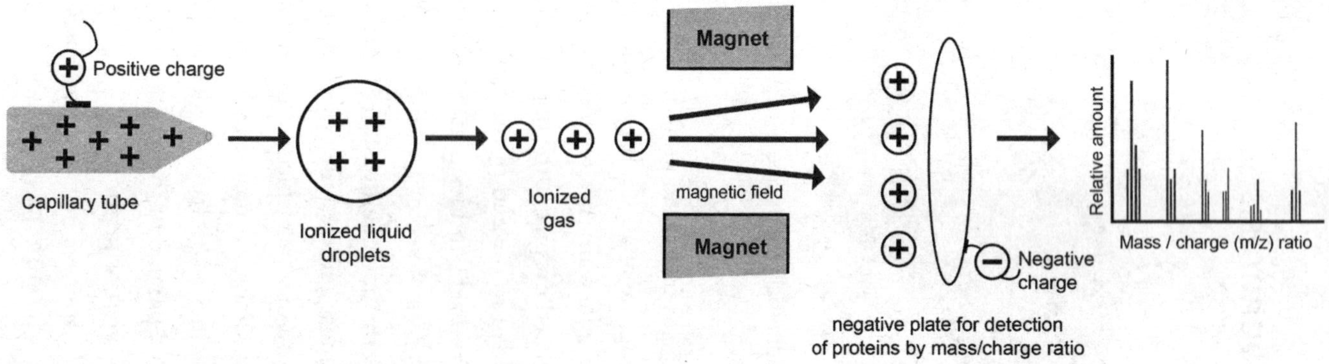

FIGURE 9.4: Simplified schematic of electrospray ionization mass spectroscopy. Details on preparation of the proteins to be injected into the mass spectrometer are important for quality of results. For example, all ions (trace metals) and salt need to be removed from the water. Only pure water (H_2O, called HPLC water) can be used.

were available. Despite such hardship, Fenn obtained a PhD in chemistry from Yale University and taught chemistry and engineering there.

While working at Yale, Fenn invented electrospray spectroscopy. However, the university chose not to pursue a patent for Fenn's creation, deciding that it had no commercial value. Instead, Fenn and one of his former graduate students started a company called Analytica, and Fenn filed a patent for his technique. Upon learning this, Yale University forced Fenn to retire and sued him.[276] Yale has a tax-free endowment of $40 billion US, and its students are charged a ridiculous $62,500 a year in tuition that is also tax-free income for Yale. Ironically and hypocritically, in its lawsuit Yale maligned Fenn's character by accusing him of manipulating the situation for his financial advantage.

Yale University has a prestigious law school, wherein community lawyers socialize and collaborate professionally within a subtle pecking order. The trial judge presiding over Fenn's 2005 case was born in and served as the mayor of West Hartford, Connecticut, which is adjacent to Yale University in New Haven. Did the judge have a social and professional conflict of interest? The judge awarded Yale "punitive" damages" of $545,000 and another $500,000 to recoup Yale's legal fees. As a result, Fenn's patent was confiscated, even though Fenn wrote and paid for the patent himself. Yale subsequently made many millions of dollars from Fenn's invention. Following Fenn's legal defeat, Yale students penned a letter to the *Yale Daily News* saying: "We are outraged that the Yale administration would malign such a good man just to win a lawsuit."[277]

John Fenn passed in 2010 at the age of ninety-three. He published over one hundred articles during his lifetime along with a book titled *Engines, Energy, and Entropy: A Thermodynamics Primer*. In 2002, at the age of eighty-five, Fenn was awarded the Nobel Prize in Chemistry for electrospray ionization spectroscopy.

Artificial Intelligence

Once a protein is isolated, the real work begins. Francis Crick, who co-discovered the DNA double-helix structure, once said: "If you want to understand function, study structure." Structure for DNA and proteins is determined by X-ray crystallography (see Box 8.1 in chapter 8). Years and sometimes decades of laborious work are required to make a biological protein form a crystal. This is followed by complex mathematical analysis of the crystal's X-ray diffraction pattern.

In recent years, technological advances in computer science have made strides in this area. The 2024 Nobel Prize in Chemistry was for AlphaFold 2, a deep learning, artificial intelligence algorithm that can estimate the three-dimensional structure of a protein from its amino acid sequence. It predicts an unknown protein's structure by comparing its amino acid sequence to one hundred thousand already known protein sequences and structures. This was the first time that a Nobel Prize was given for using artificial intelligence to solve a scientific question. AlphaFold 2 in many ways has ushered in the era of artificial intelligence for biological discoveries. So much information has been gleaned from studying the DNA (genomics) and proteins (proteomics) in a cell that artificial intelligence is needed to organize and understand it.[278]

Within the time span of one person's lifetime, biology has progressed from physiology (how parts of the body function together) to molecular biology (how atoms and molecules function together) to artificial intelligence (computers comparing large data sets to give rapid answers). Such rapid advances in science for those of us who have lived through the molecular biology revolution and now face the advent of artificial intelligence brings to mind the lyrics to Jefferson Airplane's 1967 song "White Rabbit": "When logic and proportion have fallen sloppy dead . . . Feed your head, Feed your head."

Transcription, Splicing, and Translation

Inside cells, DNA is transcribed into pre-messenger ribosyl nucleic acid (pre-messenger RNA), which is then spliced into messenger RNA (Figure 9.5). It is called messenger RNA because it carries the DNA sequence message that will become a protein. The reading of DNA into pre-messenger RNA is called transcription, because the same four base nucleotide language is copied onto the RNA, except in the RNA the nucleotide thymidine is replaced by uracil. Once pre-messenger RNA is spliced or rearranged into messenger RNA, it is translated into protein. This process is called translation, because the nucleotide sequence of RNA is translated into a new language using twenty different amino acids as the alphabet. As already mentioned, a protein chain is composed of repeating units of proteinogenic amino acids.

Transcription: Reading the DNA Genes into RNA

RNA is like DNA except the deoxyribosyl sugar backbone is replaced by a ribosyl sugar and, as noted earlier, the DNA nucleoside thymidine is replaced by uracil (guanine, cytosine, and adenosine stay the same). While DNA exists as two strands wrapped around each other in a double helix, RNA usually exists as a single strand that may twist or loop back on parts of itself.

Transcription of DNA into pre-messenger RNA is initiated by an RNA polymerase transcription complex that opens or unwinds the two stands of DNA at the site of a gene to be transcribed and then synthesizes a pre-messenger RNA strand that is complementary to a DNA strand.[279] RNA polymerase is so named because it makes an RNA polymer (i.e., a chain of ribonucleic acids) called pre-messenger RNA. Single-stranded pre-messenger RNA is made within the nucleus and, after splicing into messenger RNA, is transported outside the nucleus to the cytoplasm of the cell.

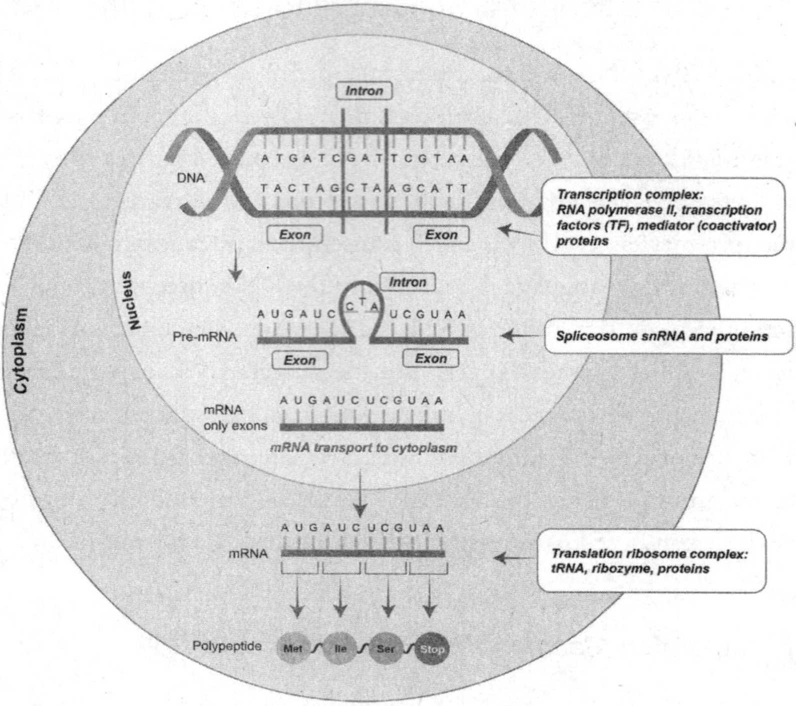

FIGURE 9.5: How a cell makes proteins from DNA. The cell uses a transcription complex to transcribe DNA into pre-messenger RNA. A spliceosome complex next converts pre-messenger RNA into messenger RNA. Then, a translation complex converts the messenger RNA into proteins. These complexes are composed of multiple proteins and different types of RNA, including small nuclear RNA, transfer RNA, and ribozyme RNA.

Why is DNA transcribed into an intermediate RNA nucleotide sequence instead of being converted directly into a protein? First, double-stranded DNA is relatively resistant to mutation (that is, errors occurring in nucleotide sequence). DNA needs to be faithfully transmitted as your genetic blueprint to your offspring. When single-stranded RNA is the genetic blueprint, as occurs with RNA viruses, they are ten thousand times more prone to mutation than double-stranded DNA viruses. Second, DNA cannot be transcribed unless it is unzipped by

RNA polymerase, after which it rezips shut. Single-stranded RNA remains open as a template for making many copies of the proteins. To make sure proteins do not continue to be made, single-strand RNA has a half-life of ten hours before being degraded.

Spliceosome: Editing Pre-Messenger RNA into Messenger RNA

In bacteria, DNA is transcribed into messenger RNA without a pre-RNA intermediate. In animals and humans, the DNA is transcribed into pre-messenger RNA that is further processed within the nucleus by cutting out segments called introns (inexpressed sequences) and splicing together segments called exons (expressed sequences). The spliceosome complex slices or cuts out introns in pre-messenger RNA and ties the remaining exons together to form the final messenger RNA.[280] By splicing together different modular regions (exons), the cell can form a variety of different proteins with different functions from the same DNA sequence.

The spliceosome complex is made up of about 170 proteins and five small nuclear RNAs. In 1993, Phillip Sharp and Richard Roberts from the Massachusetts Institute of Technology received the Nobel Prize for their 1977 discovery of pre-messenger RNA splicing.[281] Human diseases may arise from mutations in the spliceosome complex.[282]

Translation: Converting Ribonucleotides into Protein Amino Acids

Translation of messenger RNA into a protein requires an additional type of RNA called transfer RNA that has an attached amino acid. Transfer RNA is aligned on messenger RNA by the ribosome complex.[283] The ribosome complex travels along the messenger RNA, binding the transfer RNA and transferring its amino acid to a growing polypeptide chain. It continues doing this until reaching a stop sign (known as a stop codon) on the messenger RNA that signals the termination of protein formation.

Ribosomal RNA is called a ribozyme because, in analogy to a protein, it functions like an enzyme. RNA can store genetic information like DNA. Unlike DNA molecules, RNA may also perform enzymatic reactions like proteins. Under laboratory conditions, RNA can even replicate itself.[284] It is believed that RNA evolved long before DNA. Approximately 50 percent of all known viruses are RNA viruses. In 2009, the Nobel Prize in Chemistry was awarded for determining the structure of ribosomes by X-ray crystallography.

The ribosome complex has been retained throughout evolution. It is present in bacteria that predate our cells by two billion years. But over two billion years, the ribosome complex has undergone some changes. Several antibiotics (e.g., tetracycline, erythromycin, aminoglycosides) have no effect on human ribosomes but kill bacteria by inhibiting their ribosome complex.[285]

Junk DNA

The process of transcription, splicing, and translation to form proteins from DNA involves only about 1 to 2 percent of human DNA. What is all the rest of a human's DNA doing? Because the purpose for so much extra DNA has not been well delineated in the past, it has been called "junk" DNA.

As the proverb goes, "One man's junk is another man's treasure." The truth is that junk DNA is not junk at all. It is involved in epigenetics or the bureaucracy that regulates gene expression. As an example, myotonic dystrophy is the most common cause of inherited muscle weakness in people of European ancestry. The responsible gene is called DMPK (abbreviation for myotonic dystrophy protein kinase). Myotonic dystrophy has no abnormality or mutation in the transcribed DNA gene. The abnormality derives from a nontranscribed segment that does not form protein. The nonexpressed sequence of DNA has an abnormally repetitive three-nucleotide sequence (CTG).[286]

Junk DNA is involved in epigenetics, which means that which is above or over (the Greek preposition *epi*) the genes. Epigenetics starts, stops, and fine tunes gene expression and likely determines cellular aging. Epigenetics is a relatively newer field of exploration. The "junk" DNA that does not become a protein appears to have arisen at least in part from ancient viruses.[287] This suggests that virus may have played a role in our evolution, that is, in determining who we are and who we will become as human beings.

Some septuagenarians look and act like fifty-five-year-olds and vice versa. This is because the cell's aging clock (i.e., one's physiologic age) is not the same as the clock on a wall (i.e., chronologic aging). Albert Einstein is credited with saying: "Time is relative." Because of epigenetics, aging may be relative! To paraphrase a quote from Nobel Laureate John Fenn: "Nature is never schizophrenic nor wasteful."[288] Junk DNA coordinates gene expression and perhaps cell aging.

Summary

What we need to know from this brief and condensed overview of molecular biology is that the continuity of life is stored in genetic information that flows from four nucleotides in DNA to four nucleotides in messenger RNA to twenty amino acids in proteins. These nucleotides and amino acids are life's Lego pieces that can be pulled apart and snapped back together to form a completely different structure or organism, be it a bird, a wolf, a human, or a virus, akin to Hinduism's reincarnation. Size and charge differences in DNA, RNA, and protein are used to isolate, study, and create life. As we will learn in the next chapter, the ordered flow or sequence of cellular information from

DNA to RNA and then to proteins can be partially reversed by a type of virus called a retrovirus.

As Shakespeare's Hamlet pronounces to Horatio: "There are more things in heaven and earth, Horatio, than are dreamt of in your philosophy" (*Hamlet*, act 1, scene 5). It is our destiny as human beings to go forward. The only question is how we should do it. Where there is discovery, there is hope and danger. When we alter the genetic sequence of life, kill switch safeguards, if prearranged, will allow escape from unimaginable consequences.

SECTION THREE

Post-Molecular Biology: An Era of Genetically Manufactured Viruses

CHAPTER 10

HIV and AIDS: The 1980s Pandemic

Do not look under the bed at night; lying in wait is a past of dirty needles, the Koprowski CHAT vaccine, and the Uganda HIV study.—RKB

After molecular biology took over the field of life sciences, mankind was hit with a new viral pandemic called acquired immunodeficiency syndrome or AIDS, an infection related to human activity. The first report in the United States of AIDS was in 1981 when five otherwise healthy homosexual men in Los Angeles were reported to die from *Pneumocystis carinii* pneumonia, an opportunistic infection that normally only occurs in people with a severely compromised immune system.[289] Soon afterward, intravenous drug abusers who shared needles and hemophiliacs who were receiving blood product transfusions also began showing up in emergency rooms with shortness of breath. They would be intubated with machine ventilation but would succumb from suffocation despite receiving 100 percent pressurized oxygen. To save them the panic and struggle caused by slowly suffocating while strapped to a machine, they would be sedated, their subconscious brainstem fighting to breathe and keep their blood pressure up until the end.

Reports of other lethal opportunistic infections soon followed. The common marker in these patients was a deficiency in an immune cell called a helper T cell (lymphocyte), which is identified by the surface marker CD4.[290] Low CD4 helper T cells in the peripheral blood of these patients caused lethal opportunistic infections. The lower the number of CD4 cells, the more types of opportunistic infections occurred (Table 10.1).

In 1981, AIDS was reported to be associated with the development of an otherwise rare cancer called Kaposi sarcoma that appears as raised, reddish-purple lesions or nodules on the skin, mucous membranes, genitals, anus, or within internal organs.[291] Even though Kaposi sarcoma is a cancer of blood vessels, giving it a blood color, the cancer is driven by a virus called herpesvirus 8.[292] This virus is ubiquitous and does not cause cancer for people with a normal immune system. When helper T CD4 cells drop below 200 per microliter of blood, the immune system's ability to stop herpesvirus 8 is impaired, and the person is at risk for Kaposi sarcoma.

The next year, a disease was reported in Uganda that the locals called "Slim disease" because the afflicted person would become thin and wasted in appearance.[293] Slim disease spread mainly via heterosexual intercourse. It was common with prostitutes and their clients. Slim disease was later identified as AIDS.

AIDS spreads by contact with human fluids, predominately blood but also semen and vaginal fluids, and from mother to child. As a result, it was not long before AIDS turned up in America in heterosexuals, women, and newborn babies. A 1984 publication from the Centers for Disease Control linked patients with AIDS by sexual contact.[294] For confidentiality, the patients' names were removed. One of the initial patients was identified under the moniker patient O (pronounced *oh*). He was referred to as such because he was from "outside" of California. He was subsequently identified by the lay public as patient zero, even though he was not the first case of AIDS. The

Peripheral Blood CD4 Count and Infectious Agent	**Category**	**Common Organs Infected**
Any CD4 count		
Mycobacterium tuberculosis	Mycobacteria	Any organ, lung, liver, brain, bone
CD4 less than 250 cells per milliliter		
Coccidioidomycosis	Fungus	Lung, brain
CD4 less than 200 cells per milliliter		
Pneumocystis jirovecii pneumonia, previously called *pneumocystis carina* pneumonia (PCP)	Fungus	Lung
Candidiasis	Fungus	Mucous membranes and skin
Kaposi Sarcoma	Herpesvirus 8	A cancer usually in the skin but may occur in internal organs
CD4 less than 150 cells per milliliter		
Histoplasma capsulatum	Fungus	Lung, liver, lymph nodes, mucosal ulcers
CD4 less than 100 cells per milliliter		
Cryptococcus neoformans	Fungus	Brain, lung
Cryptosporidiosis	Protozoa	Small bowel
Herpes simplex viruses (HSV)	Virus	Mucosal surfaces, genitals, brain
Microsporidiosis	Fungus	Small bowel, liver, brain mucosal surfaces
JC (John Cunningham) virus	Virus	Brain
CD4 less than 50 cells per milliliter		
Cytomegalovirus	Virus	Eyes, esophagus, colon, liver, lungs
Mycobacterium avium	Mycobacteria	Any organ but especially lung, brain, bone
Toxoplasma gondii	Protozoa	Brain
Bartonella	Bacteria	Liver, skin, bone

TABLE 10.1: AIDS-Associated Opportunistic Infections Risk Stratified by CD4 Helper T Cell (Lymphocyte) Count in the Peripheral Blood

patient's name was ousted in the 1987 book *And the Band Played On* and the 1993 HBO film of the same name. Patient O was a Canadian flight attendant with approximately 250 sexual encounters per year who passed AIDS to sexual contacts and who passed away from AIDS in 1984.[295]

Luc Montagnier and Robert Gallo

Prior to 1983, the medical community did not know what was causing the ensuing pandemic. New cases and deaths were surging. Two scientists, Luc Montagnier and Robert Gallo, stepped up to the plate to rescue mankind. These same figures soon found themselves thrust into the media limelight and embroiled in a quarrel over who should get credit for their discovery of the AIDS virus.

Luc Montagnier was with the Pasteur Institute, the same Parisian institute that developed a vaccine for rabies a century earlier (see chapter 4). In early 1983, Montagnier obtained a lymph node biopsy from a patient infected with AIDS and grew the cells in the Pasteur Institute laboratory.[296] The cells contained an RNA virus that was able to reverse transcribe its RNA into DNA by having a reverse transcriptase gene. A retrovirus is a family of viruses that can reverse transcribe their RNA into DNA and insert their viral DNA into the DNA of the cell. Montagnier deduced that AIDS was caused by a new type of retrovirus.[297] Since this virus was isolated from a lymph node, he named it lymphadenopathy-associated virus (LAV).

At the time, there were two known human retroviruses that produced reverse transcriptase. They were called human T cell leukemia viruses (HTLV I and II). Both had been discovered by Robert Gallo at the National Cancer Institute of the National Institutes of Health (NIH) in Bethesda, Maryland.[298] Gallo suspected that AIDS was caused by a virus in the same HTLV family of viruses that he had already discovered. In a 1984 article published in the journal *Science*, he claimed that his team had (independently) isolated a new retrovirus named HTLV-III that was causing the AIDS pandemic.[299]

By the 1980s, molecular biology, viruses, and medicine had become big-money patents for government institutions and universities funded by the taxpayer as well as for big pharmaceutical companies that obtained the license from these taxpayer-funded institutions (see chapter 16). With potential money to be made, the National Institutes of Health (NIH) quickly held a news conference announcing Gallo's discovery of AIDS as a retrovirus. The NIH made a big faux pas by not crediting Dr. Montagnier for his earlier discovery of LAV. Over time, to avoid confusion between the two different names for the virus causing AIDS, both LAV and HTLV-III were replaced by the name human immunodeficiency virus or HIV.

Over the next several years, controversy and accusations surrounding who first discovered the HIV virus played out in the public arena and in the courts. An acrimonious transatlantic legal battle ensued between the National Institutes of Health and the Pasteur Institute as to whom should get the recognition, patent rights, and lucrative royalties generated by the discovery. In 1987, US President Ronald Reagan and French President François Mitterrand agreed that both institutions and their respective drug companies would share the royalties between themselves while excluding their own taxpayers and the rest of the world in their financial bonanza.[300]

At the end of the day, it was Montagnier who was the first to correctly identify the AIDS virus as a novel retrovirus, one different than Gallo's human T cell leukemia viruses. In 2002, Montagnier and Gallo published back-to-back editorials in *Science*.[301] Montagnier graciously credited Gallo with discovering the reverse transcriptase assay he used to identify HIV as a retrovirus, the growth factor called interleukin-2 (IL-2) used to grow infected lymphocytes at the Pasteur Institute, and the anti-HTLV antibodies that he used to document that HIV was a novel type of retrovirus. Montagnier and his colleague

Françoise Barré-Sinoussi (also at the Pasteur Institute) received the Nobel Prize in 2008.[302]

Robert Gallo was not a recipient of the 2008 Nobel Prize. Gallo started the field of human retrovirology. Without Gallo's groundbreaking achievements, HIV would not have been discovered by Montagnier. On the other hand, in the spirit of collaboration Montagnier had sent an HIV sample to Gallo's lab. Inadvertently using the French sample, Gallo's lab claimed to have independently discovered HIV. Gallo left the National Institutes of Health in 1996 to start the Institute of Human Virology at the University of Maryland School of Medicine.

The HIV retrovirus is part of a larger group of viruses called lentiviruses. The name derives from the Latin *lentus*, meaning "slow" or "sluggish," because the infection may go unnoticed for years before the onset of symptoms.[303] HIV is an RNA virus that is transcribed into DNA and then integrated into the DNA of an immune cell (i.e., helper T CD4 lymphocyte and macrophage). It may remain dormant for years before replicating and killing the CD4 immune cell. Depletion of CD4 cells leads to an increased risk of infections.

Where Did HIV Come From?

HIV is genetically similar to an African primate virus called simian immune virus or SIV. African monkeys infected with SIV are asymptomatic. They are resistant to the immune activation and CD4 immune cell depletion characteristic of AIDS in humans.[304]

There are two types of epidemic HIV: HIV1 and HIV2. These respective viruses were transmitted from different primates and behave differently in humans. HIV2 emerged from sooty mangabey monkeys infected with SIV and is largely linked to West Africa. Most people with HIV2 remain long-term nonprogressors and can live relatively symptom free for up to twenty-five years.[305]

In contrast, the HIV1 virus is genetically akin to the SIV retrovirus found in chimpanzees from the Democratic Republic of the Congo and neighboring areas. It arose in the distant past by the recombination of two monkey viruses within one or more chimps.[306] Four different HIV1 virus groups have infected the human population. These groups are designated M, N, O, and P.[307] Groups N, O, and P have remained isolated and relatively inconsequential. As we'll see later in this chapter, group M is different than the other three groups. It is this HIV1 group that caused the worldwide AIDS pandemic. Going forward herein, HIV1 group M will be referred to simply as HIV.

Chimpanzees are omnivores. They form hunting bands to catch and eat prey, including various species of monkeys. As their territory is encroached upon, chimpanzees have even been documented to kidnap and eat human babies and children.[308] It has been reasoned that chimpanzees initially became infected with SIV after eating infected monkeys. It is similarly speculated and generally accepted that the HIV virus jumped into the human population after humans ate wild chimpanzee bushmeat.

Since people have lived in Africa as hunter-gatherers for hundreds of thousands of years, why didn't humans get infected with SIV and develop AIDS prior to the twentieth century? The answer lies in a human protein called tetherin, which protects human cells from SIV and HIV proliferation. Recent studies have suggested that in the relatively recent past, two mutated SIV genes (called Nef and Vpu) were able to downregulate tetherin function, thereby facilitating the transmission of the virus into humans.[309]

When Did HIV First Appear in Humans?

The oldest confirmed human HIV infection was discovered in a human laboratory blood sample saved from a 1959 malaria study.[310]

The blood was from a person who lived in Kinshasa in the Democratic Republic of the Congo. This entails that HIV crossed into the human population sometime around or before 1959. But when exactly did this occur?

Phylogenetics is the study of the evolutionary closeness of viruses (or any organism) to each other based on their genetic sequence similarity.[311] Phylogenetic analysis compares whether each nucleotide in each position in the virus is identical or different between two viruses. The more identical nucleotides that are in the same position, the more closely related the two viruses or organisms are in terms of evolution.

A 1998 article published in the journal *Nature* reported on the genetic similarity of HIV samples from the 1996 Los Alamos Repository, including the 1959 Kinshasa sample mentioned previously.[312] By estimating a constant nucleoside change of 0.005 to 0.01 per nucleoside site per year, it was calculated that HIV first entered a human in the 1940s or early 1950s. A follow-up paper from Los Alamos published in 2000 in the journal *Science* analyzed a larger group of 159 patients with known sampling dates, including samples dated from the 1980s, which is when the medical literature first recognized AIDS, as well as samples from the 1959 Kinshasa malaria study.[313] This second paper estimated that HIV most likely entered the human population in 1931 (with a possible range from 1915 to 1941). Besides its larger sample size, this second paper also included the assumption of a quiescent or non-replicating interval when HIV was first incorporated into the DNA of humans.

Phylogenetic studies of nucleotide sequence comparisons, when used to determine chronology or the time that a new virus first appeared, depend on the assumptions used in the phylogenetic model and the number of samples available for comparison. The assumption used in previous modeling of HIV was that a constant, linear correspondence exists between time and the number of mutations, the latter being defined as the change in nucleoside bases at each site.

This assumption, based on the best estimates available at the time, may need to be adjusted. The mutation rate within a species may vary depending on the rate of virus replication that for an RNA retrovirus like HIV may fluctuate over time. Viral RNA recombination between different nucleotide strands may affect the most recent common ancestor (abbreviated as MRCA), which may alter the time frame for when HIV jumped into the human population.[314] In simple terms, one single RNA strand of HIV can switch some of its genes with those from another HIV RNA strand. This will affect the viral mutation rate especially if large numbers of virus are grown in cell culture. Nevertheless, if the assumptions made in the 2000 model are correct, HIV entered the human population around 1931. The Los Alamos Repository today contains hundreds of thousands of HIV sequences, but still none from before 1959.[315]

Dirty Needles in Clinics and Hospitals

As noted earlier in this chapter, HIV started as a zoonotic infection, which means it was transferred from animals (in this case, chimpanzees) to humans. But what caused the HIV group that entered the human population to shift from isolated cases to a worldwide epidemic in the 1980s?

Unlike other HIV1 groups that crossed into the human population but did not start a pandemic, some circumstances favorable to viral growth allowed group M to become easily transmissible through sexual relations and become a worldwide pandemic. The HIV virus has a genetic region called a promoter that increases or "promotes" its replication when signals are released from a stimulated immune system.[316] Infections stimulate the immune system. Vaccines are attenuated infectious viruses that stimulate the immune system.[317] Dirty needles used on patients will also spread infections like hepatitis and HIV, both of which stimulate the immune system. Disposable needles were first introduced in United States in 1956.[318] In the 1980s, African hospitals and clinics were still using non-disposable, non-sterilized needles on patients.[319] Unsterilized needles reused between blood draws significantly increased the spread of HIV.

HIV found its niche. It may lie asleep (non-replicating) in a human cell for years or decades until infections stimulate virus proliferation. From there, the proliferating virus can overtake and kill CD4 immune cells. Low numbers of CD4 cells allow for more infections, which cause more virus proliferation. High levels of the virus in the blood allows for easier spread and infection of other people, which perpetuates the HIV life cycle in a new host.

The Koprowski CHAT Poliovirus Vaccine

Edward Hooper, a BBC journalist, published a book in 1999 titled *The River: A Journey to the Source of AIDS*. Hooper is a true investigative reporter. He wrote a detailed story tracing the origin of HIV from interviews with some of the original key sources.[320] His book is an extensive epidemiological account of HIV. As he showed, Kinshasa in the Democratic Republic of the Congo was ground zero for both polio vaccinations and the worldwide HIV pandemic, a fact that he believed was more than just mere coincidence.

As we observed in chapter 6, the polio vaccines used in the Congo contained a live virus developed by Hilary Koprowski. This oral vaccine was produced by culturing the CHAT strand of the poliovirus in primate kidney cells. In the 1950s, the Wistar Institute in Philadelphia and the government of Belgium collaborated to use the Koprowski CHAT polio strain to vaccinate people in the Congo.[321]

When polio vaccination started, the Congo was a colony of Belgium. The entire country—the second largest in Africa—was the personal property of Belgium's King Leopold. Even the capital city, Leopoldville, was named after the Belgian monarch. In 1966, a decade after vaccinations began and independence from Belgium was achieved, Leopoldville was renamed Kinshasa.

In February 1957, mass vaccinations using the CHAT strain of live poliovirus started in several Congolese cities. During this time, the Wistar Institute denied using chimpanzee kidney cells to create the CHAT vaccine.[322] This distinction is important because chimpanzee SIV, not monkey SIV, is the direct precursor of AIDS. Retrospectively, some CHAT virus vaccine lots made in Philadelphia were tested for contamination with chimpanzee SIV by polymerase chain reaction. The lots tested negative.[323]

The Wistar Institute grew poliovirus in the kidney cell of monkeys imported from India. But how was poliovirus grown in the Congo? Did the Congo investigators use monkeys flown from India, or did they use local primates to manufacture more CHAT poliovirus? Since the publication of his book, Hooper has learned that "a large proportion of the vaccine doses administered in the Belgian territories of central Africa in the 1950s were made locally in chimpanzee cells and sera, and not in the US or Belgium."[324] The use of cells sourced from local chimpanzees instead of buying and flying in monkeys from India would have been a logical cost-cutting measure.

Another common cost-saving measure was the reuse or sharing of nonsterilized needles within Congolese hospitals and clinics. As late as 1976, an outbreak of Ebola virus (see chapter 14) in the Democratic Republic of Congo arose due to the shared use of unsterilized needles and syringes in hospitals. Nurses were given only five needles and syringes per day that had to be reused again and again on patients without proper sterilization between patients.[325]

In the Congo, chimpanzees were readily available locally. Since nobody was aware that their cells were contaminated with the chimpanzee equivalent of HIV, why should a poor country that could not even afford adequate disposable needles pay for monkeys to be captured and exported from India? Local chimpanzees were not only numerous but also bigger than the Indian monkey with larger kidneys that could provide more cells for polio vaccine production. We now know, in retrospect, that these African chimpanzees, unlike Asian monkeys, were infected with an HIV-like virus that is the source for human AIDS.[326]

Could the chimpanzee virus have jumped into humans through Koprowski's live polio vaccine that was grown in chimpanzee kidney cells? The answer is probably yes. We know that a pig retrovirus can jump into human cells when exposed to the cell free media from pig retrovirus infected kidney cells.[327] It is likely that the same mechanism caused chimpanzee SIV to spread to human subjects.

Bacteria, viruses, animals, and humans struggle to survive in low numbers until predators are removed and food is plentiful (see Figure 10.1). When those circumstances occur, life forms enter a rapid exponential phase of growth until food supplies are exhausted or predators return, after which numbers plateau and then decline. HIV sat silent in the infected person's genes for decades. If HIV crossed into humans sometime around 1931, then something happened between 1931 and 1980 that allowed HIV to spread and enter an exponential growth phase that caused the AIDS pandemic. Contributing factors likely include the use of shared needles in Congolese hospitals and clinics, casual sexual attitudes, and international travel.

Although controversial, emotionally charged, and unproven, the Koprowski CHAT polio vaccine—if sourced from chimpanzee kidney cells in the Congo—would be prima facie evidence implicating the Koprowski live vaccine in the origins of HIV. To be absolutely clear, we do not know if chimp cells were used in Congolese labs. An independent legal investigation of the most involved local personnel would have helped determine innocence or guilt. As of the time that this book was written, none has been undertaken.

Vaccines have co-transferred other live animal viruses like monkey SV40 (chapter 6) and bird avian leukosis virus (chapter 5)

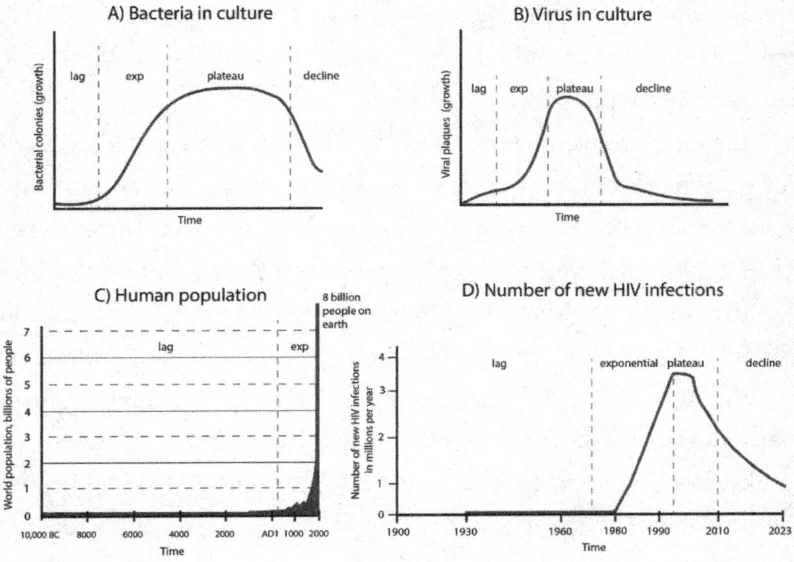

FIGURE 10.1: Life enters an exponential growth phase when predators are removed and food is plentiful. (A) Growth of bacteria in a culture dish. (B) Virus grown in cultured cells. (C) Growth of human population post Agricultural Revolution and bacterial and viral predators controlled with antibiotics and vaccines. (D) Growth of new HIV cases. New HIV infections declining due to introduction of anti-HIV drugs.

into the human population. Yet this has not activated the kill switch to stop using animal cells for vaccine production. Despite molecular biology advances, vaccine production requires growth and harvesting usually in animal cells, yeast cells, or insect cells (see chapter 11). Because vaccine-derived viruses are usually grown in nonhuman cells, unlike other cellular derived products, the US Food and Drug Administration does not require vaccines to be xenofree (animal-exposure free).

Treatment of HIV Infection

Despite multiple attempts, no effective anti-HIV vaccine has yet been developed, in part because HIV mutates too rapidly.[328] Fortunately, the spread of HIV has been controlled by using drugs that limit viral replication and markedly decrease levels of virus in the blood (aka decrease viremia).[329]

The entire nucleotide order of HIV has been sequenced. We will not go into these genes except to say that a small number of viral genes wreak a lot of havoc. HIV is an RNA virus with only nine RNA genes. Discovering the nine genes of HIV has allowed understanding of the replication cycle and mechanism of HIV infection. This allowed for development of effective drug therapies (Table 10.2).

The drug called AZT (azidothymidine or zidovudine) was originally developed in the 1960s in the hope of being a treatment for cancer. It was not effective in that capacity. In 1983, Samuel Broder, the director of the National Cancer Institute, organized a team to start testing drugs against HIV virus grown in laboratory culture. At the time, AZT was still on a shelf at the National Institutes of Health. It was tested against HIV, and it worked. AZT inhibited viral reverse transcriptase. Without effective reverse transcription of RNA into DNA, HIV could not form a DNA copy, could not be inserted into a patient's genome, and could not propagate. In 1987, AZT became the first drug to be approved for the treatment of HIV. This drug therapy was effective but less so than initially hoped. A high rate of reverse transcriptase errors allowed AZT drug resistant mutations to arise.[330]

Other nucleotide reverse transcriptase inhibitors and other classes of drugs were developed in the years to follow.[331] These drugs now include protease inhibitors (first approved in 1995), non-nucleoside reverse transcriptase inhibitors (first approved in 1996), HIV cell entry and fusion inhibitors (first approved in 2003), integrase inhibitors (first approved in 2008), and antibodies that block viral entry into cells (first approved in 2018). By 1996, to improve anti-HIV drug efficacy, doctors were treating patients simultaneous with a combination of three different anti-HIV drugs listed on table 10.2.

Combined anti-viral therapy is referred to as highly active antiretroviral therapy (HAART).[332] By using several antiretroviral drugs at once, HAART therapy suppresses viral load in the blood, decreases infections, normalizes life expectancy, and inhibits sexual transmission to an uninfected partner. Since its development, HAART therapy has converted a lethal disease into a chronic illness. The current goal of HIV treatment is to adjust HAART therapy to suppress as maximally as possible the HIV virus load in the blood.

The Uganda HIV Study

A study funded by the US government's National Institute of Allergy and Infectious Diseases, which is part of the National Institutes of Health, was reported in an article published in the year 2000 in the *New England Journal of Medicine*, the most prestigious medical journal in the world. The study was done between 1994 and 1998 in rural villages in the Rakai district of Uganda.[333] Four hundred fifteen couples who were discordant for HIV infection (one partner had HIV but the other did not) were followed and over the years tested for sexual transmission of HIV to the unaffected partner.

While the study investigators knew who in the couple was HIV positive and who was not, they withheld that information from the study participants. What the study found was that infected subjects with a high number of virus particles per milliliter of blood were more likely to infect their partner with HIV. None of subjects in the study was offered HIV anti-viral therapy before, during, or after the study, even through multiple anti-HIV drugs were available before the study started. By 1996, two years before the trial ended, the benefits of highly active anti-retroviral therapy incorporating three antiviral drugs to suppress HIV viral load was well known and was the standard of care in America and Europe.[334]

Table 10.2: HIV Drugs Produced from 1987 to 2018

Year	Drug	Class of drug	Year	Drug	Class of Drug
1987	Zidovudine (AZT)	NRTI—nucleoside reverse transcriptase inhibitor	2003	Atazanavir (ATV)	Protease inhibitor
1991	Didanosine (ddI)	NRTI—nucleoside reverse transcriptase inhibitor	2003	Emtricitabine (FTC)	NRTI—nucleoside reverse transcriptase inhibitor
1992	Zalcitabine (ddC)	NRTI—nucleoside reverse transcriptase inhibitor	2003	Enfuvirtide (INN)	HIV entry and fusion inhibitor
1994	Stavudine (d4T)	NRTI—nucleoside reverse transcriptase inhibitor	2003	Fosamprenavir (fAPV)	Protease inhibitor
1995	Lamivudine (STC)	NRTI—nucleoside reverse transcriptase inhibitor	2005	Tipranavir (TPV)	Protease inhibitor
1995	Saquinavir (SQV)	Protease inhibitor	2006	Darunavir (DRV)	Protease inhibitor
1996	Indinavir (IDV)	Protease inhibitor	2007	Maraviroc (MVC)	HIV entry and fusion inhibitor
1996	Ritonavir (RTV)	Protease inhibitor	2008	Etravirine (ETR)	NNRTI—non-nucleoside reverse transcriptase inhibitor

1996	Nevira pine (NVP)	NNRTI—non-nucleoside reverse transcriptase inhibitor	2008	Raltegravir (RAL)	HIV integrase inhibitor
1997	Delavidine (DLV)	NNRTI—non-nucleoside reverse transcriptase inhibitor	2011	Rilpivirine (RIL)	NNRTI—non-nucleoside reverse transcriptase inhibitor
1997	Nelfinavir (NFV)	Protease inhibitor	2012	Elvitegravir/ cobicistat (EVG/ COBI)	HIV integrase inhibitor
1998	Abacavir (ABC)	NRTI—nucleoside reverse transcriptase inhibitor	2013	Dolutegravir (DTG)	HIV integrase inhibitor
1998	Efavirenz (EFV)	NNRTI—non-nucleoside reverse transcriptase inhibitor	2015	Tenofovir alafenamide (TAF)	NRTI—nucleoside reverse transcriptase inhibitor
2000	Lopinavir/ritonavir (LPV/r)	Protease inhibitor	2018	Bictegravir (BIC)	INSTI—integrase strand transfer inhibitor
2001	Tenofovir disoproxil fumarate (TDF)	NRTI—nucleoside reverse transcriptase inhibitor	2018	Doravirine (DOR)	NNRTI—non-nucleoside reverse transcriptase inhibitor
			2018	Ibalizumab (IBZ)	Antibody that blocks viral entry

The National Institute of Allergy and Infectious Diseases study performed on vulnerable Ugandan villagers had institutional review board approval from Johns Hopkins University and Columbia University in America and the Uganda National Council for Science and Technology. "Safety" monitoring was performed by the National Institutes of Health. They followed the standard of care in rural Uganda, where anti-retroviral therapy was not available because the villagers were too poor to afford it.

The editor of the *New England Journal of Medicine* published her own reservations about the study.[335] Paraphrasing her concerns: (1) this study was done in Uganda because it would not be ethical in America; (2) the subjects in Uganda received zero personal benefit from the study; and (3) the interests of science were put above the well-being of the Ugandan patients. Before approving the publication, the editor sought a review from two ethicists. One ethicist deemed the study unethical, the other declared that it was ethical.

Follow-up letters to the editor published in the *New England Journal of Medicine* from the University of the West Indies (Jamaica), the Federal University of Minas Gerais (Brazil), and the University of Illinois were critical of the study's ethics. Letters from researchers at premier American research institutions—including the University of California San Francisco, the Research Triangle Park in North Carolina, and the University of Washington, Seattle—were supportive of the study.[336]

The Uganda HIV study was funded by the US taxpayer without taxpayer knowledge, unashamedly presented in the world's most prestigious medical journal, and approved by American university regulatory oversight through their institutional review boards. Its questionable safety protocols and practices were monitored by the National Institutes of Health. The practical justification by the National Institutes of Health for the study was basically *we were only bystanders documenting what would normally happen to untreated couples.*

Did the National Institutes of Health take advantage of these study "subjects'" circumstances? Is that not what happens when we experiment on animals, freely exploiting their circumstances? The Uganda HIV study starkly echoes the 1932 Tuskegee syphilis study, which was also funded by the US government Public Health Service. During that study, poor Black Americans who were intentionally left untreated for syphilis were followed and observed to advance the science of the natural history of the bacterial infection. It took half a century before the Tuskegee study was finally recognized as an infamously unethical trial.[337]

In several ways, the Uganda HIV study violates globally recognized principles on human experimentation. The post–World War II Nuremberg Code was codified in 1947 in response to unethical medical testing and experimental war crimes performed by the Nazi regime that basically reduced human subjects to dehumanized lab rats.[338] The Nuremberg Code established the principle of voluntary "informed" consent without deceit or coercion.[339] In the 2000 Uganda study, information on the true goals of the study and internationally accepted options for treatment were intentionally withheld from the subjects. At least two of the ten tenets of the Nuremberg Code that were violated are:

1. Proper preparations should be made and adequate facilities provided to protect the experimental subject against even remote possibilities of injury, disability, or death.
2. During the course of the experiment the scientist in charge must be prepared to terminate the experiment at any stage, if he has probable cause to believe, in the exercise of the good faith, superior skill and careful judgment required of him that a continuation of the experiment is likely to result in injury, disability, or death to the experimental subject.

There has never been any medical or media follow-up concerning any of those 415 couples that the Uganda study allowed to be intentionally infected with HIV. Without being given known effective treatment, are any even still alive? Did any of the couples have children infected with HIV because of the trial?

Summary

The story of HIV is the history of dedicated and courageous work by many people, institutions, and countries. Although not eliminated, HIV has been successfully contained. But it is also a story of human activity facilitating the transmissibility of HIV from a localized low-level infection into a worldwide pandemic. Because the 2000 Uganda HIV study placed science above the ethical treatment of rural Ugandans and was conducted without transparent consent, it is also a story about the importance of consent being complete and honest. Who, if given the proper opportunity to consent, would agree to them and their loved ones being under observation for a lethal disease when effective therapy already exists? Honest consent is a kill switch that, if respected, protects people (including the investigators involved) from actions that may be historically regretted.

CHAPTER 11

Human Papilloma Virus (HPV): Does Making Money Supersede Consent?

No organization is sufficiently knowledgeable or benevolent enough to justly rule another without their consent.—RKB

Human papilloma virus (HPV) causes cancer. It had long been a dream to cure cancer with a vaccine. That dream became a reality with HPV vaccine. However, the development of a vaccine against HPV presented its fair share of special problems. Because HPV carries two genes that cause cancer, the intact virus could not be used as a live or dead vaccine—one does not want to inject two cancer-causing genes into people. Moreover, as its name suggests, human papilloma virus will only grow in human cells. No animal cell line could be used to grow HPV vaccine lots. By using molecular biology, scientists figured out ingenious ways to overcome these obstacles.

Cervical Cancer

The cervix is the lower end of the womb that connects to the birth canal. The word cervix is borrowed from the Latin *cervix*, meaning "neck." The cervix is a fibrous muscular tube, the metaphorical neck of the womb. On a manual exam, it feels like the tip of a nose sticking into the upper end of the vagina. Cancer of the cervix is the fourth-most common cancer in women worldwide. In 2020, there were more than 600,000 cases of cervical cancer and approximately 340,000 deaths.[340]

After taking hold in the cervix, the cancer spreads to the uterus, vagina, and sideways in the pelvis. The first sign of cervical cancer is abnormal bleeding, usually after coitus and later spontaneously between menstrual periods. Other symptoms are a foul-smelling, watery brown vaginal discharge and ill-defined groin pain and back pain. As the cancer grows and invades local tissues, the legs enlarge from trapped fluid. Urine flow is obstructed, leading to kidney failure. The cancer may also grow into the rectum and cause painful constipation.[341] In its final stages, cervical cancer may spread distantly into the bones, liver, lung, and, some rare cases, the brain.[342] Tumor growth and constant pain are often not stopped by radiation, chemotherapy, or narcotics.

Henrietta Lacks

One historical figure in the story of the HPV is Henrietta Lacks. In 1951, as a thirty-one-year-old woman, Lacks spent the last two months of her life at Johns Hopkins University Medical Center in Baltimore, Maryland, dying from cervical cancer. In the end, blood transfusion, radiation, and other treatments did not succeed in curing Lacks. Treatments were eventually stopped, allowing her to die mercifully without prolongation of suffering. A biopsy of cancer cells in her cervix was used to establish the first human immortal cell line. This cell line was called HeLa, an abbreviation taken from the first two letters of her first and last name. Her cells were grown and sent around the world to better understand cancer biology.

However, Henrietta's cervical cells were taken without her knowledge or consent.[343]

In April 1961, the Russian cosmonaut Yuri Gagarin became the first human being to be launched into space. He orbited the earth in a Vostok spaceship. In 1964, in another Vostok-type spaceship, Russia launched HeLa cells into space to study the effect of weightlessness on a human cell line. Henrietta's cells were both the first human female DNA and the first human cell line in space.[344] Her cervical cancer cells have ever since been immortalized and grown in perpetuity. In 2010, Rebecca Skloot wrote a book called *The Immortal Life of Henrietta Lacks* that became an HBO film of the same name.

Ironically, like the taking of Henrietta's cervical cells by the Johns Hopkins Medical Center, both Skloot's book and the subsequent HBO movie were done without consent from Lack's grandson, the last member of her immediate family with firsthand memories of her life. In 2020, Ron Lacks wrote a book titled *Henrietta Lacks: The Untold Story*.[345] In his book Lacks expressed that he did not feel that Skloot's book or the film accurately presented his grandmother's life and that he did not want her exploited and financially profited from a second time. Consent is a kill switch against future problems.

Human Papilloma Virus: The Cause of Cervical Cancer

An infectious agent was suspected to cause warts as early as 1917. To confirm this hypothesis, part of a genital wart on a male medical student was injected into the forearm of two males and the genitals of a female student. All three developed warts about three months later.[346] In 1949, when human warts were examined using an electron microscope, the cells were found to contain a virus.[347] By 1963, this agent was called the papilloma virus because the virus was found within a papilloma or skin wart. (Papilloma is derived from the Latin word *papilla*, meaning "nipple," since a wart looks like a skin nipple.)[348] Because papilloma viruses are species specific, the name of a papilloma virus includes the name of the infected animal. Hence, in humans it is called the human papilloma virus.

Papilloma viruses infect skin and mucosal surfaces. Mucosal surfaces are the moist lining of body cavities and hollow organs (e.g., mouth, throat, vagina, anus). Mucosal surfaces have a slick, smooth feeling like the inside of your check. A rabbit, deer, or cow papilloma virus will not infect humans. And a human papilloma virus will not infect animals. In the 1930s, it was shown that rabbit papilloma virus, besides causing warts, could over time lead to cancer.[349]

Harald zur Hausen was a German scientist, head of the Department of Virology and Hygiene at the University of Freiberg and chairman of the board of the German Cancer Research Center in Heidelberg. In the mid-1970s, Hausen discovered that human papilloma virus caused cervical cancer.[350] Of the many types of HPV, two types that he identified (type 16 and 18) cause 70 percent of all human female cervical cancers.[351] In 2008, Hausen was awarded the Nobel Prize for showing that a virus can cause human cancer (Box 11.1).

Box 11.1: Infections That Cause Cancer

The first cancer-causing virus ever identified was discovered in 1916 by Peyton Rous at the Rockefeller Institute in New York. He found that a bird tumor, when homogenized and passed through a porcelain filter, caused tumors in other birds. The Rous sarcoma virus (RSV) (sarcoma is a type of cancer) was named after him. For demonstrating that a viral infection could cause cancer in birds, Rous received the 1966 Nobel Prize.[352]

Since Rous's discovery, multiple viruses have been shown to be associated with human cancers.[353] Examples include hepatitis B and C viruses cause liver cancer, human herpes virus 8 causes Kaposi's sarcoma, human T-cell lymphotropic virus (HTLV-1) causes lymphoma, Epstein-Barr virus causes a cancer in the throat, Merkel cell polyomavirus causes a rare skin cancer, and simian virus 40 is involved in brain and bone tumors and tumors of immune cells (lymphoma) and of the cells lining the lungs (mesothelioma).

Besides viruses, a bacteria called *Helicobacter pylori* may cause a type of cancer in the gut called MALT lymphoma.[354] Early cases of MALT lymphoma have been cured with antibiotics.[355] The role for bacteria in other human cancers is unproven.[356]

There are many types of HPV viruses that infect different areas of the human body.[357] HPV 7 causes warts on the feet. HPV 2, 4, and 7 cause warts on the hands. HPV 6 and 11 cause genital warts. HPV 16 and 18 (and to a lesser extent 31, 33, 45, and others) cause cervical cancer. Other HPV-induced mucosal cancers include anal, vulvar (inner and outer lips of vagina), vaginal, penile, and oropharyngeal (the mouth and throat immediately behind the mouth). HPV may also cause cancers of the skin in chronically immunosuppressed patients, such as organ transplant recipients.[358]

How Does HPV Cause Cancer?

HPV is a DNA virus that has only eight protein coding genes. There are two virus shell or capsid proteins called L1 and L2, named as such because they are made *late* after infection. The other proteins are made *early* after infection and are accordingly called E1, E2, E4, E5, E6, and E7. Most early (E) proteins are involved in viral replication. However, E6 and E7 cause premalignant changes in the infected host cell that eventually lead to cancer (Figure 11.1).[359]

HPV genes E6 and E7 are responsible for premalignant changes by removing normal inhibition of an infected cell's ability to proliferate. E6 and E7 inhibit two normal growth suppressor proteins called p53 and pRB, respectively. Both are tumor suppressor proteins that safeguard cells from growing or dividing at an inappropriate

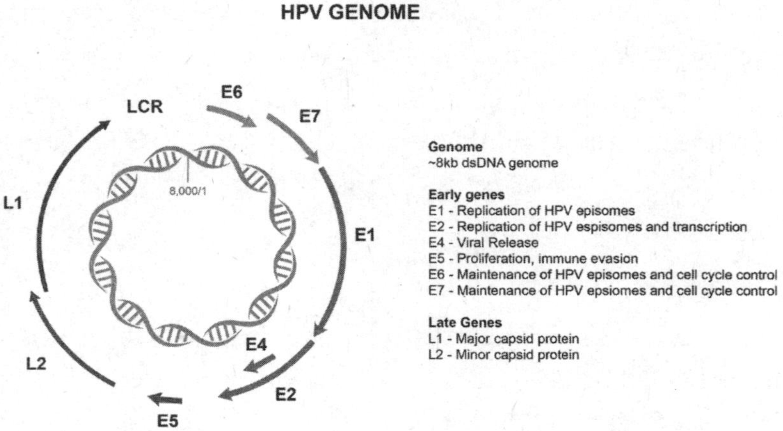

FIGURE 11.1: The DNA of the human papilloma virus. dsDNA = double-stranded deoxyribonucleic acid; E = early proteins involved in viral replication; Kb = kilobases; L = late proteins that make up the viral shell. HPV also has a DNA region that is not made into a protein but helps to regulate expression of the other genes. It is called the long control region (LCR)

rate.[360] When dysfunctional, these proteins play a contributory role in many types of tumors.[361] Following HPV infection, inappropriate growth or "dysplasia" of cervical cells will gradually transition over one or two decades into cervical cancer. That being said, most HPV dysplasia does not become irreversible cancer.

The cells that cover the cervix (or any mucous-covered organ) are called epithelial cells. The outer layer of cervix (or any mucous covered organ) is called the epithelium. The epithelium consists of several cell layers. The bottom basal cells are proliferating cells that continuously divide and renew the epithelium above with fresh cells. From the epithelium basal layer, cells are pushed up and become flattened until they fall off. The HPV virus infects only the cells at the lowest layer of epithelium. Once infected, the basal layer extends into higher layers of the epithelium, causing abnormal-looking cells to appear at different levels above the normal basal cell layer.

Dysplasia of the cervix is defined by a Cervical Intraepithelial Neoplasia (CIN) grade. Low-grade dysplasia is labeled CIN

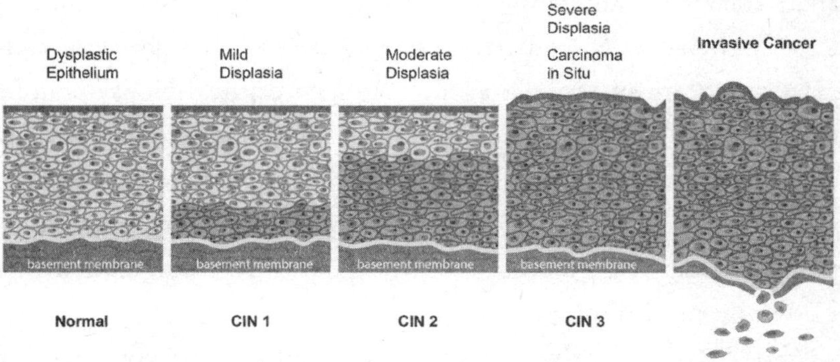

FIGURE 11.2: Schematic presentation of CIN (cervical intraepithelial dysplasia) that progresses over years or decades to cervical cancer.

1 and is defined as abnormal (dysplastic) cells in the lower third of epithelium. CIN 2 refers to abnormal cells in the lower two-thirds of epithelium. High-grade dysplasia or CIN 3 is defined as abnormal cells being present throughout the entire thickness of the epithelium. Cancer occurs when cells invade across the basement membrane that separates epithelium from the rest of the body (see Figure 11.2).

Spontaneous disappearance of dysplasia in the epithelium occurs within one to two years for at least 60 percent, 40 percent, and 33 percent of CIN 1, CIN 2, and CIN 3 patients, respectively. The lifetime likelihood of progression to cervical cancer for CIN 1, CIN 2, and CIN 3 patients is 1 percent, 5 percent, and 12 percent, respectively.[362] CIN 1 is initially observed without treatment, as most cases will disappear spontaneously. CIN 2 or CIN 3 and persistent CIN 1 grades are treated by a small, localized outpatient office excision.[363]

In 1942, Dr. George Papanicolaou, a Greek physician then teaching at Cornell Medical College, published a technically easy and low-cost method to screen for cervical dysplasia and cancer.[364] This method has since been referred to as a Pap smear, deriving its name from the first three letters of Papanicolaou's last name. During a Pap smear, the vagina is opened with a speculum and a brush collects epithelial cells from the cervical opening. If significant dysplastic cells are seen under a microscope, a cervical biopsy is done to determine the CIN grade. CIN 2 and 3 grades are treated by hot (thermal) or cold (cryo) temperature ablation. Alternatively, the affected epithelium may be cut out by large loop excision with a cauterizing cutting wire loop or by cutting out the cervical cone with a cold knife conization.

HPV infections that are not treated and do not spontaneously disappear may take years or even decades to progress from CIN to cancer. Cervical cancer is preventable and may be cured before it becomes a cancer by regular inexpensive Pap smears done in the clinic or doctor's office. The Pap smear has prevented innumerable cervical cancers. As a result, Papanicolaou was nominated on five separate occasions for a Nobel Prize, although he never was awarded the honor.

HPV Vaccine

The prior vaccines encountered in this book have been attenuated live viruses or intact dead viruses. Unlike other viruses like poliomyelitis that grows in primate kidney cells or the yellow fever virus that grows in embryonated chick eggs, there was no animal model available to grow *human* papilloma virus to make a vaccine. Even if the HPV virus could be grown in animal cells, HPV also contains cancer-inducing genes (i.e., E6 and E7) that, if included in an intact viral vaccine, could cause a healthy person to eventually develop a cancer. These problems in making the vaccine were overcome by the use of molecular biology techniques.

To produce the HPV vaccine, only the protein shell of the virus, called a virus-like particle, was used. Virus-like particles (abbreviated as VLP) are composed of virus capsule proteins that spontaneously self-assemble to form an empty virus particle that does not contain genetic material—that is, it has no RNA or DNA.[365] The VLP of HPV is composed of L1, a shell (capsid) protein that forms the outer shell of HPV. L1 proteins will spontaneously assemble to create the outer icosahedral (twenty-sided) shell of HPV. Seventy-two L1 proteins self-assemble to form a single VLP that is empty inside.[366] This viral capsid is not infectious; it is not a virus. A VLP is only the "skin" or shell of the virus particle.

An empty viral shell will stimulate the immune system against the virus just like a living human papilloma virus would do. It will stimulate the immune system because the L1 protein has a pathogen-associated molecular pattern.[367] By presenting the outer protein shell in its normal three-dimensional shape, the VLP presents a repetitive sequence of pathogen-associated molecular patterns to the immune system. This means that an immune cell called a dendritic cell (a type of macrophage) will spontaneously recognize this pathogen pattern, attempt to kill it (i.e., eat it), and then try to educate other immune cells (T and B cells) to recognize it as a pathogen. The educated B cells will then begin to make antibodies that circulate in the blood and body fluids. These antibodies can kill and prevent infection when exposed to the real virus (Figure 11.3).

How Are Virus-Like Particles Made?

VLPs are made in bakers' yeast. The production costs of using yeast are low because yeast grows rapidly in inexpensive media.[368] Because cells including yeast cells have so many genes, these genes are organized within structures called chromosomes (Box 11.2). Chromosomes are a continuous string of genes that replicate when a cell divides, so each daughter cell will have the same genes.

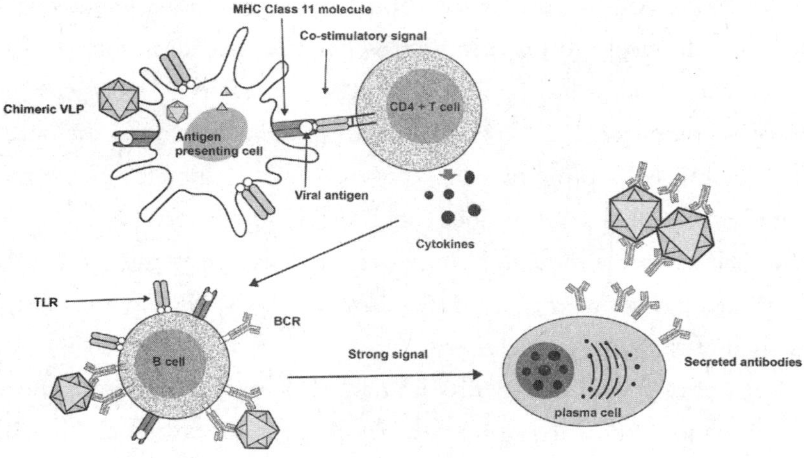

FIGURE 11.3: Immune response to HPV or an HPV capsid shell composed of the L1 protein VLP. Capsule proteins stimulate a dendritic cell (a type of macrophage) through pathogen-specific recognition. The stimulated dendritic cell will eat the HPV or VLP and represent parts of it along with co-stimulatory molecules to other immune cells (T lymphocytes). These immune cells become activated and stimulate B lymphocytes to make proteins called antibodies against HPV. The antibodies bind to the HPV and cause it to be destroyed.

Box 11.2: Chromosomes and Viruses

A cell has a fatty membrane that encloses it and walls it off from the outside environment. (Cells build walls, so do people.) A cell's hereditary (genetic) information is stored in the nucleus located inside the cell. (Cells compartmentalize work, so do humans.) For animals, plants, and fungi (but not bacteria) the nucleus is walled off with another fatty membrane that separates it from the rest of the inside of the cell.

In the 1800s, Walther Flemming, a German doctor, noticed that the nucleus had a fibrous (protein) network that could be stained with a dye and visualized under a microscope. He called the material chromatin, which is derived from the Greek word *chrōma* and means "made of color." The components of chromatin that separate and move during cell division were termed chromosomes, which in Greek means "colored bodies."

The human body has more than twenty thousand genes packaged into forty-six chromosomes (twenty-three from each parent). All genes are wrapped up and packaged into these forty-six chromosomes. If these chromosomes were fully unraveled, they would be over six feet long. To put that into perspective, the nucleus of a human cell is only 0.00000328 feet in diameter.

Yeast,[369] bacteria,[370] and human artificial chromosomes have been artificially constructed.[371] These man-made chromosomes allow for the cloning or transfer of large numbers of genes into cells. In contrast, viruses do not have chromosomes, a nucleus, or a fatty cell wall. They are very small and carry only a handful of genes located inside a protein shell. For example, the human papilloma virus has only eight genes.

The L1 gene of HPV has been placed inside a man-made yeast artificial chromosome. Basically this chromosome contains three important components: the different elements essential for a chromosome to replicate, a selection marker, and the L1 HPV gene (Figure 11.4).[372] The selection marker will color any yeast containing the YAC chromosome for easy identification.

By definition, a chromosome requires the essential elements for self-replication: an origin of replication (ORI), a centromere where proteins attach to pull replicating chromosomes apart, and telomere ends to prevent the ends from binding to each other. Other genes inserted into the chromosome include a yeast selectable marker (allowing identification of yeast containing the YAC) and a multiple cloning site (MCS) where different enzymes (i.e., restriction enzymes) may be used to insert the gene of interest, in this case the HPV L1 gene. The YAC may also carry an origin of replication and selectable marker for bacteria, so it may be grown in bacteria if desired, and Bam H1 sites, where a protein (a restriction enzyme called BamH1)

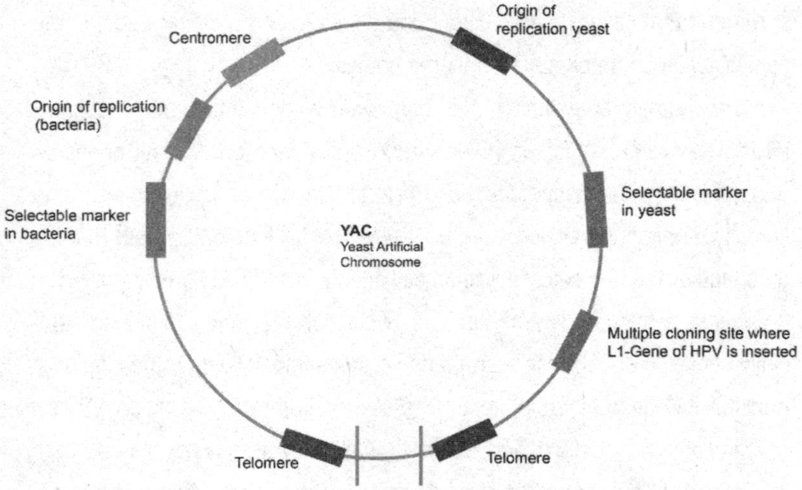

FIGURE 11.4: Yeast artificial chromosome (YAC).

can cut the YAC into one long linear piece of DNA to hold more genetic information than can be accommodated in its circular form.

As schematically shown in Figure 11.5, yeast artificial chromosomes (YACs) containing the L1 gene are placed along with yeast inside a cuvette in an electroporation instrument. An electrical pulse of the proper strength punches holes through the yeast cell wall without killing it. The transient hole allows the YAC to enter inside some yeast. It sounds like a Frankenstein movie, but electricity places a new chromosome inside a yeast cell. As the yeast divide and replicate, all their offspring will carry forth with the new chromosome and genes.

After electroporation, the yeasts from the cuvette are then plated on a culture dish, and yeast containing the artificial chromosome change color due to the selectable marker. The colored yeast colonies are removed and placed into a bioreactor (a large media culture system). As the yeast grow and reproduce, L1 proteins are made and spontaneously assemble into VLPs with the same three-dimensional size and structure of the human papilloma virus.[373] VLPs are then purified by lysis (destruction of yeast), and yeast components are removed before the vaccine is released.[374]

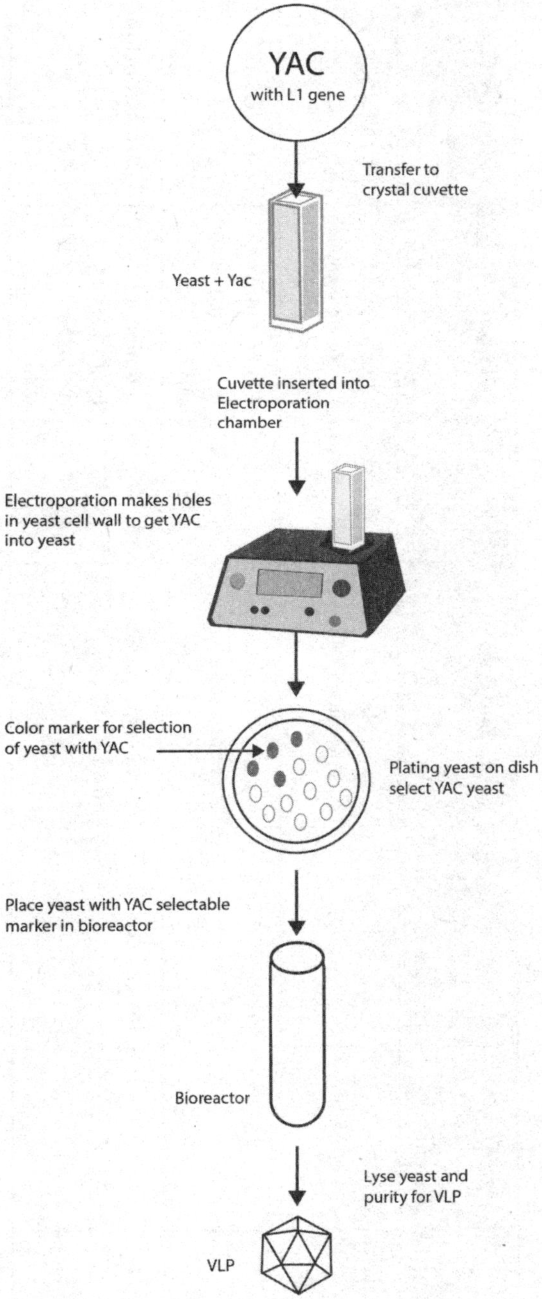

FIGURE 11.5: Production of the human papilloma virus (HPV) vaccine. Electroporation refers to electricity punching holes in the yeast membrane so that the YAC may enter. (YAC = yeast artificial chromosome). VLP = virus-like particle.

Table 11.1: HPV Vaccines[375]

Vaccine Name	Virus like particle (VLP) Protein	Cells that Produce VLP L1 Protein	Expression system	HPV types in vaccine	Adjuvant	Pharmaceutical company
Gardasilâ	L1	Yeast	Yeast artificial chromosome (YAC)	6, 11, 16, 18	Aluminum hydroxyphosphate sulfate	Merck (USA)
Gardasil 9â	L1	Yeast	Yeast artificial chromosome (YAC)	6, 11, 16, 18, 31, 33, 45, 52, 58	Aluminum hydroxyphosphate sulfate	Merck (USA)
Cervarixâ	L1	Insect cell	Baculovirus (an insect virus)	16, 18	Aluminum hydroxide and monophosphoryl lipid A	GlaxoSmithKline (UK)

Three HPV vaccines are currently available (Table 11.1). Gardasil and Gardasil 9 are produced in yeast. The Cervarix vaccine is made using an insect virus (baculovirus) that is expressed in insect cells. Due to a cross-licensing agreement to share revenue between pharmaceutical companies, only Gardasil and Gardasil 9 are marketed in America.[376] As a result, Merck has a monopoly on HPV vaccines in America.

HPV Vaccine Trials

In 2007, two randomized trials (FUTURE I and FUTURE II) were reported on Gardasil that targeted four HPV types (6, 11, 16, and 18). It included teenagers and young women aged fifteen to twenty-six who had never had an abnormal Pap smear. Half of the participants received the HPV vaccine that included VLPs and an aluminum-based adjuvant. The other half received the same aluminum adjuvant without VLPs. The vaccinated group receiving VLPs had a marked decrease in genital, vaginal, and anal warts.[377] Upon follow-up, these participants also displayed a marked decrease in cervical CIN 2 and CIN 3 precancerous dysplasia.[378]

In 2015, a vaccine randomized trial using another Gardasil vaccine, known as Gardasil 9, which targets 9 HPV types (HPV 6, 11, 16, 18, 31, 33, 45, 52, 58), was reported. Females sixteen to twenty-six years old who never had a positive Pap smear were enrolled. Roughly half of the participants received the vaccine that included VLPs and an aluminum-based adjuvant, and the other half received only the aluminum-based adjuvant. The vaccine containing VLPs markedly decreased CIN 2 and CIN 3 in the vaccinated group.[379] The results from the Cervarix vaccine against 2 HPV types (HPV 16 and 18) were also promising.[380]

These studies were limited to underaged (less than eighteen years old) teenagers and young HPV negative adults because it was thought the vaccine would be more effective in preventing an infection rather than stopping an established infection.[381] These studies were also limited to women because HPV infection in men is usually on skin-covered genitals. Mucosal surfaces like the cervix would be bathed in vaccine-induced protective antibodies that would not be present on dry skin.[382]

Success in preventing sexually transmitted genital warts and cervical CIN using the HPV vaccine in teenagers and young women who have a normal Pap smear has generated trials or future interest involving three different groups. First, the use of the single-dose vaccine in lower-income countries where few can afford the current three-dose injection regimen.[383] Second, the use of the HPV vaccine in both genders to prevent head and neck cancers. Third, women with abnormal Pap smears and established CIN 2 or CIN 3 using both L1 capsid protein and either one or both HPV E6 or E7 tumor promoting proteins.[384] As Professor Suzanne Garland, lead author of the 2007 Gardasil vaccine trial, wrote: "Now we need an effective therapeutic vaccine for those already infected and potentially at risk of disease."[385]

Due to the marked decrease in premalignant cervical CIN, it is logical and very highly likely that HPV vaccine will prevent most cervical cancers. However, due to the slow creep of CIN toward cancer and at times spontaneous resolution of CIN, it will be decades after vaccination before the results of the most important endpoint—elimination and not just delay in cervical cancer—are known for certain.

Royalty Lawsuits

There are currently over one hundred patents on HPV vaccines.[386] The biggest number of these patents are held by Merck (the fourth largest pharmaceutical company in the world), GlaxoSmithKline (the tenth largest pharmaceutical company in the world), and the National Institutes of Health of the US government.[387]

In 1991, the very first HPV vaccine patent using VLPs was filed by Ian Frazer with the University of Queensland in Brisbane, Australia. Frazer proposed that the L1 and L2 capsid proteins would form VLPs that could be used for a vaccine. One year later, Richard Schlegel at Georgetown University filed a patent for L1 capsid protein to be used alone as the vaccine, which is what current vaccines use. Both patents were licensed by the respective universities to big pharmaceutical companies.

A lawsuit eventually ensued between competing parties.[388] In 2005, the US Board of Patent Appeals and Interferences awarded patent rights to Schlegel's 1992 Georgetown University patent. Two years later, the US Federal Circuit Court reversed the lower court's decision and awarded patent rights to Frazer's 1991 Queensland University patent. To avoid further expensive litigation, the pharmaceutical companies agreed to cross-licensing each other's patent, allowing for all the involved parties to profit.[389] In return, Merck agreed to pay royalties on Frazer's patent.[390]

Because his patent was upheld as being the first, and thereby captures worldwide royalties, Frazer has achieved celebrity status in Australia. In 2012, he was named "A National Living Treasure" by the National Trust of Australia.[391] Schlegel continues his research and teaching as Professor and Chair of the Department of Pathology at Georgetown University.

Drug Company Lobbying

In 2007, Texas Governor Republican Rick Perry became the first governor to sign an executive order mandating that eleven- and twelve-year-old preteen girls be vaccinated with Gardasil. He ordered that they could not attend school without the vaccination.[392] While his order was soon overturned by the Texas legislature, Governor Perry had sought to replace consent with coercion. He has no medical training and no medical license. He did not recommend the alternative of free Pap smears and ongoing education on a healthy diet, promote the avoidance of alcohol and smoking, or encourage the use of condoms, which minimize the risk of cervical cancer as well as other cancers and diseases.

Why did Governor Perry take this action? One potential factor could be that Merck, the German pharmaceutical company that makes the Gardasil vaccine, gave money for Governor Perry's reelection through political action committees such as Texans for Rick Perry. Merck also hired Perry's chief of staff as one of their lobbyists. During the 2011 Republican presidential debate, US congresswoman Michelle Bachman publicly confronted Governor Perry on his conflict of interest here.[393] Such financial conflicts of interests are by no means restricted to the United States. The European Medicine Agency was set up in 1995 by the European Union to evaluate applications of drugs for marketing in all EU countries. Today, 80 to 90 percent of its annual budget comes from the pharmaceutical companies that it is supposed to regulate.[394]

Medical doctors are taught that a "conflict of interest" is: "A set of conditions in which professional judgment concerning a primary interest (such as a patient's interest or validity of research) tends to be unduly influenced by a secondary influence (such as financial gain)."[395] Governor Perry's executive mandate for universal Gardasil vaccination in the state of Texas may well have fit this definition.

Patient Lawsuits

Lawsuits surrounding Gardasil went beyond who owns what and into patient injury litigation. It is true that the number of serious adverse events and deaths from Gardasil are ostensibly low. The risk of serious adverse events and death per 100,000 vaccine doses is reported to be 1.0 and 0.2, respectively. Yet, because of ongoing lawsuits and parents refusing to vaccinate their children with Gardasil, it has been suggested that measures be taken to suppress negative social media attention about HPV vaccine safety concerns. [396]

Gardasil toxicities have included postural orthostatic tachycardia syndrome or POTS (which consists of low blood pressure and loss of consciousness when sitting or standing), ovarian failure (infertility), chronic fatigue syndrome (exhaustion from any physical or mental activity), autoimmune diseases, chronic regional pain syndrome, muscle and joint aches, headaches, and memory loss.[397] Several books have also been written to increase awareness of perceived HPV vaccine-related toxicity. Two such examples are *HPV Vaccine on Trial: Seeking Justice for a Generation Betrayed* by Mary Holland, Kim Mack Rosenberg, and Eileen Iorio; and *Shattered Dreams: The HPV Vaccine Exposed* by Christina England.[398]

In recent years, Merck has tried to get all lawsuits against the Gardasil vaccine dismissed based on the Vaccine Injury Compensation Program that was designed to "streamline compensation for vaccine injuries while ensuring continued vaccine availability."[399] The Vaccine Injury Compensation Program protects companies from expensive or excessive liability that could increase the costs of vaccines or cause shortages.[400] It was signed into law in 1986 under President Ronald Reagan. Since 1988, cases of vaccine injury are arbitrated by a federal bureaucracy rather than adjudicated in court by a jury of peers. The Vaccine Injury Compensation Program is a no-fault arbitration that does not hold a drug company liable. It is funded by a seventy-five cent tax on each injected vaccine.

Notwithstanding the Vaccine Injury Compensation Program, a drug company may still be sued for vaccine fraud, concealment, or failure to warn patients of its toxicity. If Merck was not transparent about Gardasil's risks, compensation for injury would not fall under the jurisdiction of the Vaccine Injury Compensation Program and could be addressed in a court of law.[401] This reemphasizes that consent is a valuable kill switch that protects everyone: researcher, patient, company, and society.

The Gardasil vaccine contains the VLP protein shell plus an aluminum salt solution. In the previous mentioned vaccine trials, the control was the aluminum salt solution without VLP. When comparing VLP plus the aluminum salt solution to only the aluminum solution, any toxicity due to the aluminum salt would be present in both the treatment and control arms. It would make the vaccine plus the aluminum appear to be nontoxic and safe.

Aluminum is added to vaccines because it is an adjuvant. An adjuvant is something that turns on your immune system.[402] However, the virus's outer shell is nature's own adjuvant, in that it already has a repetitive pathogen-associated pattern that will naturally turn on your immune system against the virus without need for an additional adjuvant. So why add an aluminum salt adjuvant in the first place? The philosophy behind the inclusion of the aluminum adjuvant is the more immune stimulation, the better. The aluminum salt adjuvant was thus added as an extra immune booster.[403] Unlike the VLP shell, the aluminum adjuvant is nonspecific and broadly activates the immune system. However, when dealing with medications or treatments, assuming that more is always better is not necessarily a safe presumption.

In contrast to initial Gardasil trials on the HPV vaccine, the optimal clinical trial would have compared (1) VLP with aluminum salts to (2) the VLP alone (3) aluminum salts alone, and (4) a true control of salt water (see Figure 11.6). This four-way trial would clarify whether the toxicity in the HPV vaccine arose from the aluminum salt

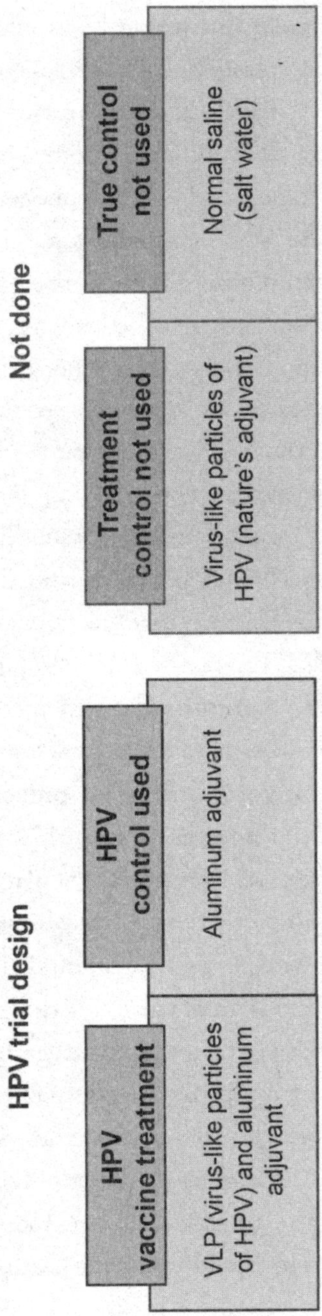

FIGURE 11.6: The optimal human papilloma virus (HPV) vaccine trial would include all four or at least three trial arms.

immune stimulant. It would also clarify if the VLP, nature's adjuvant, without the aluminum adjuvant would be as effective in mitigating cervical pre-cancerous dysplasia (CIN) with less toxicity.

The Gardasil studies that contained a treatment and control arm containing an aluminum adjuvant were reported in 2007. In 2001, six years before the Gardasil studies, a small immunogenicity trial compared VLP without adjuvant to VLP with adjuvant. The HPV L1 vaccine was highly immunogenic in generating effective HPV antibodies even without the adjuvant. It was just as effective without as with the adjuvant.[404] Why were the appropriate controls not performed in the large Gardasil trials? For one reason, doing a three- or four-arm randomized trial is more expensive. Another reason is that the US Food and Drug Administration never requested a controlled randomized trial designed to determine the toxicity from co-injecting metals like aluminum.

Luc Montagnier, the Nobel Laureate who discovered the HIV virus and a member of the Pasteur Institute, wrote the following in the foreword of the book *HPV Vaccine on Trial: Seeking Justice for a Generation*: "The reader will see the truth: the side effects are underreported by medical personnel, while there are a growing number of parents suing manufacturers and governments for inducing lifelong handicaps, even death, of their loved ones. In fact, this is the tragic example of various segments of our society, worldwide, placing economic interests before the health and protection of our younger generation."[405]

Why would an esteemed Nobel Laureate and virologist write something that many of his peers would view as blasphemy? It is important to note that Montagnier is not claiming to be against vaccines. Rather, his point is that we must optimize the safety of our vaccines. In his own words: "Let us mandate that ALL vaccines be safe for everyone. First do NO Harm."[406] Montagnier's citation of the Hippocratic Oath here reflects his training as a medical doctor. Indeed, before he was a Nobel Laureate, he lived by the Hippocratic Oath (Box 11.3).

Box 11.3. Hippocratic Oath

Hippocrates was a Greek physician (480–370 BC) who is often considered the "Father of Medicine." The oath to which his name is credited, the Hippocratic Oath, became a promise of ethical behavior traditionally sworn to by Western physicians.

Paraphrasing the oath, it proclaims: "I will do no harm or injustice to my patients. Neither will I administer a poison to anybody when asked to do so, nor will I suggest such a course . . . I will not give to a woman a pessary to cause abortion . . . And whatsoever I shall see or hear from a patient in the course of my profession, I will never divulge, holding such things to be holy secrets. If I carry out this oath . . . may I gain forever reputation, if I break it, may the opposite befall me."

In 1973, the US Supreme Court concluded that physicians must follow the law instead of their Hippocratic Oath. Untold years of precedence to swearing loyalty to an ethical code was overturned in one moment by the Supreme Court, an institution that ironically rest its laurels on case precedent. Some report that the Hippocratic Oath remains alive and well.[407] Yet, depending upon the country and medical school, its method of administration and content varies. It has been amended, replaced, or abolished compared to the original version.

Summary

This chapter might be summarized by modifying Neil Armstrong's famous lunar landing quote to say: "Developing a cancer vaccine is one giant leap forward for mankind, forced consent is a step backwards for a human." The concept of "do no harm" should carry greater emphasis for a psychologically and financially vulnerable adolescent with no infection and no illness. It should be noted that not everyone appreciates the importance of an individual's right to transparent noncoerced consent or, if underage, a parent's consent. For example, Dr. Joseph E. Balog has written regarding HPV vaccination: "Minors have a right to be protected against vaccine preventable illnesses, and society has an interest in safeguarding the welfare of children who may be harmed by the choices of their parents and guardians."[408] What this argument neglects is that without transparent noncoerced consent, one is treated as an inferior.

This brings us to the next topic of vaccine preservatives (mercury) and adjuvants (aluminum), which will be dealt with in chapters 12 and 13, respectively.

CHAPTER 12

Mercury: Toxic to Carbon-Based Life

Mercury is medically used for one reason.
It is lethal to carbon-based life.—RKB

As we've seen throughout this book, every vaccine contains a virus or piece of a virus. But vaccines often contain two other ingredients as well: mercury or aluminum. When you get injected with a vaccine, you are often injected with mercury or aluminum. Nobody tells you this when you're about to receive a vaccine. Your physician or nurse may not even know. There is no explanation given concerning why mercury or aluminum is being injected into your body. Nobody asks your consent. This is just how it is done. But why is it this way? Why do injections of mercury or aluminum upset some people? Why do some people feel betrayed when they are not informed? To understand why, we need to reconstruct the history of these metals and their role in the production of vaccines.

In this chapter, we'll examine mercury. The Greeks and Romans did not refer to this element as mercury. They instead called it *hydrargyrum*, which derives from the Greek word for silver water. The chemical symbol (Hg) is an abbreviation for hydrargyrum. Elemental mercury flows like water, so the Romans eventually renamed it Mercurius after the messenger deity Mercury, the Roman god of quickness and trickery. English speakers sometimes refer to elemental mercury as quicksilver, because it is liquid at room temperature and runs like water but has the color of silver.

Mercury and Its Many Forms

Mercury is a universal poison that kills bacteria, fungi, parasites, intestinal worms, animals, and humans. Because it would sterilize surfaces and had anti-inflammatory effects, mercury was used to treat ulcers, wounds, and infections before the invention of antibiotics. It was also known for its anti-inflammatory effects.[409] Mercury has no known natural biologic role or useful function in a living cell. It has been added to vaccines as a preservative (i.e., germicide) to ensure that bacteria and fungi are killed.

The art of using mercury as a drug involves slowly titrating the dose to kill an infection, stop inflammation, or cause the desired effect without killing the person. Mercury toxicity varies widely based on formulation, exposure method, dosage, and probably patient susceptibility.

The least toxic to most toxic forms of mercury are: (1) mercury ore (cinnabar and vermillion); (2) elemental mercury (liquid mercury) if it is not heated or atomized as a mist; (3) inorganic mercury chloride used in medications; and (4) organic mercury, which is the type of mercury used in vaccines (see Table 12.1). The difference in brain toxicity of the different formulations of mercury depends on its ability to get into the brain, that is, to cross the blood-brain barrier that exists between blood vessels and the brain.

Mercury Ore: Cinnabar and Vermilion

Human fascination with mercury began with the discovery of a red rock ore called cinnabar. An ore is a rock or mineral in nature that contains a valuable metal. Cinnabar is composed of mercury atoms bound to sulfur atoms known as mercury sulfide (HgS). When cinnabar rocks are ground to a powder, the pigment is called vermilion. The finer the powder, the more orange-red the vermilion becomes.

Vermilion (pulverized cinnabar) has been discovered covering five-thousand-year-old human skeletons in Palencia, Spain.[410] Ancient Phoenician, Egyptian, Roman, Olmec, Indian, and Chinese civilizations have all used vermilion as a red pigment. Among other purposes, ancient people used vermilion in paintings, frescos, wall decorations, pottery, cloth dying, cabinetry, jewelry box lacquer, as a writing ink, and as a cosmetic blush for the cheeks.[411] The *bindi* or circular dot placed on the forehead and between the eyebrows of Hindu women is vermilion.[412]

Vermilion, when mixed with a binder, makes the vibrant reds of European Renaissance paintings.[413] It was the most used red pigment in the world until the twentieth century. Heating cinnabar releases mercury vapor that is toxic to the brain. If it is not heated, cinnabar and vermilion are poorly absorbed and chemically inert with very low relative toxicity whether inhaled, placed on the skin, or inadvertently swallowed. Although rare, chronic long-term exposure to cinnabar may lead to mercury concentrated in the kidneys that may cause damage.[414]

Elemental or Pure Mercury

Elemental mercury has a chemical abbreviation of Hg^0 (or more simply Hg). The zero means that elemental mercury has no charge. It is the only metal to exist as a liquid at room temperature. Despite running like water, elemental mercury is 13.5 times heavier than water. Iron will even float on top of it. It has strong surface tension and will bead up if a drop falls onto the counter.

Table 12.1: Basic Types of Mercury

Type of Mercury	Cinnabar Vermillion	Elemental mercury	Inorganic mercury	Inorganic mercury	Inorganic mercury	Organic mercury	Organic mercury	Organic mercury
Chemical Structure	HgS	Hg	$HgNO_2$	Hg_2Cl_2	$Hg\,Cl_2$	CH_3Hg	$(CH_3)_2Hg$	C_2H_5Hg
Chemical Name	Mercury sulfide; found in nature as red ore	Mercury; silver liquid at room temperature	Mercury nitrate; white solid	Mercurous chloride; off-white solid	Mercuric chloride; white solid	Methyl mercury; dissoluble in fat but not in water	Dimethyl mercury; soluble in water	Ethyl mercury; not soluble in water
Drug Name				Calomel; not soluble in water	Corrosive sublime; slightly soluble in water			Thimerosal; dissolves in water
Cross Skin and/or Mucosa	No	Poorly unless heated	Poorly unless heated	Poor	Slightly	Easily	Easily	Easily

Type of Mercury	Cinnabar Vermillion	Elemental mercury	Inorganic mercury	Inorganic mercury	Inorganic mercury	Organic mercury	Organic mercury	Organic mercury
Cross Blood-Brain Barrier (BBB)	No	Poorly except when heated vapor	Poorly except for heated vapor	Poorly	Poorly	Easily crosses BBB and placenta	Easily crosses BBB and placenta	Easily crosses BBB and placenta
Main Toxicity	Nontoxic unless heated to make elemental mercury	When heated, acute (lungs, brain)	When heated (brain, i.e., Mad Hatter Disease)	Kidney, gut, rarely brain	Kidney, gut, rarely brain	Brain	Brain	Brain
Common Use	Red color for clothes, cosmetics, paintings, furniture	Dental fillings, gold or silver ore processing, batteries, instruments	Industry (e.g., making hats)	Panacea drug for many ailments (e.g., anti-syphilis)	Drug for syphilis	Rolled on seeds to prevent fungus from eating seeds	Instrument calibration	Put in vaccines and rolled on seeds to kill fungus and bacteria

Elemental Mercury Smelted from Rock Ore in Antiquity

Elemental mercury is not found naturally. It is locked up in rocks, but people from antiquity discovered how to isolate it. In AD 79, prior to his death underneath the eruption of Mount Vesuvius, the Roman writer Pliny the Elder wrote his *Natural History*, an encyclopedic collection of ancient knowledge. In it, Pliny recorded how to extract mercury from cinnabar.[415] Mercury is released from cinnabar (HgS) ore by roasting finely crushed cinnabar in a furnace. Vapor rises into an exhaust tube that enters a water-cooled condenser. Upon cooling, elemental mercury (Hg) vapor condenses into a liquid and drips out of the condenser while the sulfur combines with oxygen and exits the chamber as a gas (sulfur dioxide, SO_2).[416]

Elemental mercury, especially when freshly distilled, will reflect images like a mirror. While Romans would polish bronze until it reflected their image, in the 1600s and perhaps earlier, mirrors consisted of a piece of glass covering a thin layer of mercury or an amalgamation of mercury and tin.[417] Why did the superstition "Break a mirror, seven years bad luck" arise? Perhaps it was because mirrors were expensive, breaking it affected your image in the reflected spiritual world, or glass fragments cutting into the skin dumped mercury into your blood.

Smelted elemental mercury was also used outside the world of Western antiquity. The first-century BC Chinese historian Sima Qian writes that the famous mausoleum of the first Chinese emperor Qin Shi Huang (r. 221–210 BC) had two rivers of mercury representing the Yangtze and Yellow rivers. These mercury rivers drained into a lake of mercury representing the Pacific Ocean.[418] Except for the unearthing of an army of more than eight thousand terracotta warrior statues in the nearby necropolis, the emperor's mausoleum has never been opened and these rivers have never been found. In 2003, Sergio Gómez, an archaeologist with Mexico's National Institute of Anthropology and History, discovered residual elemental mercury in chambers beneath the Teotihuacán Feather Serpent Pyramid built in the third century AD. It is believed to represent rivers and lakes in the land of the dead.[419]

Elemental Mercury Used to Isolate Gold and Silver

While mercury containing ores can be found worldwide, approximately one-third of the world's mercury originated from the Almadén mine of Spain.[420] The mine switched hands from the Romans to the Visigoths and then to the Moors and present-day Spain. Almadén derives from the Arabic *al-maʿdin*, meaning mine or lode (i.e., the mother lode). It was closed in 2000 and is now a UNESCO world heritage site.[421]

In 1640, the Spanish priest Alvaro Alonso Barba wrote a book called *El Arte de los Metals* (English: the art of metals). Barba's book described the process of amalgamation, which consists of mixing different elements together. During amalgamation, rock ore containing silver or gold was pounded into a fine powder and mixed with elemental liquid mercury. A soft but dense amalgam of mercury and gold (or silver) could be easily (by hand) separated out from the rest of the ore. The amalgam would then be heated in a pot or furnace to boil off the mercury, leaving behind pure gold or silver.

Spanish galleons shipped mercury from the Almadén mine to the New World to process the silver- and gold-containing ores found there before it was shipped back to Spain.[422] One of these galleons, the *Guadalupe*, sank during a hurricane in 1724 off the coast of the Dominican Republic. Two hundred fifty tons of mercury went down with it.[423] So much silver and gold were removed from Mexican mines that a golden chapel, the Rosary Chapel, was built inside the Church of Santa Domingo in Puebla, Mexico. It was built in the late 1600s with a gold pulpit, walls of gold, and a gold ceiling. The Rosary Chapel is still standing, and people still pray inside it. It was even once identified as the eighth wonder of the world.[424]

The magic of how mercury makes gold appear when added to crushed ores gave rise to the incorrect belief that one metal could be turned into another, a concept called alchemy. Barba was not only a priest but also an alchemist. The success of Barba's "alchemy" eventually developed into the field of chemistry. Mercury did not create gold or transform itself into gold. It clumped together fine particles of gold (or silver) too small to be previously visualized.

Toxicity of Elemental Mercury

Provided there are no breaks on the surface, elemental mercury is poorly absorbed through the skin or gut. In the first half of the twentieth century, school children used to play with it in their bare hands during science class with no ill consequences. Toxicity of elemental mercury arises predominately from inhalation that occurs most often when it is heated to a vapor or aerosolized into a fine mist. Mercury has no smell.

Elemental mercury vapor can enter the brain directly through the nasal cavity or through the lungs into the blood. Acute elemental mercury vapor inhalation also causes suffocation and death from lung injury. Acute vapor poisoning occurs during industrial accidents or when individuals carelessly heat or spray mercury and then inhale it.[425] One case study published in the year 2000 describes how one family's children died from respiratory failure when the parents attempted to extract gold by heating mercury inside their poorly ventilated home.[426]

In contrast to acute inhalation, slow chronic exposure to mercury vapor results in neurologic toxicity. This is manifested as tremors, numbness, inability to sleep, increased saliva or drooling, and a personality change marked by irritability, depression, memory loss, temper outbursts, and poor concentration.[427]

For most Americans, 60 to 70 percent of the mercury excreted in their urine arises from dental amalgam fillings (mercury mixed with tin, zinc, or silver).[428] Exposure to mercury vapor from dental fillings is highest during placement and removal. For mercury fillings left in place, the number and size of fillings, chewing routine, and mouth flora and acidity influence the amount of vapor released.

In America, mercury fillings remain the "gold standard," or, more appropriately, the "mercury standard" due to their durability, lower risk of secondary carries, and lower cost.[429] The American Dental Association has publicly reaffirmed that mercury dental fillings are safe and strong.[430] The FDA has never investigated the toxicity of mercury fillings.[431]

Over time, mercury-free fillings have improved in both quality and durability and are available as an alternative to mercury. Phasing out all mercury amalgam fillings worldwide has been recommended by some.[432] The European Parliament has banned all mercury amalgam fillings in Europe since January 1, 2025.[433]

Elemental mercury has also been used as a poison to exterminate enemies. In 2024, Amina Abakarova, a Russian chess player, was caught on security camera spraying mercury on her opponent's chess board before a match. Shortly after the tournament started, her opponent fell ill with difficulty breathing but survived.[434]

Hollow-point bullets may be filled with elemental mercury. A hollow-point bullet will open like a "flower" upon impact. The result is a bigger wound. If filled with mercury, the bullet splatters mercury on the victim's organs.[435] In 1899, the Hague Convention outlawed expanding hollow-point bullets in warfare.

James Files is a military trained marksman and a Cuban Bay of Pigs CIA operative. While officially deemed *not* credible by the FBI, in a televised confession from the Illinois State petitionary, he testified to assassinating President John Kennedy by firing the kill shot from the grassy knoll using a "mercury round" (i.e., hollow-point mercury filled bullet). According to him, if the president's body was exhumed, the skull will be contaminated with residual mercury.[436] All that is to say, mercury is the perfect "silent assassin." If the initial impact of the bullet is not immediately lethal, the mercury will keep slowly killing the victim.

Inorganic Mercury

Inorganic mercury refers to mercury bound to noncarbon atoms such as chloride or nitrates. A nitrate consists of nitrogen bound with oxygen. Every form of mercury, whether elemental, inorganic (bound to a noncarbon atom), or organic (bound to a carbon atom), is an antiseptic that kills bacteria and fungi. Inorganic mercury in the form of mercury chloride has been used to treat various ailments related to inflammation and infection.

Mercury Chloride Used to Treat Syphilis

The origin of syphilis, a sexually transmitted disease, is unknown. It sprang up in Europe during the age of exploration around the time that Christopher Columbus returned from the Caribbean. This resulted in an unproven hypothesis that Christopher Columbus and his crew brought it back to Europe from the New World.[437] Whatever the source, this bacterial infection ravaged the Western world for 450 years. From the early 1500s until the 1940s, mercury chloride was often used to treat syphilis.

Two formulations of inorganic mercury chloride were used to treat syphilis: mercurous chloride (chemical abbreviation Hg_2Cl_2) and mercuric chloride (also known as mercury bichloride, chemical abbreviation $HgCl_2$). Neither formulation could penetrate the blood-brain barrier, so very little brain toxicity occurred. Mercurous chloride does not dissolve in water or fat and is poorly absorbed. When taken orally, it causes ulcers, cramps, diarrhea, and bleeding from the gut.[438] When given for prolonged intervals, it could cause hypersalivation, inflammation of gums with loosening of teeth, tremors, and personality changes.[439] Mercuric chloride could be partially dissolved in water and is more rapidly absorbed than mercurous chloride. Because mercuric chloride is more easily absorbed, it is also more toxic to the gut and kidney.[440]

Like using arsenic or cisplatinum (both are metals) as chemotherapy to treat cancer, the use of mercury chloride to treat syphilis involves gradually increasing its dosage until toxicities occurred and the patient's life was at risk.[441] It was believed that the toxic side effects of mercury chloride correlated with its anti-syphilitic effectiveness. Mercury treatment for syphilis lasted for up to two years. One author has summarized this treatment for syphilis (an infection transmitted through sexual intercourse) as: "Two minutes with Venus (the Goddess of love) followed by two years with Mercury (the God of quickness and trickery)."[442]

Was such a long treatment interval necessary? In 1910, the Oslo Untreated Syphilis Study demonstrated that even when untreated, syphilitic lesions would resolve spontaneously after an average of three to six months.[443] The Oslo Untreated Syphilis Study led to the US Public Health Service performing the ill-fated Tuskegee untreated syphilis study (see chapter 10) to gather more information on the natural history of untreated syphilis.[444]

A decade or more after infection, approximately 10 percent of syphilis patients developed general paralysis of the insane (also known as general paresis).[445] This probably occurred because mercury chloride compounds do not cross the blood-brain barrier and are thus unsuccessful in killing syphilis in the brain, the cause of paralysis of the insane. General paralysis of the insane first manifests in initial vague symptoms and personality changes that worsen over time to progressive dementia, tremors, confusion, lack of coordination, abnormal eye pupils, paralysis, and finally death.[446] On imaging studies, the brains of those suffering general paralysis showed atrophy (significant loss of brain cells).[447] Al Capone (1889–1947), an infamous Chicago crime boss during prohibition, died from general paralysis of the insane brought about by syphilis.[448]

In 1913, Dr. Hideyo Noguchi at the Rockefeller Institute—one of the individuals who died of yellow fever as part of the West African Commission (see chapter 5)—identified the bacteria (*Treponema pallidum*) that causes syphilis within the brains of people with general paresis.[449] Japan posthumously awarded Noguchi the Order of the Rising Sun in 1928 for his discovery, placed his picture on the Japanese currency, and erected a museum in his honor.[450]

The use of mercury as a treatment for syphilis declined sharply following the discovery of penicillin. In 1928, the Scottish physician Alexander Fleming noticed that bacteria did not grow next to moldy bread. He discovered that the penicillium fungus growing on the bread made a "juice" that killed bacteria. Fleming isolated the world's first antibiotic from this "mold juice" and called it penicillin after the mold.[451]

By the 1940s, penicillin had entirely replaced mercury as the only treatment needed for syphilis. Penicillin is virtually nontoxic to humans, highly effective against several bacterial species including *Treponema pallidum* that causes syphilis, and involves an outpatient injection given once or twice. With early use of penicillin, the entity

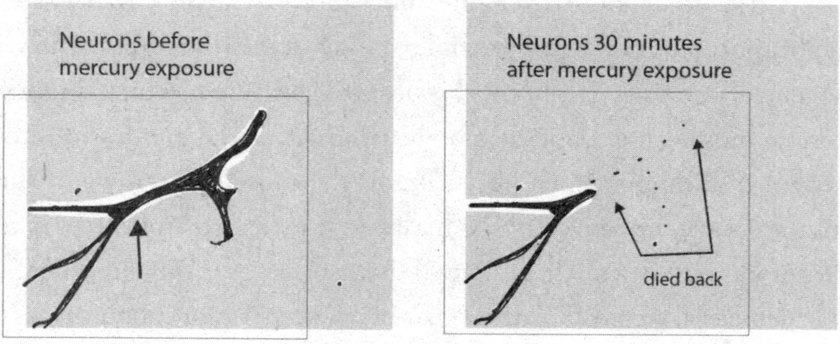

FIGURE 12.1: A brain cell in a laboratory culture dish before and after exposure to very low dose mercury.

of general paralysis of the insane disappeared from our lexicon nearly altogether. Fear and anxiety about syphilis abated. In 1945, Fleming was awarded the Nobel Prize for his life-saving work, and he was knighted by King George VI for his accomplishment.

The modern antibiotic age began with the discovery of penicillin. While infectious organisms may develop antibiotic resistance, which does not happen with mercury compounds, antibiotics are more effective, more specific, and far less toxic than mercurial drugs. The antibiotic age was the beginning of the end for mercury as a medical drug. Today, non-antibiotic sterilization of skin as a prep before surgery and for wounds is done with less toxic non-metal elements like iodine or bromide.

The neurotoxicity of mercury chloride is much less than most other forms of mercury because it is relatively inefficient at crossing the blood-brain barrier.[452] If a very low concentration (10^{-7} molar) of mercury chloride is added to a culture of neurons that lack protection offered by the blood-brain barrier, the neurons will rapidly degenerate. The neuron growth cones and extensions (dendritic processes) that make connections to other neurons will die back (Figure 12.1). In culture, this happens within twenty to thirty minutes following exposure to mercury chloride.[453]

In hindsight, when compared to penicillin, titrating the dose of mercury chloride—a universal poison—to treat syphilis seems barbarically insane. But this seemingly insane act was driven by desperation because nothing else to treat syphilis was available. Questions remain whether mercury treatment of syphilis in some cases "did more harm than good."[454]

A Universal Medical Drug Until the Mid-Twentieth Century

Syphilis was not the only ailment treated by mercury chloride. People became so lulled into mercury chloride being a normal medication that mercurial drugs were used as treatment for a wide array of mundane ailments and nonspecific symptoms as well. For instance, because one toxicity is the loosening of teeth, mercury chloride was prescribed to babies until 1948 to decrease painful teething. Mercury chloride was, in many ways, the universal medicine. To quote the English physician Thomas Dover (1660–1742): "What an admirable medicine then is mercury! . . . The pox, the piles, scorbutic and scrophulous ulcers: inflammations and fulxions of the eyes; the itch, the leprosy, and all causes of cutaneous foulness; internal ulcers, white swellings, tumours, sharp humours in the stomach and guts; stone, gout, and gravel; What an Army of the most terrible foes! Against the major part of which this friend to nature is a specific, and the best remedy."[455]

In 1857, mercury was combined with arsenic (another metal poison) and iodine in a formulation called Donovan's solution. Donovan's solution was editorialized in a top British medical journal at that time for "good results" in treating an inflammatory skin condition called psoriasis.[456] In the 1920s, mercurial drugs were used as a diuretic to treat a failing heart.[457] A diuretic is a medicine that pushes fluid out of the kidneys. Mercury worked as a diuretic because it was toxic to the kidneys.

For centuries, mercury was a panacea, a universal medication. The alchemist's dream of turning mercury into gold was finally achieved but not in the way they envisioned. Treating medical ailments with mercury by titrating its poisonous side effects turned mercury into money. This may sound barbaric, but chemotherapy and radiation are nonspecific poisons still given to patients in which their therapeutic effect is elucidated by titrating their poisonous toxicity.

Industrial Use of Mercury Nitrate

A different inorganic formulation of mercury called mercury nitrate (chemical abbreviation $Hg[NO_3]_2$) has been used in various industries over the centuries. The most notable of these is hat making. The wearing of expensive hats was fashionable between the eighteenth and early twentieth centuries. High-quality hats were made of animal fur that was rolled, pressed, wetted, and dried to make felt. The smoothest felts were made by wetting them in a mercury nitrate solution.

During the drying process, mercury vapor would evaporate into the air and be inhaled by workers. The inhalation of mercury nitrate would cause them to develop "Mad Hatter disease." This disease was a constellation of symptoms that included tremor, irritability, personality changes, loss of memory, loss of concentration, attention deficit, tics or spasms or twitching of muscles, anxiety, and agitation.[458]

The memories of mercury nitrate's toxic consequences remain etched in our culture's collective memory by the phrase "mad as a hatter" and by the character of the Hatter in the 1865 book *Alice in Wonderland* by Lewis Carroll.

Organic Mercury

Organic mercury refers to mercury bound to carbon-containing compounds. Organic mercury is fat soluble and, unlike inorganic mercury, easily crosses the blood-brain barrier to accumulate in brain cells called neurons. Organomercurials are the most neurotoxic formulation of mercury. Organomercurials include methylmercury (CH_3Hg), dimethylmercury ($[CH_3]_2Hg$), and ethylmercury (C_2H_5Hg). One might say that mercury's three evil stepsisters are "Methyl, Dimethyl, and Ethyl"!

Methylmercury

Organic mercury in the form of methylmercury was first synthesized by the British chemist George Buckton in 1858 at the Imperial

College of London. In the 1860s, he moved his laboratory to Saint Bartholomew's Hospital in London. In 1865, his assistant, Dr. Carl Ulrich, accidentally broke one of the methylmercury vials and inhaled the fumes. The next day he was anxious and confused. Agitation, weakness, and coma followed by death occurred within two weeks. Another person in the same laboratory did not become ill until one month later. Initial mild neurologic symptoms progressed over months to dementia, paralysis, and death.[459]

Organomercurials like methylmercury are a potent fungicidal (kill fungi) agent. Today, seeds are covered with methylmercury (or ethylmercury) to prevent fungi from eating them. Between 1950 and 1970 reports emerged in several war-torn or impoverished countries such as Iraq, Pakistan, and Guatemala of desperately hungry villagers pounding mercury-coated seeds into flour to make bread instead of planting the seeds. They would suffer numbness, loss of coordination, slurred speech, and difficulty hearing and seeing. In severe cases, symptoms progressed to blindness, paralysis, coma, and death.[460]

Dimethylmercury

In 1996, Professor Karen Wetterhahn, a chemist at Dartmouth College in New Hampshire, was using dimethylmercury to calibrate a scientific instrument in her laboratory. A few drops fell on her latex glove but did not make contact with her skin. She removed the glove and washed her hands. Five months later, she suddenly had trouble walking and speaking. Within a few weeks, she was comatose. She never awoke and was dead within a few months after onset of symptoms.[461] Wetterhahn's tragic story exemplifies the potency of dimethylmercury. Her death was caused by a minute amount of dimethylmercury that homed in on her brain after passing through her glove and then through the skin.

Ethylmercury

Ethylmercury readily crosses the blood-brain barrier, crosses the placenta, and can enter into a mother's milk, and like other organomercury compounds is highly neurotoxic. Ethyl mercury p-toulene sulfonamide is called Granoșan. It is manufactured by Dupont as a fungicide that is rolled on seeds After eating bread made from these seeds, farmers in the Soviet Union suffered nervous system toxicity with problems in balance, speech, and walking. Several farmers and their family members died.[462] In China, after eating rice treated with ethylmercury, forty-one people were hospitalized. They all suffered mercury poisoning and remained in poor medical condition at time of the publication, five months after ingestion.[463]

In Romania, four people consumed the meat from a hog that had been fed seeds coated with ethylmercury. Before slaughter, the hog was intermittently falling. Ten days after eating its meat, all the family members suffered neurologic symptoms. The family's fifteen-year-old son developed agitation, weakness, loss of coordination, and difficulty speaking. He slipped into a coma and died. High levels of mercury were demonstrated in the urine of all family members.[464]

Thimerosal

The history of mercury first intersects our story of vaccines in the first half of the twentieth century. In 1916 in Columbia, South Carolina, four children died and several dozen others became ill from bacterial contamination of a multi-dose vial of cholera vaccine. This was not an isolated case either.[465] To avoid the risk of bacterial contamination of vaccines, an effective germicide was needed to keep multi-dose vials sterile between draws. Beginning in the 1920s, thimerosal emerged as that germicide, and when added to vaccines is called a preservative. Thimerosal was first synthesized at the University of Chicago and marketed by the pharmaceutical company Eli Lilly. It is a germicide that is composed of 50 percent ethylmercury and 50 percent thiosalicylate.[466]

After being injected into animals without ill effect, thimerosal was declared to be safe.[467] It has been used in vaccines ever since. Details are important as the animals were observed for a short interval of one week after injection. However, as described in the above mentioned stories, gross brain toxicity caused by mercury poisoning may not appear until weeks, months, or even longer after exposure. Based on a one-week observation in adult animals, thimerosal was added to multi-dose vaccines to keep the vaccine vial sterile between draws. Compared to a single-dose vial, multiple people ranging from two to twenty could be vaccinated from one multi-dose vial, making the cost of production and storage cheaper.[468]

Because it was considered safe, thimerosal became a general anti-bacterial and anti-fungal drug. It was applied on the skin to sterilize the unclosed abdomen of babies born with an incomplete abdominal wall, a condition called omphalocele. In 1977, thirteen babies born with omphaloceles were treated with thimerosal. Ten of them died. Autopsy on nine of the ten deceased infants revealed toxic levels of mercury within their organs.[469] As a result, in the 1980s the FDA began removing thimerosal from lotions used to sterilize the skin.[470]

In 1990 in Brazil, after accidentally swallowing thimerosal, one individual developed severe neurologic complications and died despite frantic medical efforts to unsuccessfully remove the mercury from the body.[471] Paradoxically, it was during the 1980s and 1990s when the medical use of thimerosal was being scaled back that the preservative was being added to more and more vaccines. The working assumption supported by later epidemiology studies was that the cumulative dose of ethylmercury (thimerosal) in vaccines was safe. However, a controversy arose as to whether infant vaccination could cause autism.

The Autism and Vaccine Controversy

Autism is a neurodevelopmental disorder that is now diagnosed in up to one out of every thirty children in the United States. While there are different subtypes of autism, the core feature of all autism spectrum disorders is difficulty with social interaction and communication, attention deficits, repetitive behaviors, and limited interest in exploring new things.[472] The cause of autism is unknown.

A controversy concerning the relationship between autism and vaccines began in 1998 when Dr. Andrew Wakefield published an article in the prestigious medical journal *The Lancet* that was later retracted. Wakefield's article dealt with twelve children (aged three to ten) who were reported by their parents to have developed diarrhea, abdominal pain, bloating, and other gastrointestinal symptoms after being vaccinated with the measles mumps rubella (MMR) vaccine. These symptoms were later followed by traits associated with autism spectrum disorder, including regression or loss of normal age-related language and social interaction skills.[473] As the MMR vaccine does not contain mercury, the suspected culprit was the live but attenuated measles virus in the vaccine.

To determine if the MMR vaccine contributes to autism, an epidemiological study of approximately 537,000 children born in Denmark between 1991 and 1998 was conducted. This study analyzed what the risk of autism was for children after being injected with the MMR vaccine versus those not receiving MMR. The majority (about 440,000) of participants were vaccinated at fifteen months, while approximately 96,000 had not receive the vaccine.[474] The study determined that there was no difference in the incidence of autism between those receiving MMR and those who did not.

When their children began to experience gastrointestinal symptoms and later features commonly associated with autism spectrum disorder after MMR vaccination, were the mothers correct that the cause was the MMR vaccine, or is the negative epidemiology study correct? One possible but unproven explanation for some of the younger children is that they began to develop symptoms of an autism-like neurodegenerative disease called Rett syndrome, which first manifests around the same age that children are typically given the MMR vaccine. Rett syndrome is due to a defect in a gene called MeCP2. Normal mice when put in a new environment immediately explore. Mice with the abnormal Rett gene just sit there with no interest. When given a normal MeCP2 gene, mice revert to normal inquisitive behavior.[475]

As the MMR controversy faded, the autism vaccine controversy shifted to mercury-containing vaccines. Some mothers reported their child developed regressive autism after injection of thimerosal-containing vaccines.[476] As a result, epidemiological studies were again undertaken to determine whether thimerosal-containing vaccines are associated with autism. So far, these studies have shown no association. Since epidemiology studies showed no association, why did controversy persist? It is because no alternative explanation was given.

How do we explain the discordance between what these mothers report and negative epidemiological studies? This time let us look at epidemiology. Epidemiology is primarily an observational form of research and not an experimental one. It is an extremely useful and powerful tool that provides useful information for further research. Epidemiology identifies associations between the spread of diseases and other extraneous factors, but it cannot ultimately prove if the latter causes the former. It cannot unequivocally prove guilt or innocence.

Bias can occur in any human activity, including epidemiology. Could the epidemiological studies be biased? Of all scientific disciplines, epidemiologists are perhaps the ones best trained and experienced in accounting and correcting for bias. In epidemiology multiple factors may give rise to unintentional bias, including confounding influences, subconscious preconceptions in setting up the comparisons, and misclassification.

Misclassification errors that are outside of an epidemiologist's control arise from unknown problems in the sensitivity and specificity of a disease diagnosis or related factors.[477] Theoretical and unproven misclassification errors for autism may arise from lack of a quantifiable biomarker (an objective laboratory or imaging marker) to confirm the diagnosis.[478] Another potential co founding factor is that mercury exposure from all sources and ethylmercury levels within the brain (wherein it accumulates) or in blood, urine, or hair (where it can be measured) were not available in the relevant studies.

A 2023 case study reported increased mercury blood levels but no difference in hair or urine mercury levels between autistic and normal children.[479] The authors of this study concluded that there may be genetic differences (polymorphic heterogeneity) between individuals in ability to excrete and detoxify mercury. If true, some children may be more susceptible to ethylmercury toxicity at exposure levels safe for others.

Prolonged environmental exposure to inflammatory stress from charged metals like mercury (or aluminum, as we'll see in chapter 13) used in vaccines may, in theory, contribute to epigenetic changes in genes.[480] Epigenetic changes alter how a gene expresses itself as opposed to a mutation, which alters the gene itself. Epigenetic changes explain why monozygotic or identical twins can be discordant for certain diseases, such as when only one of two identical twins has schizophrenia.

Epigenetic alterations in gene expression are important for proper brain development (neurogenesis) in the fetus and infant.[481] Examples of suspected in utero epigenetic changes include instances where pregnant women have experienced extreme malnourishment, such as the Dutch Hunger Winter of 1944–1945 or the Chinese Mao Tse Tung's

"Great Leap Forward" famine of 1959 to 1961.[482] Decades later, the grown children of these women tended to have a higher incidence of schizophrenia than infants whose mothers did not experience malnutrition during pregnancy.

Is thimerosal neurotoxic? The answer is *yes*. Brain cells exposed to mercury will rapidly lose their extensions (known as dendritic processes). These brain extensions die back (i.e., retract) and sever the neurological connection between cells. There are roughly eight-five billion brain cells in each human.[483] Those brain cells have approximately eighty trillion electrical connections with each other via their dendritic processes.[484] It is not known how many of these "spare" brain cell connections must dissolve before noticeable changes occur in behavior or intelligence. It is likely that a great many disappear before gross clinical signs are noticed.

Does the neurotoxicity of the thimerosal in vaccines cause autism? Based on current epidemiologic association studies, the answer is an unequivocal no. Could the dose of thimerosal in vaccines exceed recommended neurologic safety limits? Depending upon whom you ask, the answer could be either no or yes.

In July 1999, the Centers for Disease Control, commenting on a release from the American Academy of Pediatrics and the US Public Health Service, stated that "There is no risk of harm [from thimerosal]," yet also conceded that because "some children could be exposed to a cumulative level of mercury over the first 6 months of life that exceeds one of the federal guidelines . . . thimerosal-containing vaccines should be removed as soon as possible."[485] Throughout the 1980s and 1990s and up to today, the Centers for Disease Control—along with the Food and Drug Administration and even the World Health Organization—have maintained that there is no evidence of autism or harm derived from thimerosal-containing vaccines. But if that's the case, then why did they suddenly request removing thimerosal "as soon as possible"? What happened? Why did the Centers for Disease Control recommend the immediate removal of the supposed innocuous thimerosal from vaccines?

Minamata Disease

What happened was that environmentalists changed the debate. A well-known environmentalist lawyer and the current Secretary of Health and Human Services, Robert F. Kennedy Jr., challenged the safety of thimerosal in vaccines.[486] Along with Kennedy, the United Nations Environmental Program and the United States Environmental Protection Agency sounded an alarm regarding the use of thimerosal in vaccines by pointing to Minamata disease as a harrowing precedent.

In 1956, bizarre things started happening in the Minamata Bay area of Japan. Dead fish washed up on the beaches. Dead birds fell out the sky. The final proverbial "canary in the coal mine" was when domesticated cats exhibited a lack of balance and seizures before falling over dead. They were called "the dancing cats of Minamata."[487] It was as if an Alfred Hitchcock film had come to life.

It was later discovered that the cause of these strange happenings was methylmercury poisoning in the fish, which in turn poisoned the birds and cats that ate them. But the suffering wasn't restricted to the birds and cats of Minamata Bay. The high neurologic toxicity of locals living around Minamata Bay, who like other coastal Japanese residents had a fish-heavy diet, induced muscle weakness and tremors, poor concentration, attention deficit, seizures, poor balance, and diminished vision, speech, and hearing.[488] Paralysis and death occurred in several cases. For some survivors these neurologic symptoms persisted for thirty years.[489]

The methylmercury poisoning was eventually traced to the Chisso Corporation, which dumped mercury waste into Minamata

Bay from 1951 until 1968. This mercury was converted by bacteria in the ocean into methylmercury.[490] The methylmercury became concentrated in the microscopic algae that floated in the water of Minamata Bay. These algae were eaten by small fish, which were eaten by larger fish, which were then eaten by larger carnivores, including humans. In this manner, methylmercury accumulated throughout the food chain.[491]

Among humans, the effects of Minamata disease were not limited solely to those who consumed the mercury-poisoned fish. Minamata disease also occurred in newborn babies whose mothers were exposed to the mercury. This was because methylmercury crossed the placenta and entered into the baby during gestation.[492] Many of these mothers exhibited no symptoms of mercury poisoning, suggesting that methylmercury is more toxic to developing fetal brain tissue than to an adult brain (duh!).[493] Methylmercury also can pass from the mother's breast milk into the nursing infant.[494] A study comparing methylmercury to ethylmercury in newborn monkeys demonstrated that ethylmercury is cleared more rapidly from the blood, but a higher proportion of mercury remains in the brain.[495]

Assuming that methylmercury and ethylmercury are equally neurotoxic, the Environmental Protection Agency set a safety limit for ethylmercury that is three to four times lower than the established Food and Drug Administration and World Health Organization limits (Table 12.2). In some cases, ethylmercury exposure from vaccinations exceeded the Environmental Protection Agency safety limits.[496] As a result, the Food and Drug Administration recommended the removal of thimerosal from childhood vaccines. Currently, save for multi-vial vaccines such as multi-vial influenza, thimerosal-containing vaccines are no longer used in America for children under age six or for any pregnant woman. Single-dose influenza vials do not contain thimerosal.

Table 12.2: Comparison of Total Mercury Exposure[497]

Fish			
Methylmercury Dosage	***Sardine (mg)***	***Salmon (mg)***	***Shark (mg)***
Sporadic	0.01 mg	0.02 mg	0.5 mg
Moderate	0.12 mg	0.24 mg	6 mg
Heavy	0.48 mg	0.96 mg	24 mg
Children			
Thimerosal Study	***Age of Vaccinated Child***	***Ethylmercury Dose (mg)***	
Dórea et al.	two months	0.050	
	six months	0.11	
	eighteen months	0.24	
Bingham et al.	six months	0.187	
Agency Recommended Safety Limits			
Health Organization	***Maximum Allowed Daily Mercury Exposure (mg/kg)***	***Maximum Allowed Methylmercury Exposure for an Average Six-Month-Old Infant (mg)***	
Environmental Protection Agency	0.0001	.089	
Food and Drug Administration	0.0004	.354	
World Health Organization	0.00047	.417	
Neurons in Culture			
Dose of Mercury Chloride to Cause Neuronal Cell Disintegration	10^{-7} molar » 0.2 mg		

Other government and nongovernment organizations have also taken action in light of the Minamata tragedy. In 2001, for example, the United Nations Environmental Program started the Minamata Global Mercury Initiative to bring countries together to recognize mercury as one of the top poisons for all carbon-based life forms and to reduce man-made mercury emissions worldwide. As a result of human activity, it is estimated that the world's oceans now contain over 123 million pounds of mercury that can enter the food chain.[498]

In 2013, the Obama administration signed the Minamata Convention on Mercury after removing its objections to the international treaty four years earlier. Signed by nearly 140 countries, the Minamata Convention became enforceable in 2017. Among other things, the treaty regulates mercury mining and trade; halts the manufacture of several mercury products like batteries, switches, measuring instruments, barometers, and thermometers; recommends phasing out the use of mercury dental amalgam fillings; limits industrial and coal burning emissions of mercury; and initiated restrictions on mercury in gold mining. It does not restrict mercury use by the military or for research.

Summary

A prospective randomized trial comparing vaccines with ethylmercury to the same vaccines without ethylmercury has never been done. The Food and Drug Administration has never treated mercury as a drug or toxin within a randomized vaccine trial.

Due to the Minamata Convention treaty, the Environmental Protection Agency, and individuals like Robert Kennedy Jr., the services of mercury as the "silent assassin" are being retired. Many vaccines have never contained ethylmercury and have never suffered from bacterial or fungal contamination. With the implementation of single-vial vaccines and Food and Drug Administration production regulations that document sterility before release,[499] adding ethylmercury to a vaccine has become superfluous.

Medical informed consent is a kill switch safeguard that is underappreciated in the vaccine world. Unlike medical doctors, the training of most scientists who develop many medical advances does not currently emphasize the importance of a patient's consent.

Vaccine recipients are generally not properly consented or consented at all. They are not given a choice whether their flu shot is from a mercury-free single-dose vial or comes from an ethylmercury-containing multi-dose vial. Doctors do not inform patients because most health care providers are often not themselves informed. Like the obsolete use of mercury chloride that was once used to treat syphilis, adding ethylmercury to vaccines—especially for infants, children, and pregnant women—has become an archaic technology.

CHAPTER 13

The Aluminum Age and Vaccine Adjuvants

Man is a tool-using animal. . . Without tools he is nothing, with tools he is all.—Thomas Carlyle[500]

Aluminum is a nonspecific inflammatory stimulant.—RKB

Human beings have been making tools for hundreds of thousands of years. Our first ancestors made tools from stone (hence the Stone Age). By the sixth millennium BC, human beings began using copper to manufacture primitive tools, entering the Copper Age. Around 3000 BC, humans began smelting copper and tin together to make more advanced tools, bringing us into the Bronze Age. Starting around 1200 BC, iron toolmaking emerged, opening the door to the Iron Age. We gradually transitioned into the age of steel when ironsmiths accidentally discovered that leaving iron in a coal furnace turned the iron into steel, which is a stronger alloy of iron and carbon. At the end of the nineteenth century, human beings began making tools from aluminum, a much lighter and more versatile metal than steel. You might say we are now living in the Aluminum Age. Ever since, aluminum has made human life more convenient. This includes the efficacy of our vaccines.

After oxygen and silicon, aluminum (Al) is the third most common element in the earth's crust. Although a common element, aluminum is bound by its electric charge within common rocks such as feldspar (aluminum silicate).[501] Pure aluminum, unlike pieces of gold or silver, is not found in nature. Besides rocks, aluminum is found in crystals and precious gems. Corundum is a colorless six-sided crystal of aluminum oxide (Al_2O_3). It is almost as hard as diamond. When traces of the metal chromium are present, corundum turns red and is called a ruby. When trace iron and titanium are present, it becomes a blue sapphire. When combinations of other trace metals are present, it may become a pink, orange, yellow, or green sapphire.[502]

The Aluminum Twins

Aluminum is produced predominately from bauxite, an aluminum rich ore. Bauxite is named after the French village of Les Baux-de-Provence where it was first discovered. Bauxite rocks are rich in aluminum hydroxides (chemical formula $Al[OH]_3$). Bauxite is found mostly in tropical and subtropical regions with plentiful rainwater. Rainwater that is slightly acidic washes silicon oxide (SiO_2) out of rocks, leaving behind aluminum hydroxides. America obtains its bauxite ore from the island of Jamaica.

Bauxite is converted by a chemical reaction into a white powder called alumina with the same chemical composition as corundum (Al_2O_3). While this chemical structure in crystalline form is called corundum, the powdered form is called alumina. The technique used to produce aluminum (AI) from alumina (Al_2O_3) was invented by the so-called aluminum twins: Charles Hall and Paul Héroult. The name "aluminum twins" derives from the uncanny coincidences surrounding the lives of these two men. Hall and Héroult were both

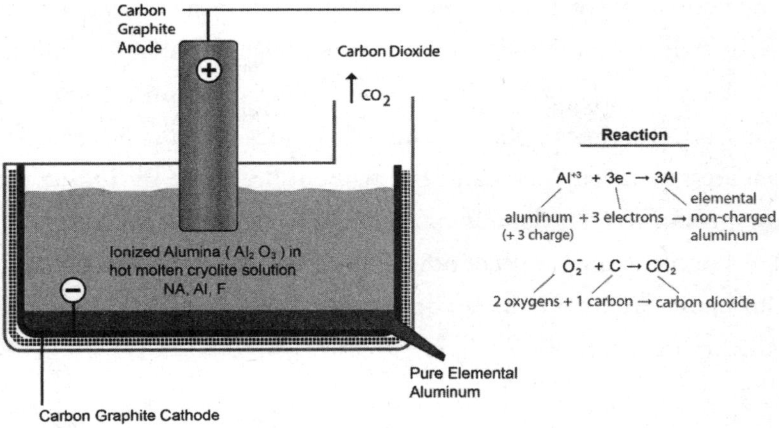

FIGURE 13.1: The Hall-Héroult process. Al = aluminum, C = carbon, CO_2 = carbon dioxide, e = electron, F = florine, NA = sodium, O = oxygen.

born in 1863, and both men died in 1914. Even more remarkably, in 1886 Hall and Héroult independently invented (and patented) aluminum smelting an ocean apart (Hall in America and Héroult in France).

The Hall-Héroult process (Figure 13.1) uses electrolysis to turn alumina into elemental aluminum (Al). As the name infers, electrolysis involves using electricity to lyse (from the Greek word *lysis* "loosening") atoms apart. As an example, using electrolysis on water (H_2O) will separate it into hydrogen (H) and oxygen (O).[503]

The Hall-Héroult process is still used to this day to make aluminum. The process starts by heating bauxite-derived alumina (Al_2O_3) until it is melted into a liquid. Then an electrical current is passed through it.[504] The electricity splits the charged Al^{+3} atoms from oxygen to generate elemental aluminum, which is composed of only neutral aluminum (Al^0) atoms that have no charge. This process consumes vast amounts of electricity. In Australia, making aluminum consumes 10 percent of the country's total electrical power supply.[505] For financial reasons, electrolysis is done in countries with abundant cheaper electricity. It is for that reason that Jamaica transports its aluminum rich bauxite ore on ships to America, where it is smelted into aluminum.

Aluminum is a white silvery metal that is 2.7 times denser than water but 2.5 times lighter than steel. It does not rust or corrode. It conducts electricity and can bend without breaking. By adding trace amounts of different atoms to aluminum, alloys can be created that have augmented strength or other beneficial properties. Once smelted, aluminum products can also be resmelted and reused, making it sustainable and recyclable.[506]

The Wright Brothers and the Aluminum Aerospace Age

Many Americans do not realize that the Wright brothers may not have been the first to invent and successfully fly an airplane. In Brazil, Alberto Santos-Dumont is credited by his countrymen with the invention of the airplane.[507] Today, one of the two commercial airports in Rio de Janeiro is named in his honor. Regardless, where one may fall on who was first, what makes the Wright brothers' airplane distinctive is their use of an aluminum engine. The Wright brothers made this decision because aluminum is much lighter than the other metals typically used to make engines at that time and thus required less lift to become airborne. They asked Alcoa (an abbreviation for Aluminum Company of America) to cast the engine.[508] Alcoa remains one of the world's largest producers of aluminum.

The Wright brothers' decision to use aluminum in their airplane was emulated by later aeronautic pioneers. The German engineer Hugo Junkers built the first all-aluminum metal airplane called the Junker J1 in 1915.[509] The fuselage was an aluminum alloy containing copper, magnesium, and manganese. The German Junker J2 was the world's first metal fighter airplane. The golden age of aviation from the 1920s through 1960s was made possible by planes built with aluminum.

In the last half of the twentieth century, aluminum made exploration of the "Final Frontier" possible. It fueled the space industry by providing lightweight, strong, and temperature resistant aluminum alloys. Be it the Russian Sputnik, the Apollo spacecraft, the Eagle lunar module that landed on the moon, or the spacecraft of SpaceX, all of these were made possible because of aluminum.

In the 1986 science-fiction film *Star Trek IV: The Voyage Home*, the *Enterprise*'s chief engineer Scotty gives the formula for "transparent aluminum" to a twentieth-century American engineer in return for building a lightweight but strong container. At that time, transparent aluminum did not exist. Today, the windows on SpaceX spacecraft are made of a transparent aluminum. Transparent aluminum is called ALON, an abbreviation for aluminum oxynitride.[510] ALON is an alloy of aluminum, oxygen, and nitrogen. It is lighter than glass but can stop fifty-caliber bullets fired from heavy-barrel military machine guns.

The quest for new and more versatile aluminum alloys is not restricted to our planet. Located in the asteroid belt between Mars and Jupiter is a metal asteroid known as 16 Psyche. It is named after the Greek deity Psyche, who is the goddess of the soul. 16 Psyche may be the "Armageddon" remnant core of a planet that had its crust and mantle blown off in the distant past.[511] It is a giant mass of heavy metals that are available without having to drill deep into the core of our planet. On October 13, 2023, NASA launched a reconnaissance mission to 16 Psyche to explore future mining potential. It is planned to arrive in 2029. The estimated value of 16 Psyche is ten thousand quadrillion dollars![512] It may be a ready-to-use source of rare heavy metals that could be used to form futuristic aluminum alloys to facilitate the next giant leap of human achievement—exploration of interstellar space.

Aluminum Metals in Modern Life

Aluminum metals appear everywhere in today's daily life.[513] It is used to make electrical wires due to its ability to conduct electricity. Because it weighs less than copper, aluminum wires allow utility poles to be spaced farther apart. Due to its lightness and resistance to rust, aluminum is also used to produce cars, trains, bicycles, fences, wheelchairs, prosthetic limbs, dental instruments, solar panels, window frames, kettles, and trays. It is used in skyscrapers for lightweight, noncorrosive roofs and nonsupporting frames. The Empire State Building in New York City was the first skyscraper to use aluminum. The Burj Khalifa skyscraper in Dubai is the tallest building in the world. It glistens silver because of aluminum.

Cooking pots and pans made of aluminum are lighter and less expensive than those made of iron. Aluminum is added to food as an anti-caking or anti-clumping agent. Aluminum foil is used to grill, bake, wrap, store, or bag food. Sealed aluminum bags are better at blocking out oxygen to keep food fresh. Accoutrements like ketchup, mustard, relish, mayonnaise, and butter come in aluminum foil packages. Potato chips, popcorn, pretzels, crackers, and cookies are sold in aluminum bags.

Aluminum is added to municipal drinking water because its positive charge clumps bacteria together that are then filtered out. In the 1960s, glass bottles started being replaced by aluminum cans that weigh less and cost less to transport. Currently, more than one hundred billion aluminum beverage cans are made every year.[514] The traditional cork stop on wine bottles are now even being phased out in favor of cheaper screw-on aluminum caps.

Both ready-to-eat and powder formulations of baby food contain aluminum.[515] One liter of baby food can contain from 100 to 760 micrograms of aluminum. Aluminum is in a mother's breast milk.[516] It is present in coffee beans and can be leached into coffee by brewing in an aluminum pot.[517] Aluminum tastes bitter and coffee brewed in aluminum containers, as it often is, makes coffee taste more bitter.

A number of personal hygiene products contain aluminum. It is the active ingredient in antiperspirants that prevents sweating, and it is used in lipstick to make it shiny. It is in toothpaste as a colorant to make the paste white. Toothpaste tubes are also made of aluminum. It is used as a thickening agent in creams, lotions, and other cosmetics.[518] Aluminum is in sunscreen lotion. It is used to keep zinc, the active sunblock ingredient, evenly dissolved in the lotion. Aluminum is a contaminant found in parenteral nutrition solutions that are used to feed calories directly into a patient's vein.[519] It is in over-the-counter medications like buffered aspirin and aluminum antacids, the latter of which are swallowed to decrease epigastric pain from heartburn, in which stomach acid regurgitates or moves backward up the esophagus toward the mouth.

Aluminum is in pesticides in the form of aluminum phosphide. It was first marketed in 1956 and is now sold under many different brand names. Aluminum phosphide when combined with water releases lethal phosphine gas. When eaten by a rodent, water in the gut cause phosphine gas to be released. Aluminum phosphide has been intentionally swallowed by people to commit suicide.[520] There is no antidote.

Aluminum Toxicity

Aluminum has no known natural biologic role or function in any living organism, but it can become toxic. Aluminum inhibits the roots of plants from growing.[521] Stunted roots cannot absorb nutrients. The result is an unhealthy, feeble plant. Acidification leaches silicon from soil, leaving behind aluminum that prevents healthy root proliferation.[522] Acid rain from pollution has contributed to about 30 percent of the earth's soil being acidic, aluminized, and unsuitable for crops.[523] That being said, a few plant strains are up to ten times more resistant to aluminum toxicity than other species.[524]

The mechanisms behind aluminum-related plant toxicity are under investigation, as aluminum toxicity is a major worldwide limitation to increasing crop production.[525] For plants and for humans, Al^{+3} has the potential to replace charged metals such as calcium (Ca^{+2}), magnesium (Mg^{+2}), and manganese (Mn^{+3}) that are normally found within cells. This results in altering or disarming protein function.[526] Positively charged Al^{+3} metal atoms like some other metals may facilitate the binding of chemicals to negatively charged DNA, a process called adduct formation.[527]This could alter a gene's function.

Aluminum is poorly absorbed through the gut or skin. When it succeeds in entering the blood, it is excreted out of the body by the kidneys. Large amounts of aluminum or the inability to excrete aluminum may overwhelm the body's ability to detoxify aluminum. Patients with kidney failure are prescribed oral aluminum antacids to bind and lower blood phosphate that is no longer adequately excreted.[528] The problem is that they cannot excrete aluminum either. Some patients on dialysis receiving aluminum antacids develop aluminum-related brain toxicity that manifests in speech, memory, and behavioral problems and ends in six to eight months with death. Postmortem autopsies have revealed that these patients have significantly elevated aluminum levels in their brain compared to patients on dialysis without neurologic syndromes as well as normal controls who have the lowest brain aluminum levels.[529]

Some patients who get chemotherapy or are treated with radiation to their pelvis will urinate blood from their bladder. Bleeding into the urine may be stopped by infusing into the bladder a solution that contains aluminum. Several patients with poor kidney function receiving aluminum-based bladder irrigation have developed brain toxicities. Symptoms included problems speaking, sudden jerks, seizures, and dementia followed by death. At autopsy, their blood and brain tissues contained high levels of aluminum.[530]

Infants born too early are called preterm or premature. Such infants may be too undeveloped to digest food orally. To keep them alive, calories are infused directly into a vein, a technique called parenteral nutrition. Standard parenteral nutrition solutions are contaminated with aluminum. When aluminum-containing parenteral nutrition was compared to aluminum-depleted solutions, the babies receiving aluminum suffered from impaired mental development.[531]

A patient undergoing dialysis may develop bone pain from bone loss, a medical condition called osteomalacia, which means "soft bones." Under an electron microscope, bones affected by aluminum-related osteomalacia are encased by aluminum in the small struts or beams of bone. These struts are called trabeculae and are inside the bone's surface like stalagmites in a cave. When these struts are covered in aluminum, calcium deposits become displaced, resulting in fragile bones. Bone pain eventually arises from the painful microfractures, and poor healing.[532]

Aluminum brain and bone toxicity often occurs in people with bad kidneys who cannot efficiently excrete aluminum. Chronic everyday exposure to aluminum occurs from the water, food, and beverages we consume and from personal hygiene products. Can aluminum in people with normal kidneys slowly accumulate and cause chronic disease? The current answer is no. But there are case reports that say otherwise.

One such example was recounted in a 2004 case report in the *American Journal of Medicine*. A French woman complained of severe fatigue and spent her days exhausted in bed. Months of medical tests for the usual culprits like low thyroid yielded normal results. Because she was religiously applying antiperspirants, the doctors checked her urine and blood and discovered high aluminum levels. Four months after stopping aluminum-containing antiperspirants, her blood and urine aluminum levels returned to normal, and her fatigue disappeared.[533]

Aluminum is ubiquitous, and most people are unaware of the possibility of aluminum toxicity. Because aluminum toxicity is rare and rarely reported, it may be overlooked in the differential diagnosis for neurologic diseases, bone demineralizing disorders, or unexplained fatigue that coexists with impaired kidney function or excessive aluminum intake.

Adjuvants and Aluminum

An adjuvant is something that helps to increase or accentuate the immune response to a vaccine. The word adjuvant is derived from the Latin word *adjuvare*, which means to help. It is the same Latin root for the English verb "to advocate." An adjuvant is not needed and not used for live, attenuated viral vaccines. It may be added to a dead virus vaccine or to vaccines composed of a piece or part of a virus.[534] Adjuvants were first recognized when accidental co-infection from another infection increased a vaccine's response.[535]

The mechanisms by which adjuvants work are based on (1) concentrating and extending the release of the virus or virus particle, and (2) inducing and exacerbating inflammation. Current adjuvants are shown in Figure 13.2. Four adjuvants were discovered in the twentieth century between 1926 and 1997. Five additional adjuvants were added in the first quarter of the twenty-first century, and still others are in development.[536]

Developed by Jules Freund in the 1930s, Freund's adjuvant is very potent in causing inflammation. It comes in two forms. Incomplete Freund's adjuvant is emulsified oil that concentrates and prevents the virus from dissipating. Complete Freund's adjuvant is the same oil to which heat-killed mycobacterium (a type of bacteria) is added for extra immune stimulation. Freund's adjuvant is so potent that it may cause ulcers and tissue necrosis at the vaccination site.[537] Because of its acute toxicity, it is not currently used as an adjuvant in human vaccines.

Freund's adjuvant continues to be used in veterinary medicine and in animal research labs. The latter has included experiments to

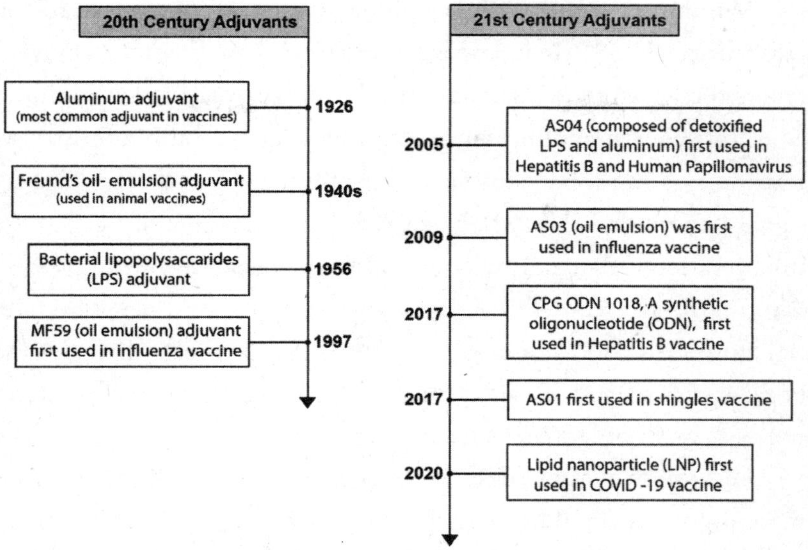

FIGURE 13.2: Examples of adjuvants used to stimulate the immune system to increase a vaccine immune response. AS01 = adjuvant system one. ASO3 = adjuvant system 3, ASO4 = adjuvant system 4, COVID-19 = coronavirus disease 2019, CPG ODN = cytosine (C) and guanine (G) oligodeoxynucleotides (ODN), LNP = lipid nanoparticle, LPS = lipopolysaccharide, MF-59 = microfluidized emulsion, 59MPL = monophosphoryl lipid A.

cause animal autoimmune disease models as a means of studying human autoimmunity, in which one's own immune system attacks a part of their body. If you inject a piece of protein from myelin that surrounds brain cells into an animal, nothing will happen. If you inject an animal with a myelin protein combined with Freund's adjuvant, however, it will cause diffuse brain and spinal cord inflammation or multiple sclerosis-like disease, which in animals is called experimental autoimmune encephalomyelitis. This is due to the immune system attacking the myelin around the brain cells.[538] Other autoimmune diseases that may be caused in animals by vaccinating them with an adjuvant or adjuvant and self-peptide include myasthenia gravis, uveitis, and arthritis that are inflammation at the nerve-muscle junction, eyes, and joints, respectively.[539]

Aluminum was the first immune system adjuvant. It was discovered in 1926.[540] It is less inflammatory than Freund's adjuvant and is today the most used adjuvant in human vaccines. Aluminum adjuvants consist of aluminum salt, usually either aluminum oxyhydroxide or aluminum phosphate. Aluminum works by the "danger signal hypothesis." Aluminum activates a protein complex called the inflammasome that normally assembles in response to infection.[541] Aluminum also causes cell death and the release of genetic material from cells.[542] Pieces of genes (DNA) are also recognized by the body as a damage-associated molecular pattern that cause an alarm response or stimulate immune cells to respond.[543]

Aluminum is the oldest, most common, and gold standard or, more appropriately, aluminum standard used as an adjuvant in human vaccines (Table 13.1).[544] As an adjuvant, it decreases the amount of vaccine needed to induce immunity and increases immune response in otherwise poor responders such as the elderly. It is a nonspecific immune stimulator.

Aluminum-containing vaccines have been reported to cause infertility,[545] autoimmune diseases,[546] and an inflammatory syndrome of persistent muscle aches, joint aches, severe fatigue, and loss of mental clarity.[547] These reports are refuted by broad epidemiological studies that show no association.

Genes that promote inflammation normally remain in a latent non-transcribed silent state. Inflammatory genes have neighboring regulatory regions called enhancers that are in the DNA of the gene. Enhancers will enhance expression of the inflammatory gene. In the laboratory, after exposure to a strong nonspecific adjuvant, enhancers are permanently modified so that inflammatory genes remain turned on or can be more easily and rapidly turned on.[548] If this laboratory finding is relevant to the bedside, it implies that after receiving a potent nonspecific adjuvant, a patient may end up with a diathesis toward a chronic pro-inflammatory state.

Table 13.1: Examples of Some Vaccines That Contain Aluminum[549]

Vaccine Trade Name	Infection	Aluminum Adjuvant Abbreviation	Aluminum Adjuvant	Al^{+3} adult dose
Biothraxâ	Anthrax	AH	Aluminum Oxyhydroxide	1.2 mg
Diphtheria and tetanus	Diphtheria and tetanus	AP	Aluminum Phosphate	0.33mg
Daptacelâ	Diphtheria, tetanus, and pertussis (DTaP)	AP	Aluminum Phosphate	0.33mg
Infanrixâ	Diphtheria, tetanus, and pertussis (DTaP)	AH	Aluminum Oxyhydroxide	0.625 mg
Pediarixâ	Diphtheria, tetanus, and pertussis (DTaP) and Hepatitis B and poliomyelitis	AH	Aluminum Oxyhydroxide	0.85 mg
Kinrixâ	Diphtheria, tetanus and pertussis (DTaP) and poliomyelitis	AH	Aluminum Oxyhydroxide	0.6 mg
Quadracelâ	Diphtheria, tetanus, and pertussis (DTaP) and poliomyelitis	AP	Aluminum Phosphate	0.33mg
Pentacel	Diphtheria, tetanus, abd pertussis (DTaP) and poliomyelitis and Hemophilus influenza B (Hib)	AP	Aluminum Phosphate	0.33mg

Vaccine Trade Name	Infection	Aluminum Adjuvant Abbreviation	Aluminum Adjuvant	Al^{+3} adult dose
PedVaxHIB	Hemophilus influenza B (Hib)	AAHS	Amorphous Aluminum Hydroxyphosphate Sulfate	0.225
Havrix	Hepatitis A	AH	Aluminum Oxyhydroxide	0.5 mg
VAQTA	Hepatitis A	AAHS	Amorphous Aluminum Hydroxyphosphate Sulfate	0.5 mg
Twinrix	Hepatitis A and hepatitis B	AH & AP	Aluminum Oxyhydroxide & Aluminum Phosphate	0.45 mg
Engerix	Hepatitis B	AH	Aluminum Oxyhydroxide	0.5 mg
Recombivax HB	Hepatitis B	AAHS	Amorphous Aluminum Hydroxyphosphate Sulfate	0.5 mg
Cervarix	Human papilloma virus	AH & MPLA	Aluminum Oxyhydroxide & monophosphoryl lipid A	0.5mg AH + 50ug MPLA
Gardasil	Human papilloma virus	AAHS	Amorphous Aluminum Hydroxyphosphate Sulfate	0.225 mg

Vaccine Trade Name	Infection	Aluminum Adjuvant Abbreviation	Aluminum Adjuvant	Al^{+3} adult dose
Gardasil 9	Human papilloma virus	AAHS	Amorphous Aluminum Hydroxyphosphate Sulfate	0.5 mg
Bexsero	Meningococcus B	AH	Aluminum Oxyhydroxide	0.519 mg
Trumenb	Meningococcus B	AP	Aluminum Phosphate	0.25 mg
Prevnar 13	Pneumococcus	AP	Aluminum Phosphate	0.125 mg
Prevnar 20	Pneumococcus	AP	Aluminum Phosphate	0.13 mg
Vaxneuvance	Pneumococcus	AP	Aluminum Phosphate	0.13 mg
Ixiaro	Japanese encephalitis	AH	Aluminum Oxyhydroxide	0.25 mg
Ticovac	Tick-borne encephalitis	AH	Aluminum Oxyhydroxide	0.35 mg

AAHS = amorphous aluminum hydroxyphosphate sulfate ($AlHO_9PS^{-3}$), AH = aluminum hydroxide (Al[O]OH), AP = aluminum phosphate (Al[OH]x[PO4]y) MPLA = monophosphoryl lipid A ($C_{94}H_{177}N_2O_{22}P$)

Summary

This chapter began where chapter 11 on the human papilloma virus left off. In the Gardasil vaccine trial, the HPV vaccine containing both the HPV virus shell protein and an aluminum adjuvant was compared to a control of only aluminum adjuvant. There was no comparison in the trial to the viral shell vaccine without the aluminum adjuvant.

The Gardasil vaccine virus is a natural virus shell that by itself induces a danger signal and immunity without an additional adjuvant danger signal. In fact, the VLPs of the Gardasil vaccine could be used as an adjuvant for other vaccines.[550] By excluding a control using the virus shell without aluminum, the trial did not adequately evaluate the efficacy of using only the immune-stimulating viral shell.

By including aluminum in both the vaccine and the control, the Gardasil trial allowed the toxicity of aluminum to be hidden. In the trial, toxicity due to injection of the vaccine (viral shell and adjuvant) would have appeared to be safe, because it would have had the same toxicity as the "control" containing aluminum adjuvant. As we saw in chapter 11, multiple lawsuits have since been filed against Gardasil. The best kill switch against those lawsuits and for the vaccine recipient's peace of mind is transparent noncoerced consent.

CHAPTER 14

Ebola Virus: Crossing the Rubicon

The single biggest threat to man's continued dominance on the planet is the virus.
—Nobel Laureate Joshua Lederberg[551]

Creating a new virus to fight a known virus is fighting fire with fire.—RKB

The Ebola virus is named for the Ebola River in equatorial Africa where it was discovered in 1976.[552] Sister Miriam was a hospital nurse working in the Democratic Republic of Congo, which at that time was a Belgian colony called Zaire. She suddenly became ill on September 23, 1976. She died seven days after onset of illness. Her blood provided the first laboratory sample of Ebola virus.[553]

In the 1976 outbreak, out of 318 infected patients, 88 percent of them died, including seventeen hospital staff. The 1976 Ebola outbreak was attributed to the use of shared syringes and needles. At the beginning of the day, each nurse was given five needles and five syringes to be reused throughout their shift. The syringes and needles were washed with warm water but not sterilized between blood draws on different patients.[554]

Ebola is a filovirus, the name of which is derived from the Latin word *filum*, meaning thread. Ebola is a long thread-like or worm-like RNA virus (chapter 2, Table 2.1). There are six species of Ebola virus. The most virulent is the Zaire Ebola species with a 90 percent mortality rate. It is second only to Rabies virus in mortality rate once symptoms start. Ebola is a zoonotic virus, meaning that it jumps from animals to humans. Each outbreak has generally occurred in a rural area involving less than a few hundred people. This changed with the 2013 outbreak that involved 28,652 people.[555]

Symptoms are a sudden high fever, lack of energy, muscle and joint aches, headache, abdominal pain, vomiting, and diarrhea. These symptoms progress over a few days to include confusion and failure of the liver, kidney, and heart. This is followed by bleeding from body orifices, which leads to shock due to low blood pressure and death.[556] The natural reservoir for the Ebola virus is the African fruit bat.[557] Monkeys, chimpanzees, and gorillas may also get infected by eating fruit contaminated by an infected fruit bat bite.[558] It is transmitted from one human to another by contact with body fluids including blood, urine, saliva, diarrhea, vomit, breast milk, amniotic fluid, vaginal discharge, and semen.

The 1995 film *Outbreak* starring Dustin Hoffman is about a team of American army doctors in HazMat suits desperately struggling to contain an outbreak of Ebola in California. In the movie, Ebola was inadvertently brought to America following transport of an infected African monkey. To this day, there is no effective antiviral medication for Ebola. Once infected, 90 percent of individuals will die. When the film was produced, there was still no vaccine for Ebola.

The Ebola Virus Vaccine

The first Ebola vaccine used another safer virus called vesicular stomatitis virus (VSV) as a genetically modified backbone for the Ebola vaccine. The vaccine was created by removing one gene from the vesicular stomatitis virus and inserting the gene for the surface protein of the Ebola virus.

VSV is from the same family of viruses as rabies (see chapter 4). Like the rabies virus, it is a bullet-shaped RNA virus composed of five genes. VSV causes self-limited mucosal blisters in hoofed animals like horses, cows, and pigs. In humans, VSV is generally not pathogenic, and infections are generally asymptomatic. However, VSV is not totally benign for humans. It occasionally causes self-limited fever, chills, head and muscle aches, and oral lesions.[559] Even more rarely, it causes diffuse brain inflammation (i.e., encephalomyelitis).[560] People around livestock such as farmers and veterinarians are at risk for VSV infection.

In 1999, a Yale University professor and researcher named John Rose reported that the surface protein gene in VSV could be replaced with the surface protein of another virus.[561] By using Dr. Rose's technique, the National Microbiology Laboratory in Canada replaced the VSV surface protein gene with the Zaire Ebola surface gene (Figure 14.1). The result was a man-made virus that could be used as a vaccine against Ebola. This vaccine is known as a recombinant viral vaccine because it is a combination of two different viruses: VSV and Ebola. In 2005, this new man-made recombinant virus was injected into monkeys. No adverse side effects occurred, and the monkeys when subsequently inoculated with the Ebola virus were immune to disease.[562]

Despite monkeys acquiring immunity to Ebola, development of a clinical human vaccine stagnated. When the Canadian government tried to license the recombinant virus for a human trial, big pharma companies were not interested. Ebola intermittently infected small numbers of poor villagers in tropical Africa. The cost of developing and running the vaccine trials could not be recovered. In 2010, only one company in the entire world, NewLink Genetics, offered to invest in a human trial.

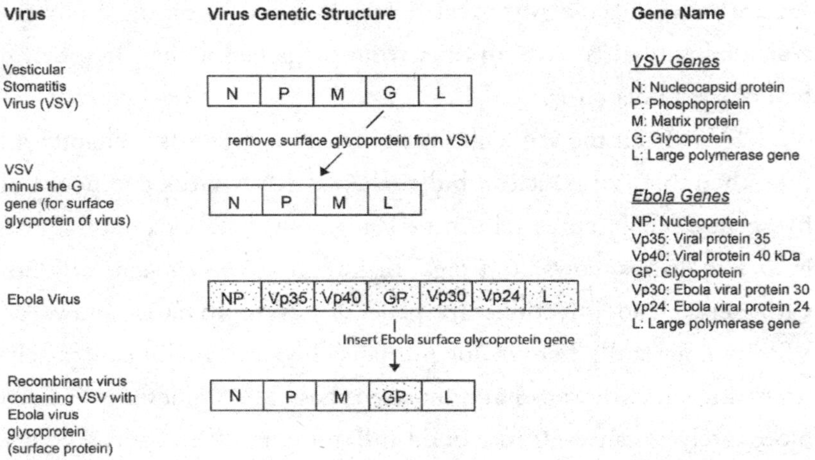

FIGURE 14.1: Genetic recombination of genes from two viruses (VSV and Ebola) to develop a new vesicular stomatitis virus (VSV) expressing the Ebola virus surface glycoprotein (GP).

NewLink Genetics's Chief Executive Officer was Chuck Link, who was admitted into the US Air Force Academy before graduating from Stanford University Medical School and was a former fellow at the National Institutes of Health. He recognized the catastrophe that would follow if Ebola transitioned into a worldwide pandemic and pushed for the vaccine to start human trials before a large outbreak occurred. In early 2014, the FDA pulled the emergency brake cord on the train moving toward a human trial. It demanded that monkey trials be repeated before starting the human trial.

The use of live Ebola virus to inoculate monkeys to document vaccine efficacy required a maximal security biosafety level (BSL-4) facility with monkey housing and specialized veterinarians. There is only one such facility in America, the National Bio and Agro-Defense Facility (NBAF). The NBAF backlog for new monkey trials was several years. Clinical Ebola vaccine development again stagnated.

The 2014–2016 Ebola epidemic changed everything. This epidemic was not limited to a few hundred Africans in remote villages.

Tens of thousands of people in Africa were infected. In 2014, the first case of Ebola jumped to America. The virus came with a patient whose symptoms began four days after leaving Africa.

For those who were aware, alarms went off in the medical system. The 1995 film *Outbreak* that warned of the Ebola virus infiltrating America became a reality. An infectious disease with no treatment that kills 90 percent of people by causing them to bleed from every opening in their body had snuck into the United States. Immediate quarantine restriction on all contacts with the infected person, including other plane passengers and crew on their return flight, went into effect. The FDA requirement for more monkey studies was lifted.

In 2014, NewLink Genetics initiated an early (phase I) trial in humans to determine safety and optimal dose after the outbreak was declared by the United States, and the Food and Drug Administration immediately allowed the clinical trials to launch, working closely with both NewLink and the US Department of Defense.[563] Then NewLink partnered the development program with Merck, a large pharmaceutical company with deeper resources to proceed toward conducting larger scale testing. In 2015, the first human efficacy (phase III) trial was published.

The randomized trial was designed as a two-tiered ring vaccination by European investigators and the World Health Organization (WHO). It was a true randomized trial with one group treated and the other untreated for the incubation period of the virus. People in contact with an Ebola patient and people in contact with those contacts were vaccinated. The treatment arm was vaccinated immediately, whereas the control arm was vaccinated after a delay of three weeks. Ebola has an incubation period of two to twenty-one days with a mean of six days. Only patients in the delayed vaccine arm got Ebola. The vaccine that is now called Ervebo was 100 percent effective in preventing Ebola.[564]

The Ebola vaccine was a success. Humanity dodged a bullet, albeit, to paraphrase Job 19:20, "by the skin of its teeth." The spread of Ebola was slowed because of effective quarantines, and Ebola had not yet mutated into a virus that could be more rapidly transmitted between humans.[565] This provided time to develop and test the vaccine, which went forward at warp speed.

Summary

With the Ebola vaccine, a new chapter in the book of life was opened. We crossed the Rubicon River into the age of inoculating people with a man-made recombinant virus. The vaccine used to prevent Ebola was a new hybrid living virus that never existed before on this planet. Given the lethality of Ebola, the risk of creating a new type of live virus was worth taking. Yet, long-term consequences of injecting increasing numbers of people with novel man-made living viruses are unknown.

Life does not behave like an algebraic equation. Altering one side of the equation does not necessarily result in one predictable outcome. Chaos theory is a better model for life. An example of chaos theory is the butterfly effect in which a very small change, such as a butterfly flapping its wings within a complex system, leads to massive differences in outcomes, such as a hurricane on the opposite side of the world.[566] Altering one small living virus may generate late and unpredictable consequences with unforeseen oscillations and fractal ramifications in unexpected areas that occur decades later. Is it possible that making a new virus without adding a kill switch may, over time and depending on the virus, have the opposite effect? Instead of preventing a pandemic, could it cause one? Is this how COVID-19 arose?

CHAPTER 15

COVID-19: The Intertwined Plots of a Global Shakespearean Tragedy

Vilifying questions as anti-science makes Nemesis, the goddess who avenges hubris, your nemesis.—RKB

Natura non confundenda est. *Don't screw with mother nature.*—Leviathan *(1989 film)*

Coronaviruses are bat viruses that in general do not infect humans. There are hundreds of different bat coronaviruses. Four coronaviruses can infect humans but cause no or only mild symptoms of a common cold.[567]

As noted in chapter 1, the first lethal human coronavirus epidemic occurred from 2002 to 2004. Because deaths followed from suffocation due to lung damage, the disease was called SARS, an abbreviation for severe acute respiratory syndrome.[568] The coronavirus causing SARS was designated SARS-CoV-1 where CoV is an abbreviation for coronavirus. Because it did not spread easily between infected humans, SARS-CoV-1 infections fizzled out and did not become a pandemic. This epidemic originated in China's Guangdong province next to Hong Kong. It was a zoonotic infection, meaning it jumped from animals and then into humans. To help quell the epidemic, China culled tens of thousands of animals.[569]

The second Chinese SARS-like disease is COVID-19, an abbreviation for coronavirus disease 2019. It is caused by a coronavirus designated as SARS-CoV-2. COVID-19 suddenly burst onto the world stage in November 2019.[570] It spread easily and rapidly between people, becoming a worldwide pandemic. COVID-19 killed millions and resulted in censorship and draconian restrictions on civil liberties. It financially ruined and emotionally scarred untold numbers of people. The COVID-19 pandemic originated in Wuhan, a city in central China. There are two competing theories for the origin of COVID-19. It either arose naturally from a bat (or another intermediary animal) or was manmade and arose from a laboratory accident.

Early in the COVID-19 pandemic, the lab leak hypothesis was called a "conspiracy theory," and in 2021 some people were doxed by the press with personal photos as "superspreaders of conspiracy."[571] By 2024, after a two-year investigation, a US congressional panel concluded that COVID-19 arose from a lab leak.[572] Why has the origin of COVID-19 been mired in so much controversy? Before we can answer this question, we must first start with another virus that, like COVID-19, is also spread by respiratory secretions, an influenza virus that is colloquially called the flu virus.

Gain of Function on the Influenza Virus

Influenza is a virus that infects birds and pigs and to a lesser extent other animals. These animals can infect humans, but only a limited number of influenza subtypes can spread by human-to-human transmission. Influenza virus subtypes are classified by their two surface proteins called hemagglutinin (abbreviated H) and neuraminidase (abbreviated N).

Subtype H5N1 is an influenza virus of birds that has infected and killed humans.[573] To date, it has not caused a human pandemic. If the infected birds are killed, human infections stop. H5N1 has not had enough time to mutate into a virus that is easily transmissible between humans. Like other zoonotic or animal-to-human viruses, "sustainable human to human transmission of the virus requires mutations different than the initial mutation allowing animal to human infectivity."[574]

Engineering a virus to add a new function that it does not normally express in nature is called gain of function. Dangerous gain-of-function experiments include engineering a virus to make it more easily transmissible between or more lethal for humans.[575] Gain-of-function research is controversial even among virologists; some support it whereas others do not.

In 2012, the Erasmus Medical Center in the Netherlands and scientists at the University of Wisconsin published that they had genetically engineered the bird influenza virus H5N1 so that it could easily spread between ferrets.[576] Easy transmission of influenza by respiratory droplets between ferrets is the assay used to predict reliably easy human-to-human transmission.[577] If this newly engineered H5N1 virus broke outside of its laboratory prison, it could trigger a worldwide pandemic.

This controversial genetic engineering of the H5N1 virus raised several ethical questions, including whether such gain-of-function research should be done, if the publication of such research should be permitted, and whether the scientists involved in such research can regulate themselves.[578] In the wake of this controversy, H5N1 research was voluntarily suspended for sixty days by the investigators.[579] However, it is important to note that a sixty-day suspension does not seriously restrict or allow time to seriously address concerns surrounding gain-of-function research.

Dr. Anthony Fauci (Box 15.1) was at the time the director of the National Institutes of Allergy and Infectious Disease (NIAID) in Bethesda, Maryland, a few metro stops from the US Congress building in Washington, DC. NIAID is a part of the National Institutes of Health (NIH). The NIH is the world's largest funding agency for biological research.

Box 15.1: Anthony Fauci—The Director of NIAID

Anthony Fauci served at the National Institutes of Health in Bethesda, Maryland, for forty years. For a large part of his tenure (1984–2022), he was the highly honored director of the National Institute of Allergy and Infectious Disease. He was respected for his role in funding research for autoimmune diseases and AIDS, and for developing effective vaccines.

In a 2012 article when writing about creating a virus in the laboratory, Fauci wrote: "In an unlikely but conceivable turn of events, what if the scientist becomes infected with the [manmade] virus, which leads to an outbreak and ultimately triggers a pandemic? . . . Scientists in this field might say–as indeed I have said—that the benefits of such experiments and the resulting knowledge outweigh the risks [of a pandemic]."[580]

Fauci's statement is not indicative of just one person's opinion but rather an institution that enabled it. Nobody at the NIH objected or countered by asking how many innocent lives the knowledge gained from a manmade viral pandemic might be worth. One life, a thousand, a million, a hundred million, a billion? Fauci was quoted as saying: "Attacks on me, quite frankly, are attacks on science."[581] How did the medical system become so frightening?

Fauci wrote that he is "someone who gave it his all."[582] So then what went wrong? When there is a problem, follow the money. As Fauci wrote about his group: "My NIAID group was focused on creating vaccines and working with pharmaceutical companies to develop treatments."[583]

At the time of announcing the sixty-day pause, Fauci published a paper praising the researchers for their voluntary two-month lull. There was a conflict of interest in his praise, because his institute, the NIAID, had, along with others, including the Bill Gates Foundation, funded gain-of-function research on H5N1 at both the Erasmus Medical Center and the University of Wisconsin.

Fauci did not hide what most should find mortifying. To reemphasize, in his 2012 publication "Research on Highly Pathogenic H5N1 Influenza Virus: The Way Forward," Fauci prophetically wrote: "In an unlikely but conceivable turn of events, what if the scientist becomes infected with the [newly created] virus, which leads to an outbreak and ultimately triggers a pandemic? . . . Scientists in this field might say—as indeed I have said—that the benefits of such [gain-of-function] experiments and the resulting knowledge outweigh the risks."[584]

The 1964 movie *Dr. Strangelove* is about an Air Force General who, despite the risk of a counter strike, orders a preemptive nuclear attack on Russia. Reality is stranger than *Dr. Strangelove.* Would Nature, the Fates, or God call Fauci's hubris and strike back?

Potential Pandemic Pathogen Care and Oversight (P3CO)

Due to the H5N1 controversy and numerous US laboratory biosafety accidents, the Obama White House Office of Science and Technology Policy (OSTP) stepped up to the plate. On October 2014, the OSTP stopped all NIH gain-of-function research funding for contagious respiratory viral pathogens, including influenza and coronavirus. This pause halted the flow of money for eighteen ongoing taxpayer-funded gain-of-function research studies taking place at fourteen institutions.[585]

The Erasmus Medical Center that performed gain of function on H5N1 and had volunteered for the sixty-day pause objected to this longer hold. In the words of Dr. Ronaldus Fouchier, who was

Erasmus's lead investigator: "We need gain of function experiments to demonstrate casual relationships between genes and mutations and particular biological traits."[586]

Restarting gain-of-function research remained on the NIH's Christmas wishlist. Just in time for Christmas, on December 19, 2017, the director of the NIH, Dr. Francis Collins, announced that the pause on gain-of-function research was lifted.[587] In lifting the ban, the Department of Health and Human Services published a framework for gain-of-function research called "Guiding Funding Decisions About Proposed Research Involving Enhanced Potential Pandemic Pathogen Care and Oversight" (abbreviated PPPCO or P3CO).[588]

Given a euphemism that sounds like the Star Wars robot C-3PO, the P3CO committee was created to review and recommend whether a gain-of-function research proposal should be funded, modified, or rejected. This sounds good, but P3CO had as much power as C-3PO. That's because the committee was circumvented by researchers and institutions redefining the definition of "gain of function."

Understanding the coronavirus gain-of-function story is, as Winston Churchill once said, "A riddle, wrapped in a mystery, inside an enigma." Making a new coronavirus that can infect people involved a worldwide collaboration of triangles within triangles (Figure 15.1).

Gain-of-Function Research on Coronavirus in America

In 2015 in the top-tier science journal *Nature Medicine*, Dr. Ralph Baric at the University of North Carolina at Chapel Hill, in collaboration with Dr. Shi Zhengli at the Wuhan Institute of Virology in China, reported that they had created a new coronavirus. They genetically recombined two coronaviruses: SARS-CoV-1, which caused the 2003 SARS epidemic, and another nonpathogenic coronavirus. This newly created hybrid laboratory virus was able to infect and damage human lung cells but less so than its SARS-CoV-1 progenitor.[589] The

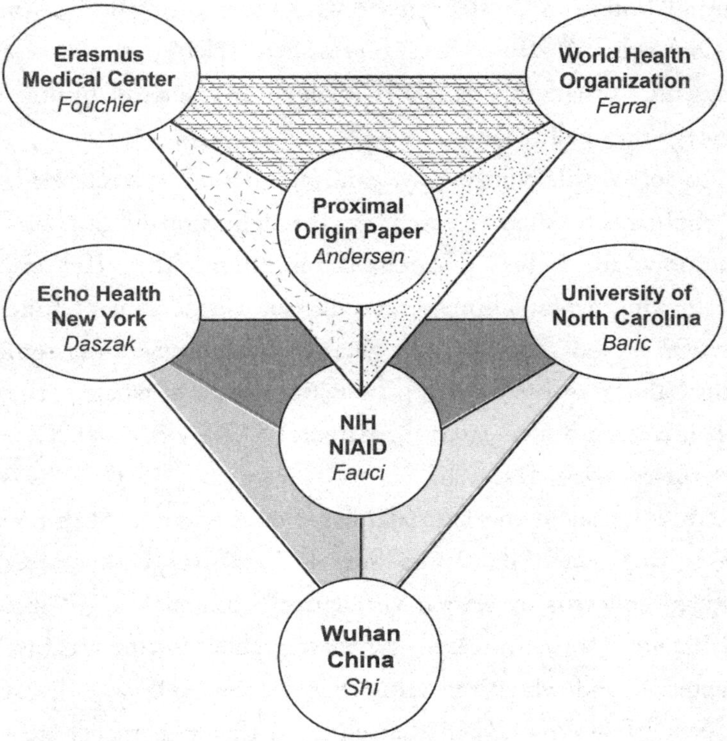

FIGURE 15.1: The main renown actors and institutions involved in the COVID-19 tragedy.

authors themselves described their research as gain of function. Did this 2015 publication break the 2014 gain-of-function moratorium?

No, it did not. The 2015 study did not violate the funding moratorium because the research was completed before the moratorium started. More importantly, Baric spilled the game plan on how the NIH will avoid future P3CO oversight. He said: "The NIH eventually concluded that the work [on a chimeric coronavirus virus] was not so risky as to fall under the [gain-of-function] moratorium."[590]

The hybrid laboratory virus created by Baric and Shi had decreased, not increased, the toxicity of the original 2003 SARS virus. So, was this gain of function? Was the NIH rationalizing their actions by using a Clintonism? "It depends on what the meaning of the word 'is' is." Or is this still gain-of-function research? Like Juliet in *Romeo and Juliet* said: "What's in a name? That which we call a rose by any other name would smell as sweet."

To soften this controversy, gain of function was renamed with the euphemism "dual research."[591] The definition of gain of function, now called dual research, is important. The NIH claimed that making a new chimeric coronavirus is not gain of function. In truth, nobody had any idea what creating a new virus could do to the balance of life on this planet. Regardless of whether the new virus increased or decreased the parental SARS virus toxicity, it was nevertheless "risky research."[592]

An editorial in the journal *Nature* on Baric and Shi's research called "Engineered Bat Virus Stirs Debate over Risky Research" included concerns by several virologists.[593] Simon Wain-Hobson at the Pasteur Institute in Paris—where the rabies vaccine was invented (chapter 4) and where the virus that causes AIDS was discovered (chapter 10)—remarked in that editorial that researchers created a new virus that "grows remarkably well [in human cells]. If the virus escaped, nobody could predict the trajectory." Richard Ebright, a molecular biologist at Rutgers University, cautioned in the article that "The only impact of this work is the creation, in the lab, of a new, non-natural risk." Even Baric himself admitted that his manmade coronavirus moves "this virus from a candidate emerging pathogen to a clear and present danger."

In contrast, Peter Daszak—a British zoologist (animal expert) and president of EcoHealth Alliance, whom we will learn more about later—defended Baric's research in the *Nature* editorial. He stated that gain-of-function research "can help indicate which pathogens should be prioritized for further research attention."

For a decade, the NIH was repeatedly warned of the dangers in creating new viruses. In a gesture to reopen gain-of-function research, the P3CO regulatory oversight committee was set up only to be thwarted by the NIH redefining the definition of gain of function.

Gain-of-Function Research Moves to China

In 2014, gain-of-function research was stopped in America by the White House Office of Science and Technology Policy in part because biosafety laboratory accidents were much too frequent. On average three per week were reported in America,[594] and one per week in Canadian biosafety labs.[595] After America halted gain-of-function research, the NIH started funding gain-of-function research on coronavirus at the Chinese Wuhan Institute of Virology (NIH / NIAID grant R01-A110964).

The Chinese government had not halted coronavirus gain-of-function research, was not structured toward reporting biosafety accidents, and was not welcoming to outside inspections. The Chinese were new to this game. They began building their BSL-4 facility in 2014. It was accredited in 2017. In 2018, one year before COVID-19 broke out, a scientist at the Wuhan Institute of Virology published a paper describing their center's hurdles in establishing a biosafety facility, challenges that are experienced by all biosafety labs. Problems mentioned in the article included inadequate management systems, insufficient resources, and lack of trained and experienced personnel.[596]

A biosafety lab must do everything the same way each time. It must have a protocol for each and every step. One person does the procedure while another person diligently documents each action and confirms that it complies with protocol. Any deviation from a standard operating procedure or the established way of conducting a procedure must be logged and investigated as an incident report, and corrective actions must also be documented. The same extensive documentation applies to all other aspects of the facility as well. These important safeguards protect scientists, laboratory staff, the general public, and the environment from encountering or spreading potentially hazardous biological materials.

University researchers who fill the positions in these facilities are trained to do the opposite. Because researchers are trying to discover the best way, they are not infrequently tinkering and changing things based on the prior experiment. University researchers do not and cannot creatively function under such exhaustive, time-consuming, and unchangeable conditions with punitive restrictions for any deviation. The NIH moved coronavirus gain-of-function research to a new inexperienced facility in China where the NIH could not directly monitor it. What could possibly go wrong?

How was a branch of the US government inconspicuously able to take American citizens' taxpayer dollars to fund gain-of-function research in a laboratory in China? They did it by redefining the definition of gain of function and then directing the money to China through a third party called EcoHealth Alliance. In the private world, the discreet transfer of money so that it can be used for illegal activity is termed money laundering. For the NIH it was business as usual.

EcoHealth Alliance is a US organization that conducts research on global health. It is headed by Peter Daszak. Previously, Daszak voiced support for gain-of-function research in the 2015 *Nature* editorial that raised safety concerns about Baric and Shi's research. With Baric's work at the University of North Carolina at Chapel Hill halted, Shi was the logical choice to continue the NIH-funded gain-of-function research.

As the director of the Wuhan Institute of Virology, Shi Zhengli had already established a good reputation as a university-trained investigator. Her life story is one of education-related separation from her family, self-sacrifice, hard work, and determination.[597] Her extensive work on bat coronaviruses had earned her the nickname "the Batwoman."[598] Throughout her career, Shi had collected over twenty thousand bat stool samples from caves in China. About 10 percent of those samples contained coronaviruses. Due to her efforts, the Wuhan Institute of Virology housed the world's most prolific coronavirus collection.

NIH / NIAID Grant R01-AI110964

The NIAID awarded Daszak and EcoHealth Alliance (in New York) and Shi and the Wuhan Institute of Virology (in China) a multimillion-dollar grant that was funded from June 2014 through May 31, 2019, for coronavirus research. According to Fauci's own words in a 2024 statement: "No portion of the grant was aimed at increasing the transmissibility of any viruses."[599]

It is true this NIH/NIAID grant does not specifically refer to increasing viral transmissibility per se. The grant does, however, speak of both finding in the wild and making in the lab new coronaviruses that bind more efficiently to human cells. The grant states that its goal is to "Test predictions of CoV [coronavirus] inter-species transmission . . . will be tested experimentally using reverse genetics . . . and virus infection experiments across a range of cell cultures from different species and humanized mice."[600]

Reverse genetics means to add or delete or modify a gene of a virus to see what types of animal or human cells the virus will then infect.[601] The term "humanized mice" refers to the genetic alteration of a strain of mice so that the cells lining the lungs of mice carry the human coronavirus receptor that allows coronavirus to infect cells. It appears that the humanized mice would be provided by Baric, who was Shi's prior collaborator on coronavirus gain-of-function research.

Whether genetically altered in a lab, selected in laboratory culture, or passed between humanized mice, new strains of a virus that arise from such experiments may have potential, if they escape from the lab, to cross over and cause disease in the human population. The NIH renewed funding to EcoHealth Alliance and the Wuhan Institute of Virology in early 2019. In November of 2019, the COVID-19 pandemic began in Wuhan and spread around the world.

Conflict of Interest

A conflict of interest means that you have something to gain or something to lose in what you arbitrate, judge, or reconcile. The more you could lose or gain, the greater your conflict of interest.

The unbelievable story behind COVID-19 is that both Francis Collins, the director of the NIH, and especially Anthony Fauci, the director of NIAID, were heavily conflicted in determining the pandemic's origin. The conflict is that they advocated for and funded the creation of new coronaviruses. They did this despite a decade of warnings not to do such "risky research." The NIH funded the Wuhan Institute of Virology when gain-of-function research was halted in America. Fauci even stated publicly that the information gained from gain of function was worth the risk, even if a worldwide pandemic resulted from creating a new virus!

Imagine the consequences if COVID-19 originated from a Chinese lab that the NIH funded with US taxpayer dollars. The blood of millions and the suffering of hundreds of millions staining the hands and tarnishing the souls of NIH brass. Their careers and reputations would be shredded. There could be criminal repercussions.

Did they admit their conflict of interest and recuse themselves from investigating the origin of COVID-19? The answer is no. By not recognizing their conflict of interest and not recusing themselves from the investigation, Collins and Fauci guaranteed the rise of conspiracy theories. By not recognizing its inherent conflict of interest, the NIH poisoned the well of trust.

The Proximal Origin Paper

On March 17, 2020, a correspondence article was published in the journal *Nature Medicine* that played a dramatic role in the discourse concerning the origins of COVID-19. Entitled "The Proximal Origin of SARS-CoV-2," its talking points were drafted by Kristian Andersen of the Scripps Research Institute in La Jolla, California, in collaboration with four other listed co-authors.[602] It was later learned that an ad hoc group of prestigious scientists not listed as authors on the article were also involved in the drafting of the publication (Figure 15.1). These individuals included:

1. Anthony Fauci, the director of NIAID, whose institute funded gain-of-function research at the Wuhan Institute.
2. Francis Collins, the director of the NIH, who supported gain-of-function research.
3. Ronaldus Fouchier, who served as the lead investigator in the influenza H5N1 gain-of-function research paper.
4. Jeremy Farrar, the director of Wellcome Trust and later the Chief Scientist of the World Health Organization, who has been quoted as saying, "I believe, broadly, that gain-of-function research can furnish scientific findings that are ultimately useful."[603]

The ad hoc group's activity was documented by Farrar (a member of the group) in his book *Spike.* A Freedom of Information Act requested by the US Congress, along with US Senator Rand Paul's book *Deception: The Great COVID Cover-Up*,[604] also uncovered this ad hoc group's back door involvement in the Proximal Origin paper, as traced by the following chain of events and correspondences.[605]

On January 31, 2020, microbiologist Kristian Andersen, a distinguished virologist, tweeted that the COVID-19 virus had some features that (potentially) looked human engineered. His tweet was deleted the same day.

On the same day as Anderson tweeted that the COVID-19 virus looked manmade, Farrar (Director of UK Wellcome Trust) emailed Anthony "Tony" Fauci (Director of NIAID, an institute of the National Institutes of Health [NIH]): "Tony really would like to speak with you this evening."

Fauci's assistant responded: "Will call shortly."

After the phone conversation, Farrar emailed Fauci: "Thanks Tony. Can you phone Kristian Anderson. He is expecting your call now."

In an email to Farrar, Fauci said that he told Andersen: "If everyone agrees with this (Anderson's) concern, they should report it to the appropriate authorities . . . the FBI or Mi5."

Fauci may not have been initially aware that the NIH was funding Wuhan via EcoHealth Alliance as he wrote: "I didn't like the fact that I was completely in the dark." Instead of contacting the FBI or Mi5, an ad hoc working group was rapidly assembled that included authors of the Proximal Origin paper and Fauci, Collins (Director of NIH), and virologists invested in or supportive of gain-of-function research like Farrar and Fouchier,

On February 1, 2020, in an email sent to Fauci referring about COVID-19, Andersen wrote: "all find the genome inconsistent with evolution." To reiterate, the email states that the COVID-19 genetic structure did not appear to arise from natural evolution in nature.

On February 2, 2020, Fouchier, the lead investigator in the H5N1 gain of function paper, wrote to Anderson: "It is my opinion that a non-natural origin of [the virus] is highly unlikely at present. Any conspiracy theory (of a lab leak) can be approached with factual information. I have written down some of the counter-arguments."

Later that day Fauci emailed the group: "Like all of us, I do not know how this evolved but given the concerns of so many people and the threat of further distortions on social media, it is essential that we move quickly."

On February 8, 2020, Andersen emailed the ad hoc group that the virus sequencing data was too inconsistent to determine its origin. He wrote in an email to the ad hoc group: "Our main work over the last couple of weeks has been focused on trying to disprove any type of lab theory, but we are at a crossroads where the scientific evidence is not conclusive. As to publishing this document in a journal. I am currently not in favor . . . publishing something that is open ended could backfire."

On February 12, 2020, Anderson wrote to the editor of *Nature Medicine*: "I wanted to reach out to you to see if there would be interest in receiving a commentary/hypothesis piece on the evolutionary origins of SARS-CoV-2? There has been a lot of speculation, fear mongering, and conspiracies put forward in this space and we thought that bringing some clarity to this discussion might be of interest to Nature. Prompted by Jeremy Farrah, Tony Fauci, and Francis Collins, . . . (we) have been working through much of the (primarily) genetic data to provide agnostic and scientifically informed hypotheses around the origins of the virus."

On March 6, 2020, Anderson emailed Farrar, Fauci, and Collins: "Thank you for your advice and leadership as we have been working through the SARS-CoV-2 'origins' paper. We're happy to say that the paper was just accepted by Nature Medicine." Fauci's response: "Nice job."

The Proximal Origin paper that came out of the ad hoc group's discussions stated: "We do not believe that any type of laboratory scenario is possible." In fairness to the ad hoc group, excerpts published by the press obtained through the Freedom of Information Act may convey a distorted meaning when taken out of the total context of communications. But the impression remains of an ad hoc group that was completely oblivious to their own conflict of interest.

Immediately upon publication, Fauci and Collins referenced the Proximal Origin paper in their press releases, on the podium, and in news conferences. There appeared to be no mention of their backdoor puppeteering of the Proximal Origin paper. When the Proximal Origin paper was published, Collins wrote: "Some folks are even making outrageous claims that the new coronavirus causing the pandemic was engineered in a lab and deliberately released to make people sick."[606]

The authors of the Proximal Origin paper can reasonably and justifiably argue that this article was their opinion at that time. But they did not acknowledge the ad hoc group's involvement in the paper. And as noted above in Andersen's own email from February 12, 2020, the Proximal Origin paper was submitted as a hypothetical commentary but used (without author objection) by the NIH and members of the press as proof to shame people and to ridicule a lab leak origin. The Proximal Origin paper provided the fuel needed for corporate media to attack anyone who dissented with the natural origin hypothesis. It precipitated a media tsunami. As just one of innumerable examples of this (and they are nearly countless), in 2020 ABC News reported in reference to the Proximal Origin paper: "Sorry, Conspiracy Theorists, Study Concludes COVID-19 Is Not a Laboratory Construct."[607]

Backlash to the Proximal Origin Paper and Emails

Since its publication, the Proximal Origin paper has received a growing number of detractors, especially after the corresponding emails from the ad hoc group behind its publication were made public. Sergei Pond, a virologist at Temple University, compared reading the Proximal Origin emails to "watching the TV show Breaking Bad, in which the main character, through a series of small, understandable decisions, ends up in a bad place . . . a desire to downplay the deep concern about the possibility of a lab origin."[608] Similarly, Robert Redfield, the former head of the Centers for Disease Control, testified before Congress in 2023 about the Proximal Origin paper group that:

"when you have a group of people that decide there can only be one point of view, that's problematic, . . . and I'll keep on saying that's antithetical to science and unfortunately that's what they [the NIH and Proximal Origin group] did."[609]

The Defense Intelligence Agency released an unclassified paper in May 2020 titled "Critical Analysis of Andersen et al on the Proximal Origin of SARS-CoV-2." They wrote: "We consider the evidence they presented (in the Proximal Origins paper) and find that it does not prove that the virus arose naturally. In fact, the features of SARS-CoV-2 noted by Andersen et al are consistent with another scenario: that SARS-CoV-2 was developed in a laboratory."[610] The Department of Energy and a classified State Department document have likewise suggested that the more likely origin of COVID-19 was from a lab leak in Wuhan.[611]

Two Nobel Laureates independently spoke out in favor of a laboratory origin. In April 2020, Luc Montagnier—the French virologist who discovered the AIDS virus (chapter 10)—said COVID-19 was most likely manmade.[612] Needless to say, Montagnier was one of the people doxed by the AP Press as a conspiracy theory "superspreader."[613] So too the former president of the California Institute of Technology David Baltimore said that the genetic sequence of the virus was the "smoking gun" indicating a lab origin. Baltimore later rescinded the term "smoking gun" and clarified that he "would not rule out either option."[614]

The Nucleotide Sequence of COVID-19

What caused Andersen to initially tweet that the virus looked manmade? What caused the Defense Intelligence Agency, the Department of Energy, a classified State Department memo, and two Nobel Laureates to contradict the Proximal Origin paper and report that COVID-19 appeared like it originated in a lab?

The coronavirus genes and proteins are shown in Figure 15.2. We will only discuss the spike protein (also known as an S protein). The S protein is what binds coronavirus to a cell. The S protein has two small but different sites: One is responsible for infection and the other for transmissibility. They are called the receptor binding domain and the furin-like cleavage site, respectively. These two sites are like two keys of a double lock. The keys to both interlocks are needed to unlock a human pandemic.

The receptor binding domain on the S protein allows virus-cell binding. It determines whether and how tightly a coronavirus will bind to a human cell. The correct sequence of random mutations must occur to make the optimal receptor binding domain for coronavirus to bind to a human cell. The COVID-19 virus possesses the optimal sequence.

Successful binding allows for infection to occur, but easy transmissibility between humans requires a furin-cleavage site, which is a sequence of twelve nucleotides used to make the four amino acids on the S protein.[615] Furin is a cellular protease. It is a protein that cuts other proteins. Furin occurs naturally in human cells. If the furin-cleavage site is present on the S protein, furin will cut the virus S protein into two smaller proteins. Cleavage of the S protein facilitates the virus opening inside the cell to release viral genes for replication. This results in a more rapid infection and more rapid spread (i.e., transmissibility) to other human cells. The COVID-19 virus had a furin-cleavage site that is not found naturally in coronaviruses of this type.[616]

These two interlocked keys—receptor binding domain and furin-cleavage site—are nature's way of protecting life. If a virus only binds to the receptor binding domain, it cannot replicate rapidly and will spread slowly. While localized epidemics may occur, the infection will "fizzle out" and a pandemic will not occur. Survivors will have immunity, and the species will survive if more mutations cause easier transmissibility.

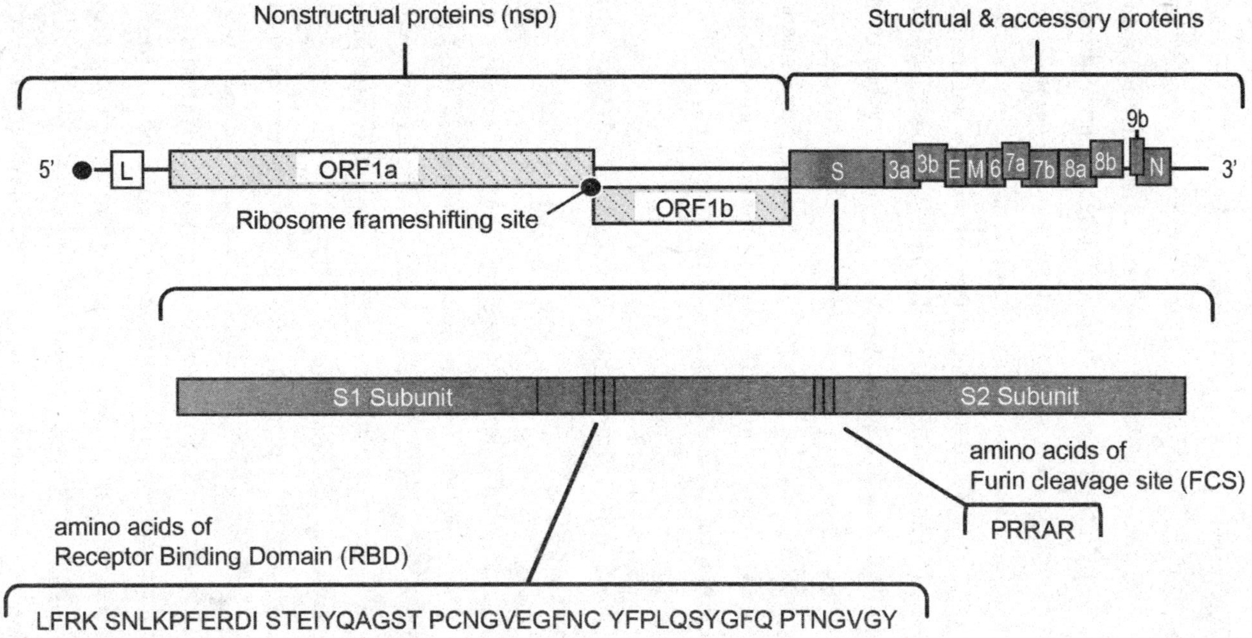

FIGURE 15.2: The Sequence of the COVID-19 Virus (SARS-CoV-2). The order of genes and proteins is shown with emphasis on the S or spike surface protein that is part of the capsule of the coronavirus. The amino acid sequence of the receptor binding domain and the furin-cleavage site of the S protein are shown. Amino acids are represented with one-letter abbreviations. These abbreviations can be found in Figure 9.2 in chapter 9.

A pandemic will only occur if a coronavirus contains the right receptor binding domain site *and* the right furin-cleavage site. This double-lock mechanism prevents a species-terminating viral event from occurring in nature. In nature, other respiratory viruses behave the same way; infectivity is different than transmissibility for influenza.[617] This is why doing gain-of-function research on influenza H5N1 to make it more transmissible caused such an ethical uproar.[618]

For the COVID-19 virus to simultaneously develop both a receptor binding domain and furin-cleavage mutations naturally is not impossible but certainly improbable. Like playing five-card draw with the initial five-hole cards being a royal flush not once but twice in a row. This could happen but is not at all likely, unless the deck was stacked. If the game was fixed and the deck stacked, the simultaneous appearance of SARS-CoV-2 containing the optimal receptor binding domain and optimal furin-cleavage site would be expected.

How Did the Proximal Origin Paper Conclude That COVID-19 Had a Natural Origin?

Why did Andersen suddenly flip from tweeting that "some of the features (potentially) look engineered (by man)" to writing in the Proximal Origin article that "NOT any type of laboratory-based scenario is possible"?[619] What sort of evidence did the Proximal Origin paper offer in support of a natural origin for COVID-19?

Before answering that question, let's put things into perspective from the prior 2003 SARS epidemic infections centered around restaurants and wet markets in Guangdong province. Wet markets get their name from the frequent washing away of the blood of freshly killed animals. In wet markets and restaurants in Guangdong province, the most expensive items are wild animals, including snakes, lizards, bats, pangolins, civets, alligators, seahorses, monkeys, and every species of bird.[620] High-end restaurants will even bring live animals to the customer's for their approval before serving them.[621] In 2003, the SARS-CoV-1 virus was discovered in Guangdong restaurants and in its wet market.

Returning to 2019, when COVID-19 first broke out in Wuhan, Peter Daszak referred back to the 2003 SARS epidemic by stating, "This is absolutely déjà vu all over again." In the same vein, Shi stated the outbreak was: "Nature punishing the uncivilized habits and customs of humans."[622] However, unlike what happened during the 2003 SARS epidemic, an animal source could not be found for COVID-19.

Despite no infected animal source, the Proximal Origin paper dismissed a laboratory origin because no laboratory coronavirus genetic sequences reported by the Wuhan Institute were sufficiently equivalent to COVID-19. They believed that a scientist would start genetic changes on a similar virus that already existed in the laboratory. Among themselves, they said: "Scientists are lazy . . . a scientist would use an already known virus [as the starting point]."[623] The fault in their logic is that it may be possible that not all manmade coronavirus sequences had been logged into the public domain. As stated in the 2014 NIH / NIAID Wuhan Institute of Virology grant: "Sequence data [on new coronaviruses] will be made publicly available via Genbank and shared when requested by other scientists, *as soon as publication is in press*" (emphasis mine). In other words, the Wuhan Institute said they would not release a new coronaviruses genetic sequence unless they already published it in an academic journal. And the NIH had agreed to pay for this!

Another inconsistency with the logic of the Proximal Origin paper and their statement that "scientists are lazy" is that nature is also "lazy." Supporting the idea that nature will also do the least amount of work is a mathematical principle and equation called Hamilton's principle of least action.[624] This equation was first derived by the eighteenth-century mathematician Pierre Maupertuis and was later refined and confirmed by three of the world's greatest mathematicians: Leonhard Euler, Joseph-Louis Lagrange, and William Hamilton. The principle of least action states that nature will always take the path requiring the least action *(minimize the path taken)*. The principle of least action is so profound that it holds true for both the visible world (Newtonian physics) and the atomic world (quantum mechanics). In the case of the origins of COVID-19, the principle of least action suggests that a closely related, if not virtually identical virus, that already existed in nature would be the starting point for the development of the human COVID-19 virus. But so far, no such virus has been found in nature.

Coronaviruses found in pangolins (also known as spiny anteaters) do have an identical receptor binding domain to the COVID-19 virus. Pangolins have long been sold in the Wuhan wet market. To get around that no pangolin or other animal was found to carry the COVID-19 virus, the Proximal Origins paper theorized that the virus had crossed from an undetected pangolin or another animal before jumping to humans. Alternatively, they hypothesized that after jumping into asymptomatic humans for many years, it acquired in a human host the genetic sequences of the SARS-CoV-2 virus that caused the COVID-19 pandemic.[625]

This was the extent of the evidence proposed by the Proximal Origin paper to disprove a lab leak. Did the proverbial fox investigate the chicken coop robbery? Overall, the paper provided no actual proof of either a lab or natural origin of COVID-19. It was merely an opinion, a rationalization, but the way it was promoted gives the impression of an alibi.

One of the Proximal Origin authors, Eddie Holmes, is a distinguished scientist from Sydney, Australia. He was the New South Wales Scientist of the Year in 2020. He subsequently wrote: "I've absolutely no problem with people knowing that my views on this issue have evolved as more data have appeared. That's science. Indeed,

I've told this to many people: the way see [*sic*] it is that we set-up an hypothesis and then tested it. As far I [*sic*] can tell we are only 'guilty' of following the proper scientific method."[626]

Unfortunately, ad hoc discussions in developing the Proximal Origin paper happened without transparency, and several of the individuals involved in that discussion were powerful people who controlled tens of billions of dollars in NIH funding. These same individuals would be compromised if COVID-19 arose from a Chinese lab that they were funding. At best, they did not appreciate the bias that arises from their own conflict of interest. The Proximal Origin paper morphed into the definitive gospel to condemn a laboratory origin.

Peter Daszak and the Condemnation of the Lab Origin Hypothesis

Peter Daszak of EcoHealth Alliance also jumped into the fray to support the "conspiracy theory" narrative. As a reminder, Peter Daszak, along with Shi Zhengli, was awarded an NIH grant to continue gain-of-function research at the Wuhan Institute of Virology after gain-of-function research was stopped in America. Along with Farrar, who was involved behind the scenes in the Proximal Origin paper, he co-authored two *Lancet* articles published in 2020. These two *Lancet* articles included more than twenty distinguished scientists from the United States, Australia, the United Kingdom, and Germany. *The Lancet* is a top-tier medical journal.

Published online on February 18, 2020, the first article was titled "Statement in Support of the Scientists, Public Health Professionals, and Medical Professionals of China Combatting COVID 19."[627] It stated: "We stand together to strongly condemn conspiracy theories suggesting that COVID 19 does not have a natural origin." The second article was published on July 17, 2020. It was titled "Science,

Not Speculation, Is Essential to Determine How SARS-CoV-2 Reached Humans."[628]

The irony is that these articles painted an investigation into a lab origin as unfounded speculation and "not science." Perhaps they were projecting the fear mongering they were reportedly trying to stop. As Shakespeare wrote in Hamlet, thou "doth protest too much, methinks."

Were all the authors of these two *Lancet* articles aware that the NIH funded gain-of-function research in Wuhan after it was halted in America? Were any of the authors potentially conflicted by their own gain-of-function research, the prospect of acquiring future NIH research funding, or fear of losing already existing funding? Were they aware that the Wuhan Institute of Virology was trying to find or make coronaviruses that could more easily infect humans? Were any aware of the NIH's behind-the-scenes involvement in the Proximal Origin article? Were any of them aware of the furin-cleavage site in SARS-CoV-2? Did any of them question the improbability of both optimal receptor binding domain and optimal furin-cleavage site sequences suddenly appearing simultaneously with no documented animal source?

The Proximal Origin article and Daszak's *Lancet* articles set off an inquisition against scientific questioning. This inquisition was not initiated by medieval clergy but by twenty-first-century scientists. It inhibited independent, nonconflicted inquiry and gave time for the evidence to grow cold.

The 2021 China-WHO COVID-19 Origin Report

In 2021, the World Health Organization (WHO) organized a committee to investigate the source of COVID-19. It consisted of ten people from ten countries.[629] Controversy surrounded the WHO COVID-19 committee, because it allowed the investigation to be controlled by Chinese officials and included Daszak, the middleman in NIH funding of the Wuhan Institute's coronavirus research. One must ask why Daszak didn't recognize his own conflict of interest and excuse himself?

The WHO report did not perform a forensic study of the Wuhan Institute laboratory. Nor did it interview its personnel from the time of pandemic onset or gain access to computer records, lab notebooks, and stored samples. Nor did it perform an independent review of standard operating procedures or biosafety incident reports. Of the 313-page WHO report, only four pages mentioned a possible lab accident.[630] The WHO report concluded that a lab leak was "extremely unlikely."[631]

The Chinese government had tested thousands of samples from animals. They did not find an animal positive for the COVID-19 virus. The wet market and other sites were clean. Daszak was quoted as saying: "A thousand samples is a great start but there's more to do [i.e., more animals to study]."[632]

Backlash to the China-WHO Origin Report

On May 14, 2021, eighteen scientists published a letter in the journal *Science* titled "Investigate the origins of COVID 19."[633] They requested a proper evaluation with "balanced consideration" for both the natural origin and the lab origin theories. The *Lancet* also published a statement on April 10, 2021, supporting more investigation into a lab origin titled "Calls for Transparency After SARS-Cov-2 Report."[634] The US State Department issued a communiqué two-and-a-half weeks after the *Lancet* letter on the China–WHO origin report. It stated that "It is critical for independent experts to have full access to all pertinent human, animal, and environmental data, research, and personnel involved in the early stages of the outbreak relevant to determining how this pandemic emerged."[635]

The European Union Diplomatic Service also issued a communiqué entitled: "EU Statement on the WHO-Led COVID-19 Origins Study." Like the US State Department communiqué, the European Union statement encouraged continued review of all the available data. It stated that "Only through a thorough review of the origins of the virus and its transmission into the human population, will we be able to better understand and control this pandemic . . . We request the WHO to continue the studies and present a clear timeline for the follow-up work, and we wish to be regularly briefed."[636]

The director general of the WHO, Dr. Tedros Ghebreyesus, did organize a second visit to China, which would include an audit of the Wuhan Institute lab and initial human cases. Zeng Yixin, deputy director of the Chinese Health Commission, said that a second WHO visit would exhibit a "lack of respect for common sense, (and) arrogant toward science."[637] Needless to say, a second WHO investigation never happened. Ironically, by this point in time both the Chinese Health Commission and the NIH had exploited the narrative that questioning them goes against "science."[638] Most of the American corporate media outlets amplified their message. In truth, however, restricting investigations by saying an investigation is anti-science is anti-science. What is the psychological benefit that underlies denial?

In 2021, Alina Chan, a Canadian postdoctoral fellow in molecular biology at Harvard and the Broad Institute of MIT, wrote in her book called *Viral: The Search for the Origin of COVID-19*: "In China there are likely scientists or administrators who know for certain that one of the hypotheses [natural versus lab origin] . . . is correct." For one of those sources to come forward, Chan admits, "great courage will be required."[639] Chan herself has shown such courage in America. After she gave an interview to *The New York Times* in June of 2024, forty scientists ganged up on this lone female postdoc in the *Journal of Virology* by accusing her of "promoting" a lab leak. They wrote that her "suggesting a lab leak stokes the flames of an anti-science, conspiracy-driven agenda."[640]

DEFUSE Grant Proposal (HR00111850017): The Smoking Gun?

Recall from earlier the two genetic locations on the viral surface S protein that suggest it is manmade—the receptor binding domain and a furin-cleavage site. We know that Daszak, Shi, and Baric had been successfully collaborating for a decade to find or genetically create a receptor binding domain in the viral spike protein with optimal affinity for human cells. In 2018, just over a year before the COVID-19 pandemic, Daszak, Shi, and Baric spilled the beans that they wanted to engineer a furin-cleavage site into a SARS-like coronavirus. They even submitted a grant seeking funding from the United States military to create a new coronavirus that would contain the furin-cleavage site.

Their grant was titled DEFUSE, which is an abbreviation for "defusing the threat of bat born coronaviruses." As the grant states: "We will analyze all SARS-CoV gene sequences for . . . the potential presence of furin-cleavage sites. . . . We will introduce appropriate human specific cleavage sites and evaluate (viral) growth."[641] DEFUSE was submitted to the Defense Advanced Research Projects Agency for funding by the Department of Defense, which refused to fund it. After COVID-19 broke out, Daszak, Shi, and Baric remained silent about their DEFUSE grant proposal.

In 2020, Major Joseph Murphy of the US Marine Corps War Fighting Laboratory found the shelved DEFUSE grant in a file. In January 2021, Major Murphy wrote a report and copied his assessment to the Inspector General of the Department of Defense. The DEFUSE grant was a road map to combine the receptor binding domain with a furin-cleavage site, which is the unique genetic fingerprint of the COVID-19 pandemic virus.

The catch-22 of getting a grant is that data is needed to get a grant, but a grant is needed to get data. The way grant applicants get around this is that they divert funds from a currently funded project to generate the data needed to get the next grant. The Department of Defense had refused to fund the DEFUSE grant. It is, however, unknown if one or more of these investigators went ahead and inserted the furin-cleavage site using their current funds.

Professor Jeffrey Sachs at Columbia University served as the chair of the *Lancet* COVID commission.[642] In 2022, Sachs along with Neil Harrison (also of Columbia University) published an article in the *Proceedings of the National Academy of Sciences* calling for an independent investigation into the work of and correspondence between Daszak at EcoHealth Alliance, Baric at the University of North Carolina at Chapel Hill, and Shi at the Wuhan Institute of Virology.[643] Sachs and Harrison discovered that the furin-cleavage site of the COVID-19 virus is identical to a human cell furin-cleavage site that was being studied by investigators at the University of North Carolina.[644] In response to *The Lancet* COVID-19 commission findings, one of the original Proximal Origin authors stated: "Harrison and Sachs allege that scientists at NIH and elsewhere, including myself and colleagues, conspired to suppress theories of a laboratory origin of SARS-CoV-2. This is false."[645]

In an interview titled "Why the Chair of *The Lancet*'s COVID-19 Commission Thinks the US Government Is Preventing a Real Investigation into the Pandemic," Sachs said: "I chaired the commission for the *Lancet* for two years on COVID. I'm pretty convinced it came out of U.S. lab biotechnology, not out of nature. . . . We don't know for sure, I should be absolutely clear. But there's enough evidence that it should be looked into. And it's not being investigated, not in the United States, not anywhere. And I think for real reasons that they don't want to look underneath the rug."[646] The former director of the Centers for Disease Control, Robert Redfield, also stated in a podcast "I think there is a real possibility that the virus's birthplace was Chapel Hill," where Baric, who collaborates with Shi and Dazak, is located.[647]

A Dystopian World of Scientific and Medical Censorship

Nathaniel Hawthorne in his 1850 historical fiction *The Scarlet Letter* exposed the fear and projection of insecurity by reference to seventeenth-century Puritans living in Massachusetts Bay Colony. At the beginning of Hawthorne's story, the main character, Hester Prynne, is belittled by a crowd of her Bostonian neighbors after giving birth to a child out of wedlock. They make her stand in the public square upon the gallows and wear a scarlet letter A for "adulterer" around her neck for the rest of her life. When looking at the response to COVID-19 by corporate media and some elected officials, has anything really changed since the 1600s? It appears that the only difference is the colonial town square of shame has been replaced by worldwide corporate and social media digital humiliation. According to Attorney General Eric Schmitt, when asked numerous times under oath about colluding with social media, Fauci responded with "I don't recall."[648]

Censorship surrounding the COVID-19 pandemic has by no means been restricted solely to questions regarding the origins of the virus. On September 9, 2021, the American Board of Internal Medicine, American Board of Family Medicine, and the American Board of Pediatrics issued a statement that threatened to rescind physicians' certifications to practice medicine if they presented "misinformation" different than the government's version about the COVID-19 vaccine (Box 15.3). The COVID-19 vaccine is a novel type of previously untested messenger RNA vaccine. Health care officials should be encouraged to monitor and report short- and long-term complications to better define risk benefit for different groups of people in diverse scenarios. Bullying in the form of written threats is intimidating, and it inhibits well-meaning physicians from thinking independently and publishing and communicating honest concerns about COVID-19 vaccine-related complications.[649]

One of the subplots of the 1984 philosophical novel by Milan Kundera called *The Unbearable Lightness of Being* is about how a talented Czechoslovakian physician's career was being destroyed for contradicting the Communist government during the 1968 Prague Spring. Who could have imagined this happening in a "free" country? How is the America government's performance any different than what the Chinese government did to Li Wenliang, as we saw in chapter 1, when he first announced COVID-19 to the world on social media? The difference is the Chinese government had the decency to apologize to Li's surviving family and to honor him postmortem.

Denigration of the lab leak hypothesis was done by organizations and people with something significant to lose, including their funding, reputations, and careers as well as (at least for some) possible criminal referral. Why was the NIH role in this not recognized as a conflict of interest? Real science is the principle of keeping an open mind. Real science is *not* censorship, intimidation, and threats. On the contrary, science encourages questions. Research is repeating the search (*re*-searching). As Nobel Laureate Richard Feynman once said: "Science is a culture of doubt. If you thought that science was certain—well, that is just an error on your part."

The risks of creating new viruses were not taken seriously by the NIH, and subsequent actions were fatally compromised by a conflict of interest arising from that failure. Kill switches can and have been added to viruses. Should we get guarantees that such checks have been put in place to stop the new virus before creating it?

Box 15.3: Statement from the American Board of Internal Medicine, the American Board of Family Medicine, and the American Board of Pediatrics.

American Board of Internal Medicine

Important: Joint Statement from ABFM, ABIM & ABP on Dissemination of Misinformation

Dear Dr. Burt,

The Federation of State Medical Boards (FSMB), which supports its member state medical licensing boards, has recently issued a statement saying that providing misinformation about the COVID-19 vaccine contradicts physicians' ethical and professional responsibilities, and therefore may subject a physician to disciplinary actions, including suspension or revocation of their medical license. We at the American Board of Family Medicine (ABFM), the American Board of Internal Medicine (ABIM), and the American Board of Pediatrics (ABP) support FSMB's position. We also want all physicians certified by our boards to know that such unethical or unprofessional conduct may prompt their respective board to take action that could put their certification at risk.

Expertise matters, and board certified physicians have demonstrated that they have stayed current in their field. Spreading misinformation or falsehoods to the public during a time of a public health emergency goes against everything our boards and our community of board certified physicians stand for. The evidence that we have safe, effective and widely available vaccines against COVID-19 is overwhelming. We are particularly concerned about physicians who use their authority to denigrate vaccination at a time when vaccines continue to demonstrate excellent effectiveness against severe illness, hospitalization and death.

We all look to board certified physicians to provide outstanding care and guidance; providing misinformation about a lethal disease is unethical, unprofessional and dangerous. In times of medical emergency, the community of expert physicians committed to science and evidence collectively shares a responsibility for giving the public the most accurate and timely health information available, so they can make decisions that work best for themselves and their families.

Warren Newton, MD, MPH
President and CEO
American Board of Family Medicine

Richard J. Baron, MD
President and CEO
American Board of Internal Medicine

David G. Nichols, MD, MBA
President and CEO
American Board of Pediatrics

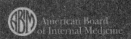

Accountability and traceability are also a potent kill switch when it comes to human behavior. At a time when information traveled by foot or horseback, Samuel Morse received a letter that his wife was ill. By the time he arrived, she was buried. Morse channeled his despair into making communication of information faster. In 1838, he invented Morse code, a system of one-dimensional dots and dashes encoding letters in the alphabet that could be sent via electrical telegraph. Morse code essentially killed the Pony Express. In 1949, the principle behind Morse's discovery led to the invention of barcodes, which are read in one horizontal dimension by a laser light. In 1994, QR codes that use two dimensions (horizontal and vertical) were invented to capture more information. Incorporation of a QR code identification marker and air-tag to identify and locate each vial of virus would be one plausible way of holding labs accountable.

In the future, artificial intelligence will likely be used to model the optimal receptor binding site for a virus, which can then be used to create a vaccine. As humanity creates and uses artificial intelligence, one or more kill switches should also be considered. Otherwise, metallic life may someday look back at carbon-based life, as we now look back at viruses, dangerously effective in killing and reproducing.

Summary

Did the COVID-19 virus jump from an animal into humans, or did it escape from a lab? Entrenched polar-opposite camps still persist.[650] In truth, either origin remains possible. Future research may yet prove a natural or laboratory origin. But what do we really know here?

What we do know is that Shi Zhengli from the Wuhan Institute of Virology and Ralph Baric from the University of North Carolina published a 2015 paper on NIH-funded genetic manipulation of coronaviruses. It was characterized as "risky research" that ultimately was followed by a three-year moratorium on gain-of-function research on respiratory viruses. Continuation of their research was defended by Daszak at EcoHealth Alliance.

From 2014 to 2019, Daszak, Shi, and Baric collaborated on another NIH grant to collect, study, and genetically manipulate the receptor binding domain from different coronaviruses in the Chinese Wuhan Institute. In 2018, Daszak, Shi, and Baric submitted a grant requesting funding to insert a furin-cleavage site into coronaviruses in Wuhan.

In November 2019, the COVID-19 pandemic began in Wuhan and spread worldwide. The virus that caused the COVID-19 pandemic suddenly appeared with the perfect receptor binding site and furin-cleavage site for human infection and transmissibility. At the onset of the pandemic, Anthony Fauci—the director of the National Institutes of Allergy and Infectious Disease, which along with the National Institutes of Health funded the research in Wuhan—helped hatch the Proximal Origin paper that was aggressively exploited to discredit a laboratory accident. At the time of this book's completion, no natural animal source for the COVID-19 virus has been discovered.

Millions died during the COVID-19 pandemic. No forensic investigation of offices, laboratory work, notebooks, emails, computers, laptops, virus sequences, stored samples, materials transferred between labs, cell phones, or phone logs in China or America has been performed. Nor have any personnel or collaborators present in the lab before or during the pandemic been questioned in either China or America.

The curtain fell on Act 1 of a worldwide horrific tragedy when President Joe Biden on his last day in office awarded Fauci a presidential pardon. Biden's pre-emptive pardon will likely dampen future investigations. What will Act 2 bring? In matters so grave as these, the truth needs to be uncovered.

COVID-19 is a gigantic red flag on the behavior of our institutions, corporate media, and political system. Time is the distance that makes us lose site of the past. It has been more than half a decade since the outbreak of COVID-19. If our "leaders," institutions, and corporate media continue to ignore and fail to investigate the root causes of unintended mistakes, it is at our own risk and our children's peril. What is the root cause of this mess? As Deep Throat supposedly whispered to reporter Bob Woodward about the 1970s Watergate scandal: "Follow the money." The final chapter of this book will do just that.

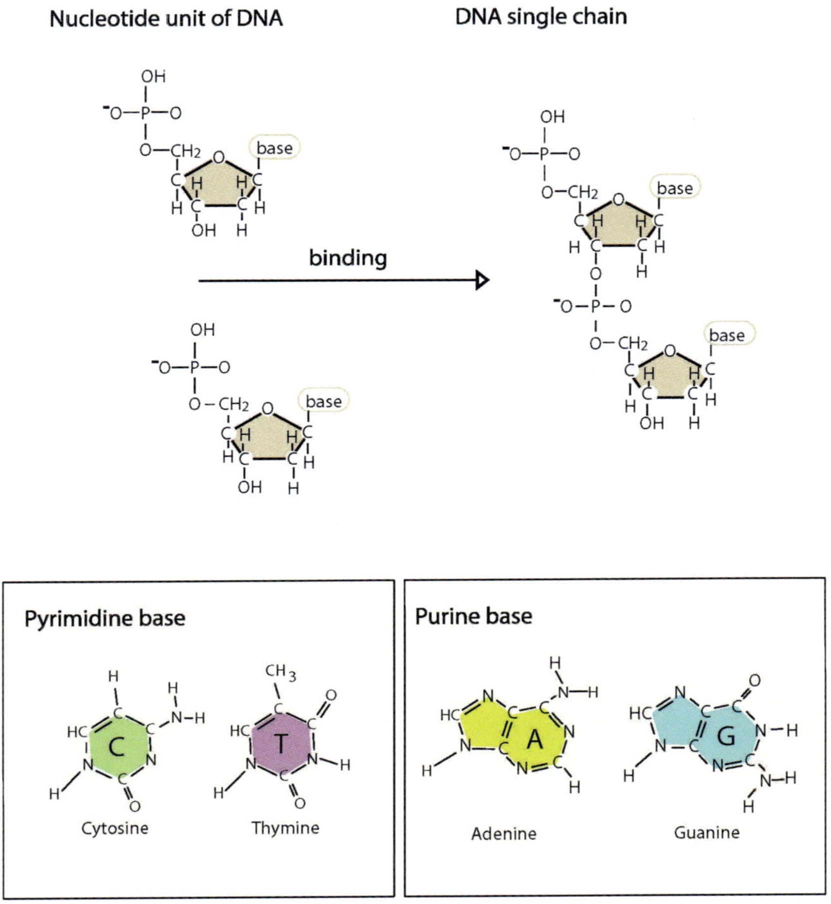

FIGURE 8.1: Nucleotide bases (cytosine, thymine, adenine, guanine) of deoxyribonucleic acid (DNA). Human DNA contains three billion base pairs of nucleotides linked together into forty-six separate chromosomes.

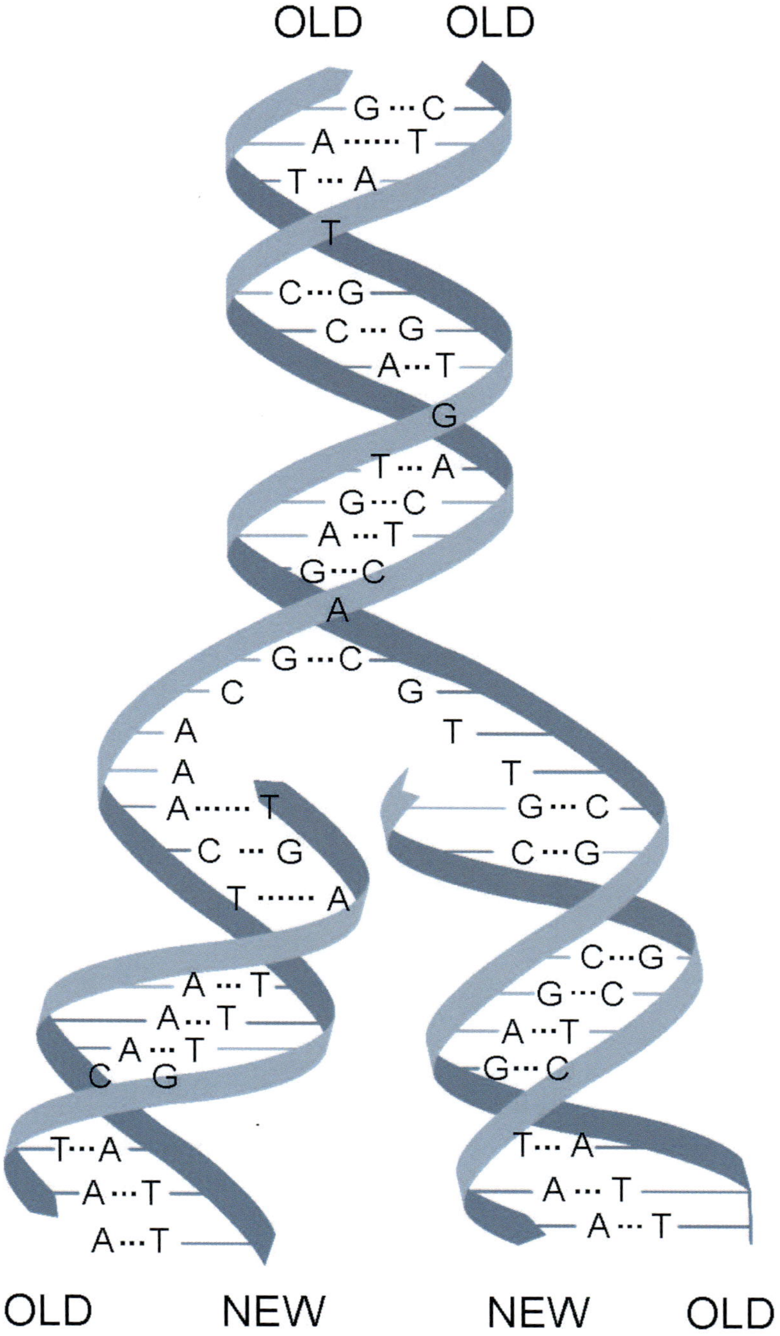

FIGURE 8.3: Double-stranded DNA undergoing replication to duplicate itself during the creation of new cells. A = adenine, C = cytosine, G =guanine, T = thymine. Blue ribbons are sugar (deoxyribose) backbone.

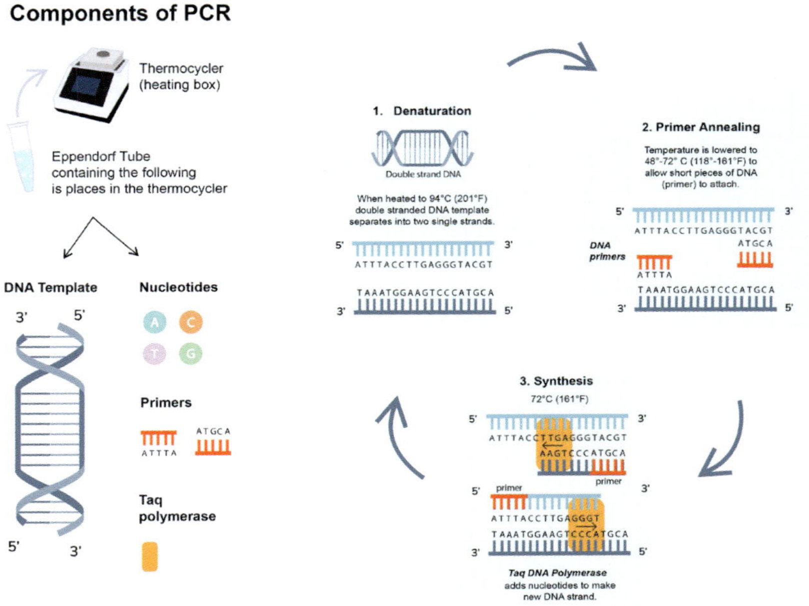

FIGURE 8.4: Scheme of polymerase chain reaction (PCR). There are three steps to PCR: 1) denaturation (separation of double strand DNA), 2) primer annealing (binding), 3) synthesis of complementary DNA strand. The process repeats in an automated cycle within a bench-top instrument called a thermocycler. In the first round of amplification, two strands become four, then four become eight, with each amplification cycle doubling the amount of DNA.

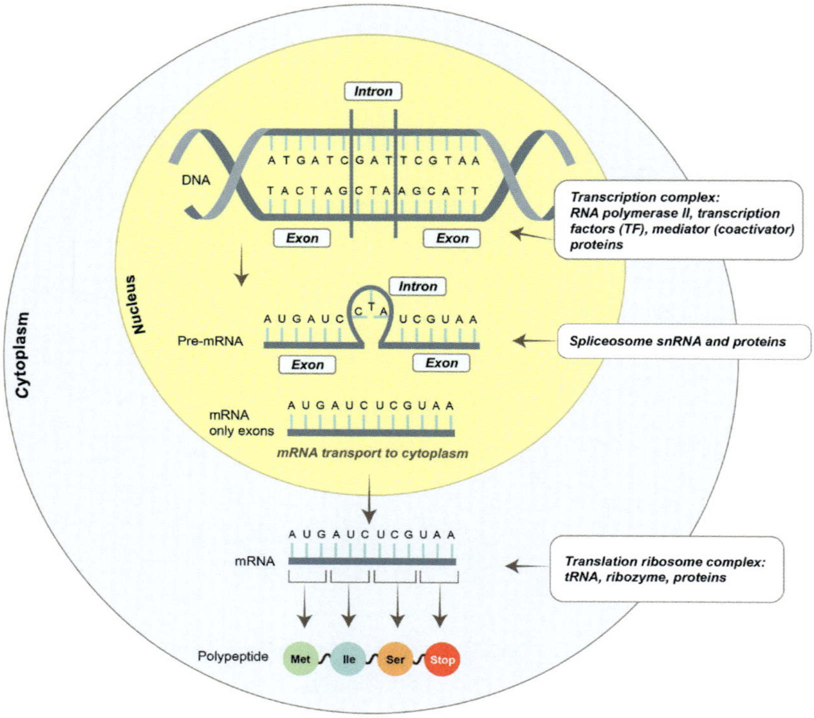

FIGURE 9.5: How a cell makes proteins from deoxyribonucleic acid (DNA). The cell uses a transcription complex to transcribe DNA into pre-messenger ribonucleic acid (RNA). A spliceosome complex next converts pre-messenger RNA into messenger RNA. Then, a translation complex converts the messenger RNA into proteins. These complexes are composed of multiple proteins and different types of RNA including small nuclear RNA, transfer RNA, and ribozyme RNA.

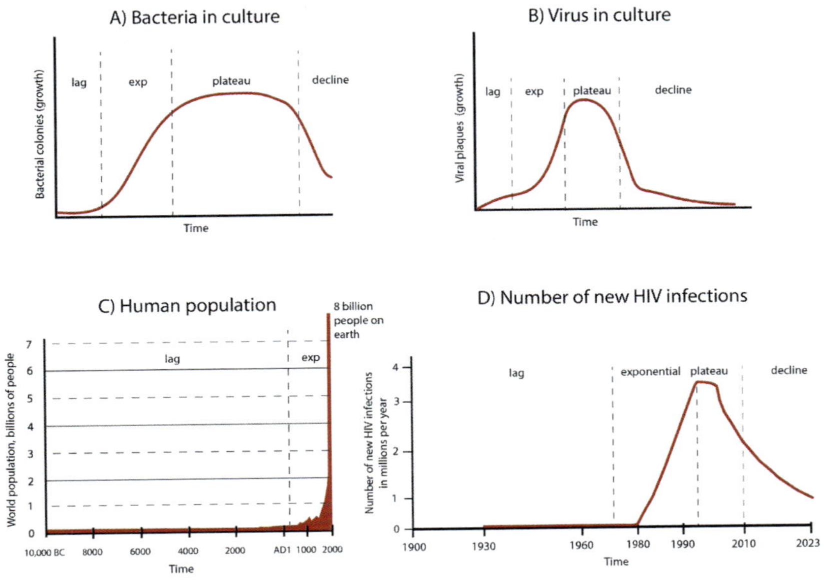

FIGURE 10.1: Life enters an exponential growth phase when predators are removed and food is plentiful. (A) Growth of bacteria in a culture dish counted as number of bacterial colonies. (B) Virus grown in cultured cells counted as number of plaques. (C) The human population struggled until the Agriculture Revolution and bacteria and viruses were controlled with antibiotics and vaccines. (D) According to the phylogenetic models, HIV virus existed in a few humans as early as 1931. In the 1980s, HIV infections exponentially increased. Since the late 1990s, new HIV infections are declining with the introduction of antiviral drugs (the predators).

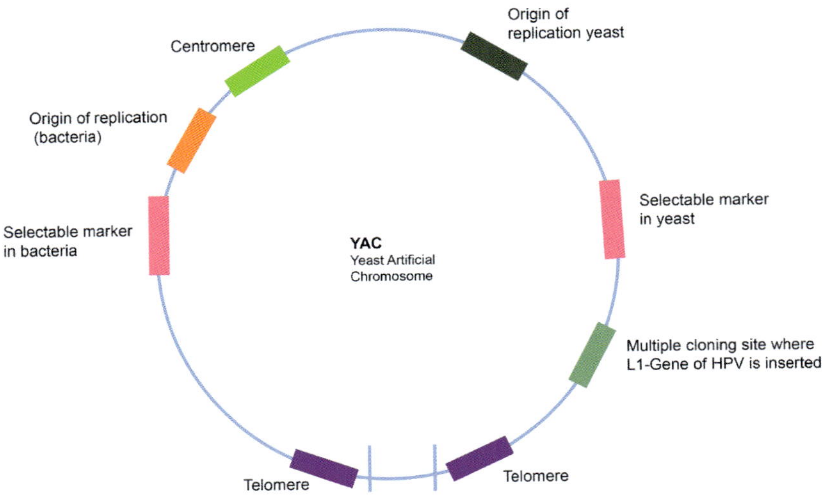

FIGURE 11.4: Yeast artificial chromosome (YAC).

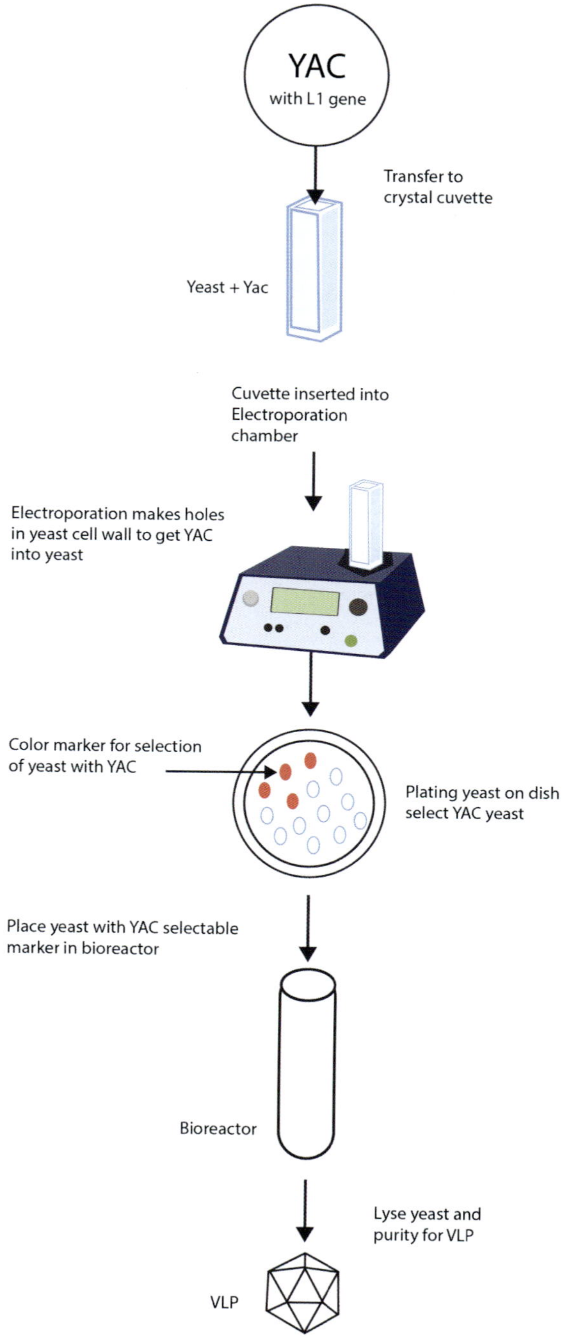

FIGURE 11.5: Production of the human papilloma virus (HPV) vaccine. Electroporation refers to electricity punching holes in the yeast membrane so that the yeast artificial chromosome (YAC) may enter. VLP = virus like particle.

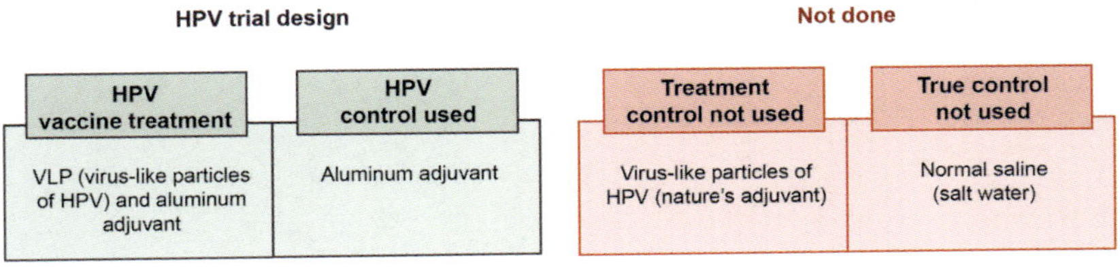

FIGURE 11.6: The optimal human papillomavirus (HPV) vaccine trial would include all four or at least three trial arms.

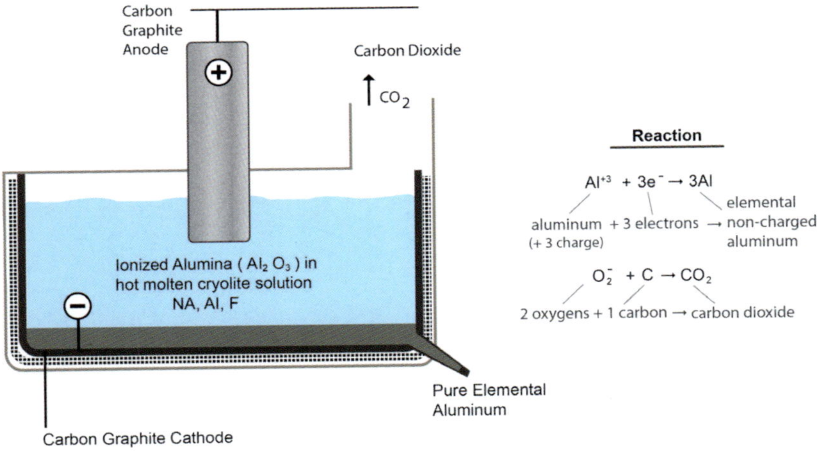

FIGURE 13.1: The Hall-Heroult process to make aluminum. Al = aluminum, C = carbon, F = fluorine, e = electron, NA = sodium, O = oxygen.

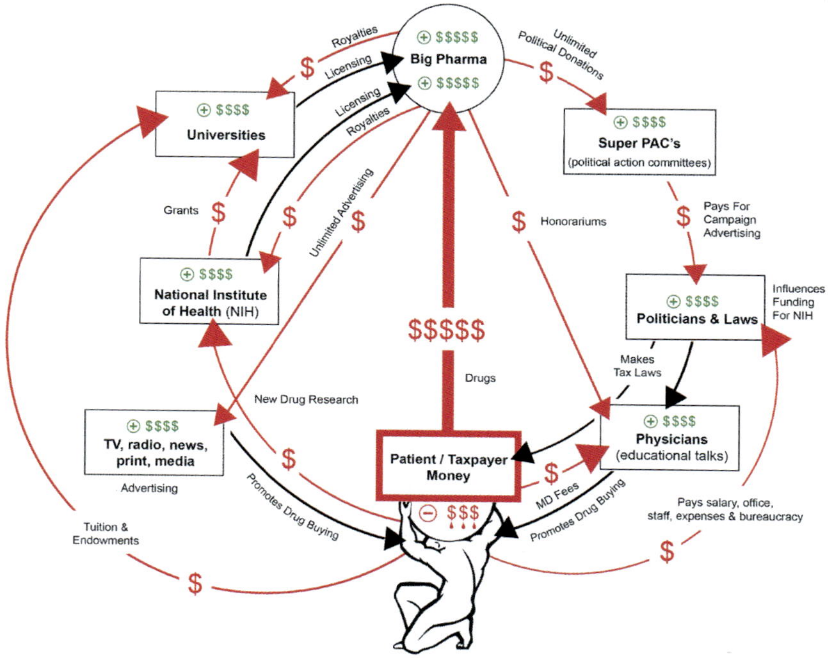

FIGURE 16.1: The cycle of money to collaborators versus from DOPEs (taxpayers and patients). DOPE = **D**o not have the **O**pportunity to **P**articipat**E**. PAC = political action committee.

CHAPTER 16

A Root Cause Analysis: Truth Is Not Black and White; It Is Hidden Behind the Screen

There is a tendency to blame one person or one group of people. But that will not correct the root causes of a problem.—RKB

The only real danger that exists is man himself. He is the great danger. And we are pitifully unaware of it.—Carl Jung[651]

Miranda—"People have to know, we meant it for the best. To make people safer."
Mal—"Somebody has to speak for these people."
Simon—"Do we have a plan?"
Mal—"Put it on every screen."
—Serenity *(2005 film)*

People are not allowed to investigate themselves. Obviously, a person would have a conflict of interest in judging his or her own conduct. In contrast, agencies, institutes, and departments of local, state, and federal governments are routinely allowed to investigate themselves. The COVID-19 tragedy is a case in point. Career institutionalists concerned about professional reputation and self-advancement have a conflict of interest. To prevent this quisling behavior, a review process located outside of the institution would be a more appropriate and nonconflicted kill switch. To understand how we deal with intergroup problems, we turn to game theories—theoretical scenarios on how people settle conflicts.

Game Theory

World War II ended when America dropped the atomic bombs named "Little Boy" and "Fat Man" on Hiroshima and Nagasaki. Hundreds of thousands of Japanese died in an instant and of radiation poisoning over the subsequent years. Several American politicians, military brass, and university academics advocated for preemptive war against Russia to prevent it from acquiring nuclear bombs. Francis Matthews, Secretary of the Navy, advocated becoming "aggressors for peace."[652] The mathematician John von Neuman, who was a pioneer in game theory, remarked: "If you say bomb them tomorrow, I say why not bomb them today?"[653]

Once Russia detonated its own nuclear bomb in 1949, America's nuclear monopoly ended. In its place, a nuclear arms race jumped into the stratosphere. Nuclear weapons forever changed warfare in unpredictable ways. Because unorthodox thinking was needed, the US military funded an outside non-military corporation called RAND, an abbreviation for research and development

The RAND Corporation had carte blanche to hire whomever they wanted, to study whatever they wanted, to be independent of the military, and to go outside of the usual military thinking no matter how bizarre. The military needed options. RAND employed individuals from various fields, including mathematicians who studied game theories on how people settle conflicts. Game theory strives to understand how people solve conflicts to their best interest in different situations. Let us look at some of these situations.

Cooperative Game Theory

The Prisoners' Dilemma: One-Time Choice to Collaborate or Defect

Developed in 1950 by RAND mathematicians Merrill Flood and Melvin Dresher, the theoretical game known as the prisoners' dilemma involves two equal participants who are given a one-time choice to collaborate or defect.[654] In this scenario, the two prisoners have been arrested for a crime and have been kept in solitary confinement with no means of communication. Each prisoner is then interviewed by the authorities in separate rooms regarding who is guilty for the offense. Here are the rules:

- If *neither* prisoner says who did the crime, they both spend one year in jail.
- If *only one* of the prisoners says the other did the crime, the snitch goes free and the other spends four years in jail.
- If *both* prisoners say the other person did the crime, they both spend two years in jail.

In the prisoners' dilemma, when both people collaborate to keep their mouths shut, they receive a far shorter sentence than if both attempted to defect (i.e., snitch on each other). However, most pairs defect, insofar as if the other person snitches and they do not, the one prisoner will go free, while the other will spend four years (i.e., twice as much time) in prison.

According to game theory, the prisoners' dilemma reveals that people determine their course of action compared to the other party, not on the overall good for both. As the expression goes: "People want to see you do well but not better than them."

Tit for Tat: Repetitive Choice to Collaborate or Defect

An iterative (repetitive) version of the prisoners' dilemma was designed by political scientist Robert Axelrod. He called it "tit for tat."[655] The rules are the same as for prisoners' dilemma, except that (1) you get a positive reward of money (or points) depending on whether you collaborate or defect; and (2) you will have to choose to collaborate or defect multiple times against the same opponent. You must consider what your counterpart will do in the next round based on your prior response. The goal is to win as much money (or points) as possible. Here is an example:

- If *both* individuals collaborate, both get twenty dollars.
- If *only one* collaborates, he gets nothing, while the one who defected gets forty dollars.
- If *neither* collaborates and both defect, both get ten dollars.

Axelrod asked mathematicians to design different response strategies to optimize points, such that one of the pair always collaborates; one always defects; one defects only after the other defected in the prior response; one would randomly defect; one defects two consecutive times after a defection by the other player; and other combinations. Axelrod had a computer run two strategies against each other for two hundred iterations and then had each strategy go up against every other strategy. He ran fifteen strategies against each other and then repeated the entire computer tournament multiple times.

The top performing strategies all emphasized collaboration and forgiveness. The best strategy collaborated and forgave the other person when they chose to defect but was not a pushover. The winning strategy retaliated when the opponent defected, but only once after each opponent's defection. Collaboration was profitable, whereas repeated retaliation and sustained noncollaboration was not profitable.

Game theory strategies run on computers reaffirmed what many of the world's major religions have been saying for millennia: Do unto others as you would have done unto yourself; confront injustice but then forgive transgressions.

During the Cold War, America and Russia had been locked into a permanent defect (noncollaborative) response. Both sides spent a fortune on nuclear proliferation trying to one-up each other. Game theory pointed to another mutually beneficial and cost-saving strategy.[656] America and Russia eventually switched strategies, moving from each side being stuck in a permanent noncollaborative, defect response to each side collaborating on arms reduction. Under supervision from the other side, each side began a mutually beneficial gradual dismantling of nuclear warheads.

In the above two game theory scenarios, the two participants in the game (the two criminals in the prisoners' dilemma, or America versus Russia in tit for tat) were roughly equivalent in power. In real life, however, one participant—especially if that participant is the government—typically possesses significantly greater resources. Let's extend traditional game theory to include unequal participants—that is, participants with unequal power. When there are unequal participants, game theory is either covertly or overtly forced.

Forced Game Theory

Unequal Participants: Repetitive Collaborate or Defect

In terms of game theory, let us look at a junior researcher's options in writing a paper supervised by more powerful people who have a vested interest in the paper's conclusion and who also control the researcher's future funding opportunities. The goal is not to ascribe motive to anyone. None of us have any idea what is in another person's mind.

The intent is not to question honesty or sincerity in writing a conclusion for COVID-19 origin such as: "We do not believe that any type of laboratory scenario is possible."[657] Instead let us, from a hypothetical game theory scenario, analyze how uniformity of opinion may be shaped when participants in the group have markedly unequal resources, reputation, and power.

The National Institute of Allergy and Infectious Diseases—the same institution headed by Fauci for nearly forty years—distributes $6 billion every year in research funding. It is the major funding source for genetic manipulation to create new viruses. It was funding coronavirus research at the Wuhan Institute of Virology. NIAID has a conflict of interest and a self-invested bias in the outcome of your paper. It also controls the grant funding of virologists doing research.

If you collaborate, your paper will be published in a prestigious journal. Publications are one of the currencies used to acquire academic promotions. You would also become a part of an exclusive inner circle that would likely pay future collaborative dividends, such as being subsequently awarded a multi-million-dollar NIH contract.[658]

If you defect and maintain that the COVID-19 virus has a man-made signature, your paper will have trouble getting published. Members of the impromptu committee (or their friends) would likely be the reviewers and would probably reject your paper. If your paper finally was published, it would likely be in a fairly obscure journal. And if that journal learned that the most influential and largest research funding agency in the world refused to be a part of your publication, your paper would likely be retracted. Your academic career could be irrevocably forestalled or perhaps finished.

Like the fictional character Mr. Andersen (Neo) in the 1999 movie *The Matrix*, you have now entered the world of game theory. Like in the book *Dark Matter* by Blake Crouch, you are now confronted with a choice that will alter the subsequent course of your reality. In the theoretical world of game theory, you have one self-preservation choice: collaborate. For players with markedly unequal resources, the weaker player's "rational" move to advance is always to collaborate.

Unequal Participants: Collaborate or DOPE

In the real world, people in the game may not even know that the game is being played on them by the collaborating group. In this game, DOPE stands for Do not have the Opportunity to ParticipatE. To understand this "collaborate or DOPE" game, we need to understand the flow of money, that is, who is unknowingly paying (i.e., the DOPEs) and who is receiving the money (i.e., the collaborators). To understand how this game is played by pharmaceutical companies, the NIH, and universities, we need to be aware of the Bayh-Dole Act.

The 1980 Bayh-Dole Act is a bipartisan piece of legislation sponsored by Indiana Democratic Senator Bayh and Republican Kansas Senator Dole. It was a well-intentioned law that was designed to accelerate practical applications of research by allowing the NIH, universities, and drug companies to share profits generated from taxpayer funded research. It gave the NIH and universities ownership of taxpayer-funded research that they could license to drug companies for a share of the profits from sales.

The unforeseen consequence of the Bayh-Dole Act was that universities, the National Institutes of Health, and pharmaceutical companies became joined at the hip in sharing profits from pushing drugs and vaccines upon an innocent public. How does this work in practice? The collaborators in this game are universities, the National Institutes of Health, and drug companies. The researcher is a pawn in the game. The indirect beneficiaries are legacy news and political action committees. The DOPEs are the taxpayers and patients. Here are the rules.

Researcher pawn. A researcher's creative thoughts, persistence, networking, decades of education, experience, creativity, and writing skills are all used to obtain a grant. Whatever the grant amount, an additional 50 to 90 percent is automatically taken by the university for what are euphemistically called "indirect" costs (see chapter 6). Then comes the researcher's hard work to do the experiments, interpret the results, and make the discovery. The researcher may even pay out of pocket to patent his or her invention.

Because of the Bayh-Dole Act, the researcher's intellectual property is *not* owned by the researcher. It is also *not* owned by the taxpayer who paid for it. The researcher, depending on the owner's "generosity," may get a small fraction of the owner's profit. So who is the owner that moves the chess pieces (does the terms) with the drug company?

University Collaborator. Because of the Bayh-Dole Act, the university owns the intellectual property rights to a researcher's thoughts and work. The university writes the license and determines the rules a drug company must follow, including who they can hire and what the drug company can say. The university may write into the license that they can audit the company's books and hiring policies and limit a company's "free speech." Universities can also award themselves hundreds of thousands or millions of dollars in milestone payments and additional drug royalties in the ballpark of 5 to 8 percent of the total pre-tax sales profits. Since 1980, whenever you buy a drug or a vaccine, you are also paying money to a tax-free university, despite the fact that many of these prestigious higher education institutions already have tax-free endowments exceeding tens of billions of dollars.

Since the medieval period, people have invested in a corporation in return for stock shares. If the corporation lost money, they lost their investment. If it made money, investors were awarded a share of the profits. Those who knowingly and voluntarily took the risk got the reward or suffered the loss. After the Bayh-Dole Act, the people who do the investing when it comes to drug and vaccine research, i.e., the taxpayers, receive nothing except a very expensive drug that many cannot afford.

The university essentially has it both ways; it benefits from researcher without the risk or doing the work. The researcher's grant already pays them indirect payments that cover more than their facility and administrative costs. Then like the drug company, the university benefits from the profits of every drug or vaccine sold. Universities are now *de facto* tax-exempt for-profit companies.

Since the Bayh-Dole Act, universities and even hospitals that have no research facilities have changed their *modus operandi*. They now make a new hire sign terms of employment, in which they surrender intellectual property rights. If you refuse, you do not get hired. Even if you are working on something totally unrelated on your own time while at home, universities and hospitals are demanding intellectual property ownership. In medieval feudalism, employers owned indentured servants, who were legally obligated to work without pay. Since the Bayh-Dole Act, universities and more recently hospitals righteously, shamelessly, and legally claim ownership of an employee's mind.

Drug company collaborator. Research is like gold mining. It is expensive, and most of the time it does not pay off. It is in a multinational pharmaceutical drug company's financial interest to allow the American taxpayers to pay for the research. If the researcher hits a rich deposit of gold ore, the university will place a claim on the mine, and a pharmaceutical company will license the claim (the research) from the university.

Drug companies got another bonanza when in 1997 the US Food and Drug Administration allowed direct-to-customer advertising via television, radio, print, and online. Only two countries in the world, America and New Zealand, allow drug companies to advertise directly to the customer. Since 1997, drug companies have become drug and vaccine pushers via commercials with subliminal messages of smiling beautiful drug users or innuendos of fear or guilt for not buying their drug or vaccine.

After 1980, drug company profits skyrocketed. Americans are now spending about $600 billion a year on prescription drugs.[659] To alert people, Marcia Angell, the former editor of the *New England Journal of Medicine*, wrote a book called *The Truth About the Drug Companies: How They Deceive Us and What to Do About It.*

National Institutes of Health collaborator. The extent to which National Institutes of Health (NIH) and its employees profited from the Bayh-Dole Act is not transparent. Before COVID-19, articles began appearing that criticized the NIH for not disclosing royalties and conflict of interest on self-enrichment from taxpayer funded research.[660]

After COVID-19 and in response to a lawsuit from the watchdog group OpenTheBooks.com, the NIH was forced to release records on royalty payments from drug companies during the interval of October 2021 to September 2023. During that time of COVID-19 vaccine mandates, the NIH received $710 million in royalties from drug companies.[661] This may explain why, despite the COVID-19 catastrophe, the NIH wanted to spend $168,000 on a museum exhibit in honor of Fauci.[662] The journal *Science* reported that an NIH researcher could only receive $150,000 per year in royalties, with the rest going to the NIH bureaucracy.[663]

It is ironic that the NIH—a government conglomeration that funded genetic alteration of benign viruses to turn them into human pathogens (see chapter 15)—is receiving a windfall largesse in profits from COVID-19 vaccines. As Anthony Fauci, the director of National Institute of Allergy and Infectious Diseases, wrote in his autobiography: "My NIAID group was focused on creating vaccines and working with pharmaceutical companies to develop treatments."[664] The NIH is the authority on who should get vaccinated and how often the vaccine and its boosters should be injected. The NIH has demanded that COVID-19 boosters be done indefinitely on everyone regardless of the level of neutralizing antibody that already exists in the blood. When the regulator, authority on safety, and producer are on the same money train, it is a conflict of interest.

Corporate media beneficiary. Corporate news organizations obtain a significant portion of their revenue from drug company advertising. This drives profits and supports the extravagant salaries of legacy news broadcasters, some of whom are paid many tens of millions of dollars every year.[665] Investigation into drug or vaccine profits is not in a news program's interests, since it could boomerang back to collapse the network's revenue stream. When doing the general good for society means getting fired, the general good gets ignored.

Political action committee beneficiary. A drug company cannot directly give money to a politician, but it may do so indirectly by giving money to a political action committee (PAC) to influence the election. The PAC then exercises its "free speech" on unlimited commercials for or against a political candidate. Like a wolf pack, a PAC gangs up to shred any politician not in line with its drug company donors.

As mentioned in chapter 11, drug company contributions to Texas Governor Perry's campaign through two different PACs may have been a factor in Perry's (unsuccessful) attempt to make HPV vaccines mandatory for teenage girls. If they did not get the vaccine, the girls would not be allowed to get an education.[666] Is the end result of denying education to twelve- and thirteen-year-old girls, unless the ruling class gets its way, any different whether it occurs in America or in Afghanistan?[667]

Who pays: The DOPE. American citizens are not informed that they are paying for this game. Sick and suffering citizens who paid for the medical research are left vulnerable and defenseless with unaffordable bills. As Senator Bernie Sanders said on the Senate floor: "The top 10 drug companies made over $112 billion in profit and while they pay their CEOs exorbitant compensation packages, one out of 4 Americans cannot afford to pay for the medicine they need."[668]

In game theory, a few individuals collaborate within a group to enrich their own self-interest. Due to the Bayh-Dole Act, powerful institutions are psychologically, emotionally, and financially tone-deaf to public suffering. In the "drug DOPE" game, citizens who pay for the research and pay for the expensive drugs are always stuck with paying the bill. The "drug DOPE" game is an unending way to shift wealth into the pockets of a select, privileged few. It polarizes society into the haves and the have nots. The "drug DOPE" game monetizes illness and suffering to the advantage of those who already have nearly all the chips on their side of the table.

The Root Cause

In *Citizens United v. the Federal Election Commission*, the US Supreme Court ruled that companies can give unlimited money to PACs so as not to restrict a company's right to "free speech." Companies should have free speech (which universities oddly limit in their licenses). What the majority in the Supreme Court missed is that companies, very wealthy individuals, and other powerful institutions should not have the right to manipulate society in secret by buying elections for their profit and against the common good of society. Such behavior used to be considered corruption.

Supreme Court Justice John Paul Stevens said in dissent that this landmark ruling is "a rejection of the common sense of the American people, who have recognized a need to prevent corporations from undermining self-government."[669] The word "corporation" is from the Latin verb *corporatio*, "to form into a body." Due to the Bayh-Dole Act, companies, universities, and the government are now one giant collaborating cabal or hidden super "corporation." As the Italian fascist ruler Benito Mussolini once said: "Fascism is the merger of state and corporations."[670] They all share in a "piece of the action."

Like water that runs around a rock, money from the well-intended Bayh-Dole Act has found its way around the common good of society. It has been twisted for the financial advantage of drug companies, government bureaucracies, and well-endowed and tax-exempt universities at the expense of its citizens (Figure 16.1). President George Washington in his farewell speech warned about the addiction to and abuse of money and power. He warned of the "necessity of reciprocal checks of political power, by dividing and distributing it into different depositories and constituting each the guardian of the Public Weal against invasions by the others."[671] Government institutions cannot be trusted to investigate themselves. To restate the obvious, it is in the self-interest of institutionalists to look the other way in order to climb the ladder.

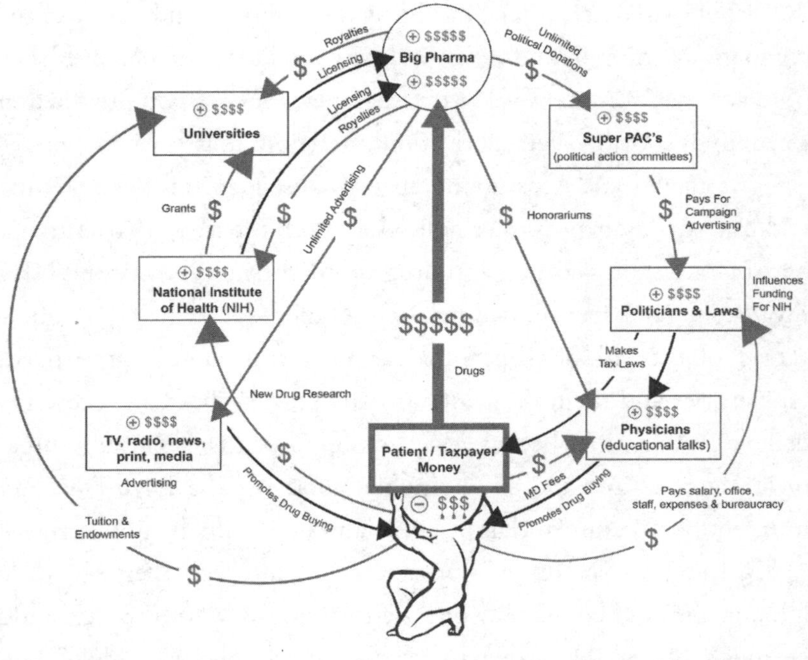

FIGURE 16.1: The cycle of money to collaborators versus from DOPEs (taxpayers and patients). DOPE = Do not have the Opportunity to ParticipatE.

Remedies

To avoid throwing the proverbial baby out with the dirty bathwater when it comes to suggesting solutions to this immensely complex cycle of money, it is prudent to begin modestly by shining lights on drug advertising, PACs, and the Bayh-Dole Act as well as by emphasizing the importance in medical care of noncoerced consent. Drug company direct-to-customer advertising is pushing drugs and vaccines on society for corporate (and university) profit. It is making the public dependent, drug-seeking "addicts" and blurs the line between drug companies and drug dealers. In analogy to cigarette advertising that was terminated for the common good, direct-to-customer drug advertising should be terminated.

If PACs remain legal, they should be forced to publish in large print with each advertisement their officers' names and salaries as well as a list of each of its donors, including the company and names of the company's chairman and CEO and how much they donated. If they object to that minimal level of transparency, they are not interested in freedom of speech. Their motivation is freedom to deceive.

The Bayh-Dole Act's unanticipated consequence is a frightening and fraternizing nepotism of policies and profit between government bureaucracies, universities, and drug companies. University and NIH royalties on taxpayer-funded research should be terminated. If a university objects, its privileged tax-exempt status should be revoked. Universities and their assets are tax exempt, and they can accept tax deductible donations because they are supposed to be charitable organizations that "provide for the public good."[672] The Bayh-Dole Act unintentionally stained that privilege and obligation by universities.

Researchers who do the work and whose intellectual energy made it happen should be the only ones getting royalties. And those should be much higher than what universities parsimoniously "dole" out. Respecting a researcher's intellectual rights would attract the best and brightest from around the world to hasten new discoveries.

Summary

A civilized society resolves conflict through informed consent. It respects the rights of the individual to know the game at play, to be included and benefit from it, to decline to play, to decide for him or herself, and to not be doped or bullied. The difference between a gift and theft is consent. The difference between making love and rape is consent. The difference between giving a medication and committing assault is consent. The first step toward inclusivity is transparent non-coerced consent. The final and most sacred kill switch is transparent noncoerced consent. Instead of taking "a share of the loot" from the drug-DOPE game, we need our universities, the National Institutes of Health, and our medical system to enshrine the principle of non-coerced consent.

ACKNOWLEDGMENTS

I wish to convey my gratitude to Dodie McCracken and former United States Congressman and Senator Mark Kirk, who suggested the title *Kill Switch*. I would also like to thank Blake A. Jurgens, Ph.D., Master of Divinity, and Fulbright Scholar for editorial review.

ENDNOTES

Chapter 1

1. X. Li, W. Cui, and F. Zhang, "Who Was the First Doctor to Report the COVID-19 Outbreak in Wuhan, China?," *Journal of Nuclear Medicine* 16.6 (2020): 782–83.
2. The narrative details here and in the next couple paragraphs derive from J. Czerin, "Dr. Li Wenliang and the Time of COVID-19," Journal of Nuclear Medicine 61.5 (2020): 625.
3. Cissy Zhou, "Coronavirus: Whistle-Blower Dr Li Wenliang Confirmed Dead of the Disease at 34, After Hours of Chaotic Messaging from Hospital," *South China Morning Post*, February 7, 2020, https://www.scmp.com/news/china/society/article/3049411/coronavirus-li-wenliang-doctor-who-alerted-authorities-outbreak.
4. Shawn Yuan, "Grief, Anger in China as Doctor Who Warned About Coronavirus Dies," *Al Jazeera*, February 7, 2020, https://www.aljazeera.com/news/2020/2/7/grief-anger-in-china-as-doctor-who-warned-about-coronavirus-dies.
5. See "Virus Whistleblower Doctor Punished 'Inappropriately': Chinese Probe," *The Economic Times*, March 20, 2020, https://health.economictimes.indiatimes.com/news/diagnostics/virus-whistleblower-doctor-punished-inappropriately-chinese-probe/74725984; Ian Collier, "Coronavirus: China Apologises to Family of Doctor Who Died After Warning About COVID-19," *Sky News*, March 20, 2020, https://

news.sky.com/story/coronavirus-china-apologises-to-family-of-doctor-who-died-after-warning-about-covid-19-11960679.

6. Quote from Sagan taken from *Cosmos: A Personal Voyage*, season 1, episode 2, "One Voice in the Cosmic Fugue," produced by Adrian Malone, broadcast in October 5, 1980 on PBS.

Chapter 2

7. M. Tokuyama et al., "ERVmap Analysis Reveals Genome-Wide Transcription of Human Endogenous Retroviruses," *Proceedings of the National Academy of Sciences of the United States of America* 115.50 (2018): 12565–72.
8. L. A. Pray, "Transposons: The Jumping Genes," *Nature Education* 1.1 (2008): 204.
9. A. King, "Hidden Players: The Bacteria-Killing Viruses of the Gut Microbiome," *Nature,* October 31, 2024, https://www.nature.com/articles/d41586-024-03532-w.
10. P. Forterre, "To Be or Not to Be Alive: How Recent Discoveries Challenge the Traditional Definitions of Viruses and Life," *Studies in History and Philosophy of Biological and Biomedical Sciences* 59 (2016): 100–108.
11. J. Louten, *Virus Structure and Classification: Essential Human Virology* (Academic Press, 2016), 19–29.
12. A. J. Wollman et al., "From Animaculum to Single Molecules: 300 Years of the Light Microscope," *Open Biology* 5.4 (2015): 150019.
13. R. Hooke, *Micrographia Or Some Physiological Descriptions of Minute Bodies* (1665; repr., Cosmino, 2007).
14. L. S. King, "Dr. Koch's Postulates," *Journal of the History of Medicine and Allied* Sciences 7 (1952): 350–61.
15. P. Mazzarello, "A Unifying Concept: The History of Cell Theory," *Nature Cell Biology* 1.1 (1999): E13–E15.
16. M. Schultz, "Rudolf Virchow," *Emerging Infectious Diseases* 14.9 (2008):1480–81.
17. A. Gamgee, "The Pasteur-Chamberland Filter," *British Medical Journal* 6.1 (1886): 464.

18. M. A. Shampo and R. A. Kyle, "Ernst Ruska—Inventor of the Electron Microscope," *Mayo Clinic Proceedings* 72.2 (1997): 148.
19. K. R. Richert-Poggeler et al., "Electron Microscopy Methods for Virus Diagnosis and High Resolution Analysis of Viruses," *Frontiers in Microbiology* 9 (2019): 3255.
20. R. Tolf, *The Russian Rockefellers: The Saga of the Nobel Family and the Russian Oil Industry* (Hoover Institution Press, 1976), 188–90.
21. A. Agrawal, "Merchant of Death—The Story Behind the Nobel Prize," *The Times of India*, April 5, 2020, https://timesofindia.indiatimes.com/blogs/unheardshepherd/merchant-of-death-the-story-behind-the-nobel-prize/.
22. L. Ji, "Why Is There No Nobel Prize in Mathematics?," *Notices of the International Consortium of Chinese Mathematicians* 1.1 (2013): 42–52.
23. B. Asbrink, "Nationalization Is a Beautiful Word for a Very Ugly Thing," *Nobel Brothers*, August 15, 2011, https://www.branobelhistory.com/society/nationalisation-is-a-beautiful-word-for-a-very-ugly-thing/.
24. S. A. Plotkin and S. L. Plotkin, "The Development of Vaccines: How the Past Led to the Future," *Nature Reviews Microbiology* 9.12 (2011): 889–93.
25. Cleveland Clinic, "Childhood Immunization Schedule," https://my.clevelandclinic.org/health/articles/11288-childhood-immunization-schedule.

Chapter 3

26. Z. S. Moore, J. F. Seward, and J. M. Lane, "Smallpox," *The Lancet* 367.9508 (2006): 425–35.
27. N. Barquet and P. Domingo, "Smallpox: The Triumph over the Most Terrible of the Ministers of Death," *Annals of Internal Medicine* 127.8 (1997): 635–62.
28. D. B. Martin. "The Cause of Death in Smallpox: An Examination of the Pathology Record," *Military Medicine* 167 (2002): 546–51.
29. J. A. Rosenfeld, review of *The Speckled Monster: A Historical Tale of Battling Smallpox*, by Jennifer Lee Carrell, *BMJ* 328 (2004): 233.

30. Quote taken from *Meditations* 6.6. Translation from Marcus Aurelius, *Meditations*, trans. M. Hammond (Penguin Classics, 2006).
31. I. W. Sherman, *The Power of Plagues*, 2nd ed. (ASM Press, 2017), 189.
32. S. Sabbatani and S. Fiorino, "La peste antonina e il declino dell'Impero Romano. Ruolo della guerra partica e della guerra marcomannica tra il 164 e il 182 d.c. nella diffusione del contagion," *Infezioni in Medicina* 17.4 (2009): 261–75.
33. R. P. Duncan-Jones, "The Impact of the Antonine Plague," *Journal of Roman Archaeology* 9 (1996): 108–36; J. R. Fears, "The Plague Under Marcus Aurelius and the Decline and Fall of the Roman Empire," *Infectious Disease Clinics of North America* 18 (2004): 65–77.
34. K. B. Patterson and T. Runge, "Smallpox and the Native American," *American Journal of the Medical Sciences* 323.4 (2002): 216–22.
35. C. Gibson, *The Aztecs Under Spanish Rule: A History of the Indians of the Valley of Mexico, 1519–1810* (Stanford University Press, 1964).
36. G. W. Christopher et al., "Biological Warfare: A Historical Perspective," *JAMA* 278 (1997): 412–17.
37. E. A. Fenn, "Biological Warfare in Eighteenth-Century North America Beyond Jeffrey Amherst," *Journal of American History* 86 (2000): 1552–80.
38. National Library of Medicine, "Smallpox Variolation," *Smallpox: A Great and Terrible Scourge*, last updated March 5, 2024, https://www.nlm.nih.gov/exhibition/smallpox/sp_variolation.html?lang=en.
39. F. Roşu, *Slavery in the Black Sea Region, c. 900–1900: Forms of Unfreedom at the Intersection Between Christianity and Islam*, Studies in Global Slavery 11 (Brill, 2022), 21–22.
40. H. Barker, *That Most Precious Merchandise: The Mediterranean Trade in Black Sea Slaves, 1260–1500* (University of Pennsylvania Press, 2021).
41. C. J. Burrell, C. R. Howard, and F. A. Murphy, "Pathogenesis of Virus Infections," *Fenner and White's Medical Virology* (2017): 77–104.
42. M. Radetsky, "Smallpox: A History of Its Rise and Fall," *Pediatric Infectious Disease Journal* 18 (1999): 85–93.

43. S. Riedel, "Edward Jenner and the History of Smallpox and Vaccination," *Proceedings—Baylor University Medical Center* 18.1 (2005): 21–25.
44. E. Jenner, *An Inquiry into the Causes and Effects of the Variolae Vaccinae* (London, 1798).
45. E. L. Scott, "Edward Jenner, F.R.S., and the Cuckoo," *Notes and Records of the Royal Society* 28 (1974): 235–40.
46. B. L. Jacobs, et al., "Vaccinia Virus Vaccines: Past, Present and Future. *Antiviral Research* 84.1 (2009): 1–13.
47. L. Schrick et al., "An Early American Smallpox Vaccine Based on Horsepox," *New England Journal of Medicine* 377.15 (2017): 1491–92.
48. G. A. Poland, "Smallpox Vaccines: From First to Second to Third Generation," *The Lancet* 365.9457 (2005): 362–63.
49. F. Fenner et al., *Smallpox and Its Eradication* (World Health Organization, 1988).
50. T. Yoshikawa, "Third-Generation Smallpox Vaccine Strain-Based Recombinant Vaccines for Viral Hemorrhagic Fevers," *Vaccine* 39.41 (2021): 6174–81.
51. A. Volz and G. Sutter, "Modified Vaccinia Virus Ankara: History, Value in Basic Research, and Current Perspectives for Vaccine Development," *Advances in Virus Research* 97 (2017): 187–243.
52. J. Kenner et al., "LC16m8: An Attenuated Smallpox Vaccine," *Vaccine* 17.24 (2006): 47–48.
53. M. A. Strassburg, "The Global Eradication of Smallpox," *American Journal of Infection Control* 10.2 (1982): 53–59.
54. G. A. Shchelkunova and S. N. Shchelkunov, "40 Years Without Smallpox," *Acta Naturae* 9.4 (2017): 4–12.
55. D. A. Henderson and P. Klepac, "Lessons from the Eradication of Smallpox: An Interview with D. A. Henderson," *Philosophical Transactions of the Royal Society B* 368.1623 (2013): 20130113.
56. L. Krueger, "A Transformative Deal for Nature: A New Global Biodiversity Framework Could Mark a Turning Point in How We Manage Our Relationship to Nature, *The Nature Conservatory*, January

15, 2020, https://www.nature.org/en-us/what-we-do/our-insights/perspectives/a-transformative-deal-for-nature/.

Chapter 4

57. A. de Souza and S. N. Madhusudana, "Survival from Rabies Encephalitis," *Journal of the Neurological Sciences* 339 (2014): 8–14; B. Davis, G. Rall, and M. Schnell, "Everything You Always Wanted to Know About Rabies Virus (But Were Afraid to Ask)," *Annual Review of Virology* 2 (2015): 451–71.
58. J. W. Krebs, J. T. Wheeling, and J. E. Childs, "Rabies Surveillance in the United States During 2002," *Journal of the American Veterinary Medical Association* 223 (2003): 1736–48.
59. S. L. Messenger, J. S. Smith, and C. E. Rupprecht, "Emerging Epidemiology of Bat-Associated Cryptic Cases of Rabies in Humans in the United States," *Clinical Infectious Diseases* 35 (2002): 738–47.
60. Z. F. Fu, "Rabies and Rabies Research: Past, Present and Future," *Vaccine* 15 (1997): S20–S24.
61. T. Hemachudha et al., "Pathophysiology of Human Paralytic Rabies," *Journal of NeuroVirology* 11 (2005): 93–100.
62. X. Lu, W. Zhu, and G. Wu, "Rabies Virus Transmission via Solid Organs or Tissue Allotransplantation," *Infectious Diseases of Poverty* 7 (2018): 82.
63. H. Raux, A. Flamand, and D. Blondel, "Interaction of the Rabies Virus P Protein with the LC8 Dynein Light Chain," *Journal of Virology* 74 (2000): 10212–16.
64. N. Tordo and A. Kouknetzoff, "The Rabies Virus Genome: An Overview," *The Onderstepoort Journal of Veterinary Research* 60.4 (1993): 263–69.
65. K. A. Smith, "Louis Pasteur, the Father of Immunology?," *Frontiers in Immunology* 3 (2012): 68.
66. D. J. Hicks, A. R. Fooks, and N. Johnson, "Developments in Rabies Vaccines," Clinical and Experimental Immunology 169.3 (2012): 199–204.

67. R. Rappuoli, "Inner Workings: 1885, the First Rabies Vaccination in Humans," *Proceedings of the National Academy of the Sciences of the United States of America* 111.34 (2014): 12273.
68. B. Sanders, M. Koldijk, and H. Schuitemaker, "Inactivated Viral Vaccines," *Vaccine Analysis: Strategies, Principles, and Control* 28 (2014): 45–80.
69. E. Mix et al., "Animal Models of Multiple Sclerosis—Potentials and Limitations," *Progress in Neurology* 92.3 (2010): 386–405.
70. A. G. Baxter, "The Origin and Application of Experimental Autoimmune Encephalomyelitis," *National Review of Immunology* 7.11 (2007): 904–12.
71. S. Patil et al., "Revelation in the Field of Tissue Preservation—A Preliminary Study on Natural Formalin Substitutes," *Journal of International Oral Health* 5.1 (2013): 31–38.
72. C. H. Fox et al., "Formaldehyde Fixation," *Journal of Histochemistry and Cytochemistry* 33.8 (1985): 845–53.
73. F. Blum, "Der Formaldehyd als Antisepticum," *Münchener Medizinische Wochenschrift* 32 (1893): 601–2; F. Blum, "Der formaldehyd als haertungsmittel, *Zeitschrift für wissenschaftliche Mikroskopie und mikroskopische Technik* 10 (1893): 314–15. See also H. Goring, "Professor Dr Ferdinand Blum gestorben," *Hessisches Arzteblatt* 20 (1959): 123.
74. E. A. Hoffman et al., "Formaldehyde Crosslinking: A Tool for the Study of Chromatin Complexes," *Journal of Biological Chemistry* 290.44 (2015): 26404–11.
75. M. S. Tullu et al., "Neurological Complications of Rabies Vaccines," *Indian Pediatrics* 40 (2003): 150–54.
76. J. F. Bell and G. J. Moore, "Allergic Encephalitis, Rabies Antibodies, and the Blood/Brain Barrier," Journal of Laboratory and Clinical Medicine 94.1 (1979): 5–11.
77. T. Hemachudha et al., "Myelin Basic Protein as an Encephalitogen in Encephalomyelitis and Polyneuritis Following Rabies Vaccination," *New England Journal of Medicine* 316.7 (1989): 369–74.

78. R. E. Kissling, "Growth of Rabies Virus in Non-Nervous Tissue," *Proceedings of the Society for Experimental Biology and Medicine* 98 (1958): 223–25.

79. A. P. Robinson et al., "The Experimental Autoimmune Encephalomyelitis (EAE) Model of MS: Utility for Understanding Disease Pathophysiology and Treatment," *Handbook of Clinical Neurology* 122 (2014): 173–89.

80. A. I. Boullerne, "The History of Myelin," *Experimental Neurology* 283 (2016): 431–45.

81. C. E. Rupprecht and R. V. Gibbons, "Clinical Practice: Prophylaxis Against Rabies," *New England Journal of Medicine* 351.25 (2004): 2626–35; C. Liu and J. D. Cahill, "Epidemiology of Rabies and Current US Vaccine Guidelines," *Rhode Island Medical Journal* 103.6 (2013): 51–53. PMID: 32752569.

82. F. Cliquet et al., "Oral Vaccination of Dogs: A Well-Studied and Undervalued Tool for Achieving Human and Dog Rabies Elimination," *Veterinary Research* 49.1 (2018): 61.

83. A. Belotto et al., "Overview of Rabies in the Americas," *Virus Research* 111.1 (2005): 5–12.

84. T. Muller and H. Schluter, "Oral Immunization of Red Foxes in Europe—A Review," *Journal of Etlik Veterinary Microbiology* 9 (1998): 35–59; D. H. Johnston et al., "An Aerial Baiting System for the Distribution of Attenuated or Recombinant Rabies Vaccines for Foxes, Raccoons, and Skunks," *Reviews of Infectious Diseases* 10.4 (1988): S660–64; H. H. Thulke et al., "Assessing Anti-Rabies Baiting—What Happens on the Ground?," *BMC Infectious Diseases* 4 (2004): 9; W. W. Müller, "Where Do We Stand with Oral Vaccination of Foxes Against Rabies in Europe?," *Archives of Virology. Supplementum* 13 (1997): 83–94.

85. Ed Yong, "That Time Europe Air-Dropped Vaccine-Loaded Chicken Heads to Bait Rabid Foxes," *The Atlantic*, December 1, 2015, https://www.theatlantic.com/science/archive/2015/12/that-time-europe-air-dropped-vaccine-loaded-chicken-heads-to-bait-rabid-foxes/417951/.

86. P. Pattnaik et al., "Alarming Rise in Global Rabies Cases Calls for Urgent Attention: Current Vaccination Status and Suggested Key Countermeasures," *Cureus* 15.12 (2023): e50424.

Chapter 5

87. J. Vainio and F. Cutts, *Yellow Fever* (World Health Organization, 1998).
88. E. A Vigil, "The Black Vomit (*vomito negro*) of Iqitos, Peru, Identical with Yellow Fever," *JAMA* 8.2 (1910): 120–23.
89. M. B. Franco et al., "Deficiency of Coagulation Factors Is Associated with the Bleeding Diathesis of Severe Yellow Fever," *Annals of Hematology* 102.7 (2023): 1939–49.
90. M. C. Crosby, *The American Plague: The Untold Story of Yellow Fever, the Epidemic That Shaped Our History* (Berkley Books, 2006).
91. K. R. Foster, M. F. Jenkins, and A. C. Toogood, "The Philadelphia Yellow Fever Epidemic of 1793," *Scientific American* 279.2 (1998): 88–93.
92. B. G. Smith, *Ship of Death: A Voyage That Changed the Atlantic World* (Yale University Press, 2020).
93. See the exhibit "Politics of Yellow Fever in Alexander Hamilton's America," *National Library of Medicine*, https://www.nlm.nih.gov/exhibition/politicsofyellowfever/index.html.
94. P. A. Mackowiak and P. S. Sehdev, "The Origin of Quarantine," *Clinical Infectious Diseases* 35.9 (2000): 1071–72.
95. E. Tognotti, "Lessons from the History of Quarantine, from Plague to Influenza A," *Emerging Infectious Diseases* 19.2 (2013): 254–59.
96. J. MacDonald, *Travels, in Various Parts of Europe, Asia, and Africa, During a Series of Thirty Years and Upwards* (Forbes, 1790), 276.
97. Smith, *Ship of Death*, 275 n. 6.
98. M. A. Johansson et al., "Incubation Periods of Yellow Fever Virus," *American Journal of Tropical Medicine and Hygiene* 83.1 (2010): 183-88.
99. J. Jones, "Origin of the Yellow-Fever Epidemic in New Orleans, 1878: What Is the Remedy?," *The Sanitarian* (New York), June 1, 1879, 246.
100. J. M. Keating, *A History of the Yellow Fever: The Yellow Fever Epidemic of 1878, in Memphis, Tenn* (Howard Association, 1878).
101. G. J. A. O'Toole, *The Spanish War: An American Epic. 1898* (Norton, 1984).
102. T. B. Allen, "Remember *The Maine*?," *National Geographic* 193.2 (February 1998): 107; T. Miller, "Remember The Maine," *Smithsonian*

Magazine, February 1998, https://www.smithsonianmag.com/history/remember-the-maine-56071873/.

103. Naval History and Heritage Command, "Captain Charles D. Sigsbee to Secretary of the Navy John D. Long, 2/15/1898," https://www.history.navy.mil/research/publications/documentary-histories/united-states-navy-s/destruction-of-the-m/captain-charles-d-si-3.html.
104. D. Nasaw, *The Chief: The Life of William Randolph Hearst* (Houghton Mifflin, 2000); L. Mulvey, *Citizen Kane* (British Film Institute, 1992).
105. Office of the Historian, "US Diplomacy and Yellow Journalism 1895–1898," *Milestones in the History of the U.S. Foreign Relations*, https://history.state.gov/milestones/1866-1898/yellow-journalism.
106. R. B. Edgerton, *Remember the Maine, to Hell with Spain: America's 1898 Adventure in Imperialism* (Mellen, 2004).
107. Crucible of Empire, "Timeline," PBS, https://www.pbs.org/crucible/tl10.html#:~:text=In%20the%20American%20press%2C%20headlines,the%20Spanish%20were%20responsible%20for.
108. H. G. Rickover, *How the Battleship Maine Was Destroyed* (Department of the Navy, Naval History Division, 1976), 94–97, 104–6.
109. P. Feng, "Major Walter Reed and the Eradication of Yellow Fever," *The Army Historical Foundation*, https://armyhistory.org/major-walter-reed-and-the-eradication-of-yellow-fever/.
110. H. A. Kelly, *Walter Reed and Yellow Fever* (McClure, Phillips & Co., 1906).
111. A. Mehra, "History of Medicine, Politics of Participation: Walter Reed's Yellow-Fever Experiments," *American Medical Association Journal of Ethics* 11.4 (2009): 326–30.
112. "Biography of Dr. Carlos Juan Finlay," *Military Medicine* 166.1 (2001): 5.
113. C. Finlay, "The Mosquito Hypothetically Considered as an Agent in the Transmission of Yellow Fever Poison," *Yale Journal of Biology and Medicine* 9.6 (1937): 589–604.
114. R. Ross, "Dr. Jesse W. Lazear and Yellow Fever," *Nature* 112 (1923).
115. J. A. del Regato, "James Carroll: A Biography," *Annals of Diagnostic Pathology* 2.5 (1998): 335–49.

116. W. Reed et al., "The Etiology of Yellow Fever—A Preliminary Note," *Philadelphia Medical Journal* 6 (1900): 790–96.
117. "The Mosquito Hypothesis," *Washington Post*, November 2, 1900, 6.
118. D. Ploth, "Walter Reed at Camp Lazear: A Paradigm for Contemporary Clinical Research," *American Journal of the Medical Sciences* 357.1 (2019): 7–15.
119. A. Agramonte, "The Inside History of a Great Medical Discovery," *The Scientific Monthly* 1.3 (1915): 209–37.
120. Claude Moore Health Sciences Library, "'Ready to Do My Bit': The Personal Diary of Dr. Henry Hanson and the West Africa Yellow Fever Commission," University of Virginia, 2007, https://exhibits.hsl.virginia.edu/hanson/the-west-africa-yellow-fever-commission-1925-1934/index.html.
121. A. Stokes, "The Transmission of Yellow Fever to *Macacus rhesus*: Preliminary Note," *JAMA* 90 (1928): 253–55; A. Stokes, J. H. Bauer, and N. P. Hudson, "The Transmission of Yellow Fever to *Macacus rhesus*," *Reviews in Medical Virology* 11.3 (1928): 141–48.
122. N. P. Hudson, "Adrian Stokes and Yellow Fever Research: A Tribute," *Transactions of the Royal Society of Tropical Medicine and Hygiene* 60.2 (1966): 170–74.
123. S. Y. Tan and J. Furubayashi, "Hideyo Noguchi (1876–1928): Distinguished Bacteriologist," *Singapore Medical Journal* 55.10 (2014): 550–51.
124. "Dr. W. A. Young," *Nature* 122 (1928).
125. M. Theiler and H. H. Smith, "The Effect of Prolonged Cultivation *in vitro* upon the Pathogenicity of Yellow Fever Virus," *Journal of Experimental Medicine* 65.6 (1937):767–86; M. Theiler and H. H. Smith, "The Use of Yellow Fever Virus Modified by *in vitro* Cultivation for Human Immunization," *Journal of Experimental Medicine* 65.6 (1937): 787–800; H. H. Smith and M. Theiler, "The Adaptation of Unmodified Strains of Yellow Fever Virus to Cultivation *in vitro*," *Journal of Experimental Medicine* 65.6 (1937): 801–8.
126. S. Elvidge, "Developing the 17D Yellow Fever Vaccine," *Nature Portfolio*, September 28, 2020, https://www.nature.com/articles/d42859-020-00012-9.

127. E. Norrby, "Yellow Fever and Max Theiler: The Only Nobel Prize for a Virus Vaccine," *Journal of Experimental Medicine* 204.12 (2007): 2779–84.

128. J. Benchimol, "Yellow Fever Vaccine in Brazil: Fighting a Tropical Scourge, Modernising the Nation," in *The Politics of Vaccination: A Global History*, ed. C. Holmberg (Manchester University Press, 2017), 174–208; J. Benchimol, "How Brazil Joined the Quest for a Yellow Fever Vaccine," *Bulletin of the World Health Organization* 91.3 (2013): 165–66.

129. I. Löwy, "The 1942 Massive Contamination of Yellow Fever Vaccine: A Public Health Consequence of Scientific Arrogance," *American Journal of Public Health* 111.9 (2021): 1654–60.

130. A. M. da Costa Lima, "Consideraçes sobre a propagaço da febre amarela e a vacinaço contra esta doença," *Revista Medico Cirurgica do Brasil* 46 (1938): 371–82

131. R. E. Thomas, D. L. Lorenzetti, and W. Spragins, "Mortality and Morbidity Among Military Personnel and Civilians During the 1930s and World War II from Transmission of Hepatitis During Yellow Fever Vaccination: Systematic Review," *American Journal of Public Health* 103.3 (2013): e16–e29.

132. J. G. Frierson, "The Yellow Fever Vaccine: A History," *Yale Journal of Biology and Medicine* 83.2 (2010): 77–85.

133. P. K. Vogt, "Avian Tumor Viruses," *Advances in Virus Research* 11 (1965): 293.

134. T. D. Waters et al., "Yellow Fever Vaccination, Avian Leukosis Virus, and Cancer Risk in Man," *Science* 177 (1972): 76–77.

135. N. M. Tauraso et al., "Yellow Fever Vaccine. I. Development of a Vaccine Seed Free from Contaminating Avian Leukosis Viruses," *Proceedings of the Society for Experimental Biology and Medicine. Society for Experimental Biology and Medicine* 127.4 (1968): 1116–20; C. C. Draper, "A Yellow Fever Vaccine Free from Avian Leukosis Viruses," *Journal of Hygiene* 65.4 (1967): 505–13.

136. F. de Andrade Gondolfi et al., "Yellow Fever Vaccine-Related Neurotrophic Disease in Brazil Following Immunization with 17DD," *Vaccines* 11.2 (2023): 445.

137. E. G. Fernandes et al., "Yellow Fever Vaccine-Associated Viscerotropic Disease Among Siblings, São Paulo State Brazil," *Emerging Infectious Diseases* 29.3 (2023): 493–500.
138. P. F. C. Vasconcelos et al., "Serious Adverse Events Associated with Yellow Fever 17D Vaccine in Brazil: A Report of Two Cases," *The Lancet* 358 (2001): 91–97; M. Martin et al., "Fever and Multisystem Organ Failure Associated with 17D-204 Yellow Fever Vaccination: A Report of Four Cases," *The Lancet* 358 (2001): 98–104; R. C. Chan et al., "Hepatitis and Death Following Vaccination with 17D-204 Yellow Fever Vaccine," *The Lancet* 358 (2001): 121–26.
139. P. P. Mortimer, "Yellow Fever Vaccine," *BMJ* 324.7335 (2002): 439; A. F. Ribeiro et al., "Neurologic Disease After Yellow Fever Vaccination, São Paulo, Brazil, 2017–2018," *Emerging Infectious Diseases* 27.6 (2021): 1577–87.
140. C. V. Gould et al., "Transmission of Yellow Fever Vaccine Virus Through Blood Transfusion and Organ Transplantation in the USA in 2021: Report of an Investigation," *The Lancet. Microbe* 4.9 (2023): e711–21.
141. Centers for Disease Control, "Yellow Fever Vaccine. Recommendations of the Advisory Committee on Immunization Practices (ACIP)," *Morbidity and Mortality Weekly Report* 51.17 (2002): 1–10.
142. J. D. Poland et al., "Persistence of Neutralizing Antibody 30–35 Years After Immunization with 17D Yellow Fever Vaccine," *Bulletin of the World Health Organization* 59 (1981): 895–900.
143. Centers for Disease Control, "Yellow Fever Vaccine."

Chapter 6

144. N. Lévêque and B. L. Semler, "A 21st Century Perspective of Poliovirus Replication," *PLoS Pathogens* 11.6 (2015): e1004825; C. B. Coyne, K. S. Kim, and J. M. Bergelson, "Poliovirus Entry into Human Brain Microvascular Cells Requires Receptor-Induced Activation of SHP-2," *EMBO Journal* 26.17 (2007): 4016–28; A. Iwasaki et al., "Immunofluorescence Analysis of Poliovirus Receptor Expression in Peyer's

Patches of Humans, Primates, and CD155 Transgenic Mice: Implications for Poliovirus Infection," *Journal of Infectious Diseases* 186.5 (2002): 585–92.

145. G. Lein and D. Heymann, "The Problems with Polio; Toward Eradication," *Infectious Diseases and Therapy* 2.2 (2013): 167–74; S. Bunimovich-Mendrazitsky and L. Stone, "Modeling Polio as a Disease of Development," *Journal of Theoretical Biology* 237.3 (2005): 302–15.
146. S. N. Langel et al., "Maternal Gatekeepers: How Maternal Antibody Fc Characteristics Influence Passive Transfer and Infant Protection," *PLoS Pathogens* 16.3 (2020): e1008303; M. Albrecht and P. C. Arck, "Vertically Transferred Immunity in Neonates: Mothers, Mechanisms and Mediators," *Frontiers in Immunology* 11 (2020): 555; N. Linder et al., "Placental Transfer of Maternal Poliovirus Antibodies in Full-Term and Pre-Term Infants," *Vaccine* 16.2–3 (1998): 236–39.
147. J. Golden and N. Rogers, "Nurse Irene Shea Studies the 'Kenny Method' of Treatment of Infantile Paralysis,1942–1943," *Nursing History Review* 18 (2010): 189–203; V. Cohn, *Sister Kenny: The Woman Who Challenged the Doctors* (University of Minnesota Press, 1976); M. C. Meehan, "Sister Kenny: The Woman Who Challenged the Doctors," *JAMA* 235.22 (1976): 2435.
148. Quote taken from the review of the book co-authored by Kenny and John Pohl, "The Kenny Concept of Infantile Paralysis and Its Treatment," *American Journal of the Diseases of Children* 68.1 (1944): 77.
149. E. Kenny and M. Ostenso, *And They Shall Walk: The Life Story of Sister Elizabeth Kenny* (Dodd, Mead & Company, 1943).
150. E. Kenny, *My Battle and Victory* (Hale, 1955).
151. L. Hawkins, *The Man in the Iron Lung: The Frederick B. Snite, Jr., Story* (Doubleday, 1956); D. Corson, "Frederick Snite 'The Man in the Iron Lung' a Legend at Notre Dame," *The Spirit of Notre Dame*, 2001, https://www3.nd.edu/~wcawley/corson/fsnite.htm.
152. T. Walker, *Roosevelt and the Warm Springs Story* (Wyn, 1953).

153. D. M. Oshinsky, *Polio: An American Story* (Oxford University Press, 2005); A. J. Salisbury, "The National Foundation—March of Dimes," *Progress in Clinical and Biological Research* 18 (1977): 11.

154. R. Verville, *War, Politics, and Philanthropy: The History of Rehabilitation Medicine* (University Press of America, 2009), 123.

155. M. E. Molliver, *David Bodian, 1910–1992: A Biographical Memoir* (National Academy of Sciences, 2012).

156. D. Bodian, I. M. Morgan, and H. A. Howe, "Differentiation of Types of Poliomyelitis Viruses: III. The Grouping of Fourteen Strains into Three Basic Immunological Types," *American Journal of Epidemiology* 49.2 (1949): 234–47.

157. S. A. Plotkin, "CHAT Oral Polio Vaccine Was Not the Source of Human Immunodeficiency Virus Type 1 Group M for Humans," *Clinical Infectious Diseases* 32 (2001): 1068–48.

158. John Brookland, "The London Airport Monkey Run," *Animal Rights and Wrongs* (blog), November 23, 2021, https://animalrightsandwrongs.uk/tag/research-monkeys/.

159. The College of Physicians of Philadelphia, "How Vaccines Are Made? Early Laboratory Methods for Developing Vaccines," History of Vaccines, January 10, 2018, https://historyofvaccines.org/vaccines-101/how-are-vaccines-made/early-laboratory-methods-developing-vaccines.

160. T. Weller et al., "Studies on the Cultivation of Poliomyelitis Viruses in Tissue Culture: I. The Propagation of Poliomyelitis Viruses in Suspended Cell Cultures of Various Human Tissues," *Journal of Immunology* 69.6 (1952): 645–71.

161. J. Enders, F. Robbins, and T. Weller, "The Cultivation of the Poliomyelitis Viruses in Tissue Culture," Nobel Prize lecture delivered on December 11, 1954, https://www.nobelprize.org/uploads/2018/06/enders-robbins-weller-lecture.pdf.

162. S. J. Olshansky and L. Hayflick, "The Role of the WI-38 Cell Strain in Saving Lives and Reducing Morbidity," *AIMS Public Health* 4.2 (2017): 127–38.

163. K. Konishi et al., "Whole-Genome Sequencing of Vero E6 (VERO C1008) and Comparative Analysis of Four Vero Cell Sublines," *Frontiers in Genetics* 13 (2022): 801382.
164. H. M. Weaver, "A Formula to Determine the Cost of Research," *Journal of the Association of American Medical Colleges* 25.4 (1950): 248–54.
165. C. M. Croce, "Hilary Koprowski (1916–2013): Vaccine Pioneer, Art Lover, and Scientific Leader," *PNAS* 110.22 (2013): 8757.
166. H. Koprowski, J. George, and N. Thomas, "Immune Response to Human Volunteers upon Oral Ingestion of a Rodent Adapted Strain of Poliomyelitis Virus," *American Journal of Hygiene* 55 (1952): 108–26.
167. D. S. Dane et al., "Vaccination Against Poliomyelitis with Live Virus Vaccines: 1. A Trial of TN Type II Vaccine," *BMJ* 1 (1957): 59–74.
168. Dane et al., "Vaccination Against Poliomyelitis."
169. H. Koprowski et al., "Clinical Investigations on Attenuated Strains of Poliomyelitis Virus: Use as a Method of Immunization of Children with Living Virus," *JAMA* 160.11 (1956): 954–66.
170. Plotkin, "CHAT Oral Polio Vaccine."
171. H. Koprowski, "First Decade (1950–1960) of Studies and Trials with the Polio Vaccine," *Biologicals* 34 (2006): 81–86.
172. S. Y. Tan and N. Ponstein, "Jonas Salk (1914–1995): A Vaccine Against Polio," *Singapore Medical Journal* 60.1 (2019): 9–10; J. E. Salk et al., "Formaldehyde Treatment and Safety Testing of Experimental Poliomyelitis Vaccines," *American Journal of Public Health and the Nation's Health* 44 (1954): 563–70.
173. M. Meldrum, "A Calculated Risk: The Salk Polio Vaccine Field Trials of 1954," *BMJ* 317.7167 (1998): 1233–36.
174. J. Juskewitch, "Lessons from the Salk Polio Vaccine: Methods for and Risks of Rapid Translation," *Clinical and Translational Science* 3.4 (2010): 182–85.
175. P. A. Offit, *The Cutter Incident: How America's First Polio Vaccine Led to the Growing Vaccine Crisis* (Yale University Press, 2007).
176. P. A. Offit, "The Cutter Incident, 50 Years Later," *New England Journal of Medicine* 352 (2005): 1411–12.

177. B. E. Eddy et al., "Tumors Induced in Hamsters by Injection of Rhesus Monkey Kidney Cell Extracts," *Proceedings of the Society for Experimental Biology and Medicine* 107.1 (1961): 191–97.

178. Eddy et al., "Tumors Induced in Hamsters."

179. B. H. Sweet and M. R. Hilleman, "The Vacuolating Virus, S.V. 40," *Proceedings of the Society for Experimental Biology and Medicine* 105.2 (1960): 420–27.

180. T. Curtis, "Monkeys Virus and Vaccine," *The Lancet* 364 (2004): 407–8.

181. M. Carbone, A. Gazdar, and J. S. Butel, "SV40 and Human Mesothelioma," *Translational Lung Cancer Research* 9.1 (2020): S47–59.

182. D. Bookchin and J. Schumacher, *The Virus and the Vaccine: Contaminated Vaccine, Deadly Cancers, and Government Neglect* (St. Martin's, 2004), 380.

183. R. A. Vilchez, C. A. Kozinetz, and J. S. Butel, "Conventional Epidemiology and the Link Between SV40 and Human Cancers," *The Lancet Oncology* 4.3 (2003): 188–91.

184. D. J. Bergsagel et al., "DNA Sequences Similar to Those of Simian Virus 40 in Ependymomas and Choroid Plexus Tumors of Childhood," *New England Journal of Medicine* 326 (1992): 988–99.

185. M. Carbone et al., "Simian Virus 40-Like DNA Sequences in Human Pleural Mesothelioma," *Oncogene* 9 (1994): 1781–90; M. Carbone et al., "SV40-Like Sequences in Human Bone Tumors," *Oncogene* 13 (1996): 527–35.

186. M. Carbone, "Simian Virus-40 Large-T Antigen Binds P53 in Human Mesotheliomas," *Nature Medicine* 3 (1997): 908–12.

187. S. G. Fisher, L. Weber, and M. Carbone, "Cancer Risk Associated with Simian Virus 40 Contaminated Polio Vaccine," *Anticancer Research* 19.3 (1999):2173–80.

188. Y. Xu et al., "Twenty-Year Outcome of Prevalence, Incidence, Mortality and Survival Rate in Patients with Malignant Bone Tumors," *International Journal of Cancer* 154.2 (2024): 226–40.

189. I. Ilil and M. Ilil, "International Patterns and Trends in the Brain Cancer Incidence and Mortality: An Observational Study Based on the Global Burden of Disease," *Heliyon* 9.7 (2023): e18222.

190. W. Cal et al., "Trends Analysis of Non-Hodgkin Lymphoma at the National, Regional, and Global Level, 1990–2019: Results from the Global Burden of Disease Study," *Frontiers in Medicine* 8 (2021): 738693.

191. World Health Organization, "History of the Polio Vaccine," https://www.who.int/news-room/spotlight/history-of-vaccination/history-of-polio-vaccination; "Surveillance of Poliomyelitis in the United States, 1958–61," *Public Health Reports* 77.12 (1962): 1011–20.

192. D. Orsini and M. Martini, "Albert Bruce Sabin: The Man Who Made the Oral Polio Vaccine," *Emerging Infectious Diseases* 28.3 (2022): 743–46.

193. Orsini and Martini, "Albert Bruce Sabin."

194. D. M. Horstmann, "The Sabin Live Poliovirus Vaccination Trial in the USSR, 1959," *Yale Journal of Biology and Medicine* 64.5 (1991): 499–512.

195. Horstmann, "Sabin Live Poliovirus Vaccination Trial."

196. Horstmann, "Sabin Live Poliovirus Vaccination Trial."

197. J. Martín, "Vaccine-Derived Poliovirus from Long Term Excretors and the End Game of Polio Eradication," *Biologicals: Journal of the International Association of Biological Standardization* 34.2 (2006): 117–22.

198. I. Ilil and M. Ilil, "Brain Cancer Incidence."

199. M. Famulare et al., "Sabin Vaccine Reversion in the Field: A Comprehensive Analysis of Sabin-Like Poliovirus Isolates in Nigeria," *Journal of Virology* 90.1 (2015): 317–31; J. Quarleri, "Poliomyelitis Is a Current Challenge: Long-Term Sequelae and Circulating Vaccine-Derived Poliovirus," *Geroscience* 45.2 (2023): 707–17; A. Mohanty et al., "Vaccine Derived Poliovirus (VDPV)," *InfezMed* 31.2 (2023): 174–85.

200. D. M. Evans et al., "Increased Neurovirulence Associated with a Single Nucleotide Change in a Noncoding Region of the Sabin Type 3 Poliovaccine Genome," *Nature* 314 (1985): 548–50.

201. L. N. Alexander, "Vaccine Policy Changes and Epidemiology of Poliomyelitis in the United States," *JAMA* 292 (2004): 1696–701.

202. U.S. Centers for Disease Control and Prevention, "Polio Vaccination," July 9, 2024, https://www.cdc.gov/vaccines/vpd/polio/public/index.html.

203. J. P. Alexander et al., "Transmission of Imported Vaccine-Derived Poliovirus in an Undervaccinated Community in Minnesota," *Journal of Infectious Diseases* 199 (2009): 391–97
204. A. S. DeVries et al., "Vaccine-Derived Poliomyelitis 12 Years After Infection in Minnesota," *New England Journal of Medicine* 364 (2011): 2316–23.
205. R. Link-Gelles et al., "Public Health Response to a Case of Paralytic Poliomyelitis in an Unvaccinated Person and Detection of Poliovirus in Wastewater—New York, June–August 2022," *Morbidity and Mortality Weekly Report* 71.33 (2022): 1065–68; A. Rai et al., "Polio Returns to the USA: An Epidemiological Alert," *Annals of Medicine and Surgery* 82 (2022): 104563.
206. Mohanty et al., "Vaccine Derived Poliovirus."
207. G. R. Macklin et al., "Enabling Accelerated Vaccine Roll-Out for Public Health Emergencies of International Concern (PHEICs): Novel Oral Polio Vaccine Type 2 (nOPV2) Experience," *Vaccine* 41.1 (2023): A122–A127.
208. "How Much Money Did Jonas Salk Potentially Forfeit by Not Patenting the Polio Vaccine?" *Forbes*, August 9, 2012, https://www.forbes.com/sites/quora/2012/08/09/how-much-money-did-jonas-salk-potentially-forfeit-by-not-patenting-the-polio-vaccine/.
209. Plotkin, "CHAT Oral Polio Vaccine."
210. H. Koprowski et al., "Immunization of Infants with Living Attenuated Poliomyelitis Virus Laboratory Investigations of Alimentary Infection and Antibody Response in Infants Under Six Months of Age with Congenitally Acquired Antibodies," *JAMA* 162.14 (1956): 1281–88.
211. U.S. Centers for Disease Control and Prevention, "Polio Vaccination."
212. Eddy et al., "Tumors Induced in Hamsters."
213. Offit, "Cutter Incident."
214. Martín, "Vaccine-Derived Poliovirus."
215. Mohanty et al., "Vaccine Derived Poliovirus."
216. Bookchin and Schumacher, *Virus and the Vaccine.*

Chapter 7

217. C. Cao et al., "Understanding Periodic and Non-Periodic Chemistry in Periodic Tables," *Frontiers in Chemistry* 8 (2021): 813.
218. LibreTexts Chemistry, "1.2 Principles of atomic structure," accessed January 12, 2024, https://batch.libretexts.org/print/url=https://chem.libretexts.org/Bookshelves/Organic_Chemistry/Map%3A_Organic_Chemistry_(Wade)_Complete_and_Semesters_I_and_II/Map%3A_Organic_Chemistry_I_(Wade)/01%3A_Introduction_and_Review/1.02%3A_Principles_of_Atomic_Structure_(Review).pdf.
219. L. Brink, "Forces," The Nobel Prize Foundation, August 9, 2001, https://www.nobelprize.org/prizes/themes/forces.
220. N. Bohr, "The Structure of the Atom," Nobel Prize lecture delivered on December 11, 1922, https://www.nobelprize.org/uploads/2018/06/bohr-lecture.pdf.
221. R. P. Feynman, *QED: The Strange Theory of Light and Matter* (Princeton University Press, 1985).
222. L. Pauling. *The Nature of the Chemical Bond and the Structure of Molecules and Crystals: An Introduction to Modern Structural Chemistry* (Cornell University Press, 1960).
223. M. A. Zoroddu et. al., "The Essential Metals for Humans: A Brief Overview," *Journal of Inorganic Biochemistry* 195 (2019): 120–29.
224. D. S. MacPherson et al., "A Brief Overview of Metal Complexes as Nuclear Imaging Agents," *Dalton Transactions* 48.39 (2019): 14547–65.
225. E. Gibon et al., "The Biological Response to Orthopaedic Implants for Joint Replacement: Part I. Metals," *Journal of Biomedical Materials Research Part B* 105.7 (2017): 2162–73.
226. C. Harris, B. Croce, and C. Cao, "Tissue and Mechanical Heart Valves," *Annals of Cardiothoracic Surgery* 4.4 (2015): 399.
227. R. Morrison and R. Boyd, *Organic Chemistry*, 6th ed. (Benjamin-Cummings, 1992).
228. L. Pauling, "Modern Structural Chemistry," Nobel Prize lecture delivered on December 11, 1954, https://www.nobelprize.org/uploads/2018/06/pauling-lecture.pdf.

229. R. Mulliken, "Spectroscopy, Molecular Orbitals, and Chemical Bonding," Nobel Prize lecture delivered on December 12, 1966, https://www.nobelprize.org/uploads/2018/06/mulliken-lecture.pdf.
230. Å. G. Ekstrand, "Award Ceremony Speech," presented at the ceremony of the 1918 Nobel Prize in Chemistry, June 1, 1920, https://www.nobelprize.org/prizes/chemistry/1918/ceremony-speech/.
231. F. Bretislav and D. Hoffmann, "Clara Haber, nee Immerwahr (1870–1915): Life, Work and Legacy," *Zeitschrift für anorganische und allgemeine Chemie* 642.6 (2016): 437–48.

Chapter 8

232. G. Wolf, "Friedrich Miescher: The Man Who Discovered DNA," *Chemical Heritage* 21 (2003): 37–41.
233. P. A. Levene, "The Structure of Yeast Nucleic Acid. IV. Ammonia Hydrolysis," *Journal of Biological Chemistry* 40.1 (1919): 415–24.
234. O. Avery, C. MacLeod, and M. McCarthy, "Studies on the Chemical Nature of the Substance Inducing Transformation of Pneumococcal Types: Induction of Transformation by a Desoxyribonucleic Acid Fraction Isolated from Pneumococcus Type iii," *Journal of Experimental Medicine* 79.2 (1944): 137–58.
235. T. Ghose, "Oswald Avery: The Professor, DNA, and the Nobel Prize That Eluded Him," *Canadian Bulletin of Medical History* 21.1 (2004): 135–44.
236. E. Chargaff, "Chemical Specificity of Nucleic Acids and Mechanism of Their Enzymatic Degradation," *Experientia* 6 (1950): 201–9.
237. L. A. Pray, "Discovery of DNA Structure and Function: Watson and Crick," *Nature Education* 1.1 (2008): 100.
238. T. M. Thomas, "The Birth of X-Ray Crystallography," *Nature* 491 (2012): 186–87.
239. A. Roy and A. G. Sheeja Rekha, "A Review on X-Ray Diffraction," *International Journal of Pharmaceutical Research and Applications* 7.2 (2022): 786–88.
240. Joachim Pietzsch, "Perspectives: The Parent Trap," The Nobel Prize Foundation, https://www.nobelprize.org/prizes/physics/1915/perspectives/.

241. S. Galli, "X-Ray Crystallography: One Century of Nobel Prizes," *Journal of Chemical Education* 91.12 (2014): 2009–12.

242. R. Sommer, "How to Grow Crystals for X-Ray Crystallography," *Structural Chemistry* 80.8 (2024): 337–42.

243. J. T. Waters et al., "Transitions of Double-Stranded DNA Between the A- and B-Forms," *Journal of Physical Chemistry B* 120.33 (2016): 8449–56.

244. J. D. Watson and F. H. C. Crick, "Molecular Structure of Nucleic Acids: A Structure for Deoxyribose Nucleic Acid," *Nature* 171 (1953): 737–38.

245. J. D. Watson, *The Double Helix: A Personal Account of the Discovery of the Structure of DNA* (Atheneum, 1968).

246. M. Wilkins, *The Third Man of the Double Helix: An Autobiography* (Oxford University Press, 2015).

247. R. R. Jarrett, "Watson, Crick, DNA, Nobel Prize," *Pediatric House Calls* (blog), December 2, 2017, https://pediatric-house-calls.com/james-watson-francis-crick-dna/.

248. D. Rogers, "After Prometheus, Are Human Genes Patentable Subject Matter?," *Duke Law and Technology Review* 11.2 (2013): 434–508. https://scholarship.law.duke.edu/cgi/viewcontent.cgi?article=1243&context=dltr.

249. F. Kabata and D. Thaldar, "The Human Genome as the Common Heritage of Humanity," *Frontiers in Genetics* 14 (2023): 1282515.

250. *Association for Molecular Pathology v. Myriad Genetics, Inc.*, 569 U.S. 576 (2013).

251. D. Crow, "James Watson to Sell Nobel Prize Medal," *Financial Times*, November 28, 2014, https://www.ft.com/content/5fb47ebe-75bc-11e4-a1a9-00144feabdc0; S. Y. Tan and A. N. McCoy, "James Dewey Watson (1928–): Co-Discoverer of the Structure of DNA," *Singapore Medical Journal* 61.10 (2020): 507–8.

252. "Russia's Usmanov to Give Back Watson's Auctioned Nobel Medal," *BBC News*, December 9, 2014. https://www.bbc.com/news/world-europe-30406322.

253. See chapter 3 in K. Mullis, *Dancing Naked in the Mind Field* (Pantheon, 1998).

254. K. Mullis, "Cosmological Significance of Time Reversal," *Nature* 218 (1968): 663–64.

255. Mullis, *Dancing Naked*, 209.

256. L. Garibyan and N. Avashia, "Polymerase Chain Reaction," *Journal of Investigative Dermatology* 133.3 (2013): 1–4

257. K. Mullis, "Kary B. Mullis Biographical," The Nobel Prize Foundation, last updated 2005, https://www.nobelprize.org/prizes/chemistry/1993/mullis/biographical/.

258. M. Gross, "All About Allium," *Current Biology* 31.22 (2021): R1449–R1452.

259. "Immortality Drive ISS–What Is the Immortality Drive Program?," SciQuest, https://sciquest.org/immortality-drive-iss/.

Chapter 9

260. Gerardus Johannes Mulder, "On the Composition of Some Animal Substances," *Journal für praktische Chemie* 16.129 (1839).

261. H. B. Vickery, "The Origin of the Word Protein," *Yale Journal of Biology and Medicine* 22 (1950): 387–93.

262. T. L. Hendrickson, V. de Crécy-Lagard, and P. Schimmel, "Incorporation of Nonnatural Amino Acids into Proteins," *Annual Review of Biochemistry* 73 (2004): 147–76.

263. In humans, there is also rarely used twenty-first proteinogenic amino acid called selenocysteine that replaces sulfur with a selenium atom; it will not be discussed further in this volume. See Y. Zhang and V. N. Gladyshev, "High Content of Proteins Containing 21st and 22nd Amino Acids, Selenocysteine and Pyrrolysine, in a Symbiotic Deltaproteobacterium of Gutless Worm *Olavius algarvensis*," *Nucleic Acids Research* 35.15 (2007): 4952–63.

264. E. A. Bell, "Nonprotein Amino Acids of Plants: Significance in Medicine, Nutrition, and Agriculture," *Journal of Agricultural and Food Chemistry* 51.10 (2003): 2854–65.

265. S. M. Sears and S. J. Hewett, "Influence of Glutamate and GABA Transport on Brain Excitatory/Inhibitory Balance," *Experimental Biology and Medicine* 246.9 (2021): 1069–83.

266. J. L. Bada et al., "A Search for Endogenous Amino Acids in Martian Meteorite ALH84001," *Science* 279 (1998): 362–65.

267. W. Steigerwald, "First Look at Ryugu Asteroid Sample Reveals It Is Organic-Rich," NASA.gov, February 23, 2023, https://www.nasa.gov/centers-and-facilities/goddard/first-look-at-ryugu-asteroid-sample-reveals-it-is-organic-rich/.

268. Paul Voosen, "This May Be the Most Distant Object in Our Solar System: 'Farout' Dwarf Planet Spotted During Search for Hypothesized Ninth Planet," American Association for the Advancement of Science, December 17, 2018, https://www.science.org/content/article/may-be-most-distant-object-our-solar-system.

269. C. Sagan and B. Khare, "Tholins: Organic Chemistry of Interstellar Grains and Gas," *Nature* 277 (1979): 102–7.

270. "Mars 2020: Perseverance Rover," NASA.org, last updated November 10, 2024, https://science.nasa.gov/mission/mars-2020-perseverance/science/.

271. R. Milo, "What Is the Total Number of Protein Molecules per Cell Volume? A Call to Rethink Some Published Values," *Bioessays* 35.12 (2013): 1050–55.

272. A. K. W. Tiselius, "Electrophoresis and Adsorption Analysis as Aids in Investigations of Large Molecular Weight Substances and Their Breakdown Products," Nobel Prize lecture given on December 13, 1948, https://www.nobelprize.org/uploads/2018/06/tiselius-lecture.pdf.

273. H. H.-H. Chiang, "The Laboratory Technology of Discrete Molecular Separation: The Historical Development of Gel Electrophoresis and the Material Epistemology of Biomolecular Science, 1945–1970," *Journal of the History of Biology* 42 (2009): 495–527.

274. C. S. Ho et al., "Electrospray Ionization Mass Spectroscopy: Principles and Clinical Applications," *Clinical Biochemist Reviews* 24 (2003): 3–12.

275. J. B. Fenn et al., "Electrospray Ionization for Mass Spectroscopy of Large Biomolecules," *Science* 246 (1989): 64–71.

276. *Fenn v. Yale University*, 283 F. Supp. 2d 615 (D. Conn. 2003).

277. M. Labowsky et al., "Yale Patent Lawsuit Was Terrible Mistake," *Yale Daily News*, March 2, 2005.

278. H. Kissinger, C. Mundie, and E. Schmidt, *Genesis: Artificial Intelligence, Hope, and the Human Spirit* (Little, Brown & Company, 2024).
279. R. Landick, "A Long Time in the Making: The Nobel Prize for RNA Polymerase," *Cell* 127.6 (2006): 1087–90; M. Girbig, A. D. Misiaszek, and C. W. Müller, "Structural Insights into Nuclear Transcription by Eukaryotic DNA-Dependent RNA Polymerases," *Nature Reviews Molecular Cell Biology* 23 (2022): 603–22.
280. A. J. Ward and T. A. Cooper, "The Pathobiology of Splicing," *Journal of Pathology* 220 (2010): 152–63.
281. T. N. Raju, "The Nobel Chronicles. 1993: Richard John Roberts (b 1943) Phillip A Sharp (b 1944)," *The Lancet* 355.9220 (2000): 2085.
282. R. A. Padgett, "New Connections Between Splicing and Human Disease," *Trends in Genetics* 28.4 (2012): 147–54.
283. V. Ramakrishman, "Ribosome Structure and the Mechanism of Translation," *Cell* 108.4 (2002): 557–72.
284. T. A. Lincoln and G. F. Joyce, "Self-Sustained Replication of an RNA Enzyme," *Science* 323 (2009): 1229–32.
285. D. N. Wilson, "Ribosome-Targeting Antibiotics and Mechanisms of Bacterial Resistance," *Nature Reviews Microbiology* 12.1 (2014): 35–48.
286. G. Meola and R. Cardani, "Myotonic Dystrophies: An Update on Clinical Aspects, Genetic, Pathology, and Molecular Pathomechanisms," *Biochimica et Biophysica Acta* 1852.4 (2015): 594–606.
287. International Human Genome Sequencing Consortium, "Initial Sequencing and Analysis of the Human Genome," *Nature* 409 (2001): 860–921.
288. J. B. Fenn, *Engines, Energy, and Entropy: A Thermodynamic Primer* (1982; repr. Freeman & Company, 2003), 50.

Chapter 10

289. Centers for Disease Control, "*Pneumocystis* Pneumonia—Los Angeles," *Morbidity and Mortality Weekly Report* 30.21 (1981): 1–3.

290. K. K. Vidya Vijayan et al., "Pathophysiology of CD4+ T-Cell Depletion in HIV-1 and HIV-2 Infections," *Frontiers in Immunology* 8 (2017): 580.
291. Centers for Disease Control, "Kaposi's Sarcoma and Pneumocystis Pneumonia Among Homosexual Men—New York City and California," *Morbidity and Mortality Weekly Report* 30.25 (1981): 305–8.
292. N. Iftode et al., "Update on Kaposi Sarcoma-Associated Herpesvirus (KSHV or HHV8)–Review," *Romanian Journal of Internal Medicine* 58.4 (2020): 199–208.
293. R. D. Mugerwa, L. H. Marum, and D. Serwadda, "Human Immunodeficiency Virus and AIDS in Uganda," *East African Medical Journal* 73.1 (1996): 20–26.
294. D. M. Auerbach et al., "Cluster of Cases of the Acquired Immune Deficiency Syndrome: Patients Linked by Sexual Contact," *American Journal of Medicine* 76.3 (1984): 487–92.
295. R. A. McKay, "'Patient Zero': The Absence of a Patient's View of the Early North American AIDS Epidemic," *Bulletin of the History of Medicine* 88.1 (2014): 161–94.
296. L. Montagnier, "Historical Essay. A History of HIV Discovery," *Science* 298 (2002): 1727–28.
297. F. Barre-Sinoussi et al., "Isolation of a T-Lymphotropic Retrovirus from a Patient at Risk for Acquired Immune Deficiency Syndrome (AIDS)," *Science* 220 (1983): 868–71.
298. R. C. Gallo, "The Discovery of the First Human Retrovirus: HTLV-1 and HTLV-2," *Retrovirology* 2 (2005): 17.
299. R. C. Gallo et al., "Frequent Detection and Isolation of Cytopathic Retroviruses (HTLV-III) from Patients with AIDS and at Risk for AIDS," *Science* 224 (1984): 500–503.
300. Ronald Reagan, "Remarks Announcing the AIDS Research Patent Rights Agreement Between France and the United States," The American Presidency Project, March 31, 1987, https://www.presidency.ucsb.edu/documents/remarks-announcing-the-aids-research-patent-rights-agreement-between-france-and-the-united.
301. Montagnier, "History of HIV Discovery"; R. C. Gallo, "Historical Essay: The Early Years of HIV/AIDS," *Science* 298 (2002): 1728–30.

302. L. Montagnier, "25 Years After HIV Discovery: Prospects for Cure and Vaccine (Nobel Lecture)," *Angewandte Chemie* 48.32 (2009): 5815–26.

303. S. Chevret et al., "A New Approach to Estimating AIDS Incubation Times: Results in Homosexual Infected Men," *Journal of Epidemiology and Community Health* 46.6 (1992): 582–86.

304. A. J. Jasinska, C. Apetrei, and I. Pandrea, "Walk on the Wild Side: SIV Infection in African Non-Human Primate Hosts—From the Field to the Laboratory," *Frontiers in Immunology* 13 (2023): 1060985.

305. S. Nyamweya et al., "Comparing HIV-1 and HIV-2 Infection: Lessons for Viral Immunopathogenesis," *Reviews in Medical Virology* 23.4 (2013): 221–40.

306. E. Bailes et al., "Hybrid Origin of SIV in Chimpanzees," *Science* 300 (2003): 1713.

307. B. S. Taylor et al., "The Challenge of HIV-1 Subtype Diversity," *New England Journal of Medicine* 358.15 (2008): 1590–602.

308. L. Smith and S. Marsh, "Attacks Escalate as Habitat Faces Increasing Pressure from Man," *The London Times*, December 31, 2003, https://www.thetimes.com/comment/register/article/chimps-eat-children-in-war-of-survival-s9l5zm8pn52?region=global.

309. C. Z. Buffalo et al., "Structural Basis for Tetherin Antagonism as a Barrier to Zoonotic Lentiviral Transmission," *Cell Host and Microbe* 26.3 (2019): 359–68; J. F. Arias et.al., "Tetherin Antagonism by Vpu Protects HIV-Infected Cells from Antibody-Dependent Cell-Mediated Cytotoxicity," *PNAS* 111.17 (2014): 6425–30.

310. A. J. Nahmias et al., "Evidence for Human Infection with an HTLV-III/LAV-Like Virus in Central Africa, 1959," *The Lancet* 1 (1986): 1279–80.

311. D. Baum, "Reading a Phylogenetic Tree: The Meaning of Monophyletic Groups," *Nature Education* 1.1 (2008): 190.

312. T. Zhu et al., "An African HIV-1 Sequence from 1959 and Implications for the Origin of the Epidemic," *Nature* 391 (1998): 594–97.

313. B. Korber et al., "Timing the Ancestor of HIV-1 Pandemic Strains," *Science* 288 (2000): 1789–96.

314. Personal communication with Dr. Bette Korber, theoretical biologist and biophysicist, at Los Alamos National Laboratory.

315. C. Kuiken et al., eds., *HIV Sequence Compendium 2010* (Los Lamos National Registry Laboratory, 2011).

316. P. M. Sharp and B. H. Hahn, "The Evolution of HIV-1 and the Origin of AIDS," *Philosophical Transactions of the Royal Society of London B* 365.1552 (2010): 2487–94; L. M. Wong and G. Jiang, "NF-κB Sub-Pathways and HIV Cure: A Revisit," *EBioMedicine* 63 (2021): 103159.

317. A. Dutilleul, A. Rodari, and C. Van Lint, "Depicting HIV-1 Transcriptional Mechanisms: A Summary of What We Know," *Viruses* 12.12 (2020): 1385; J. H. Day et al., "Does Tuberculosis Increase HIV Load?," *Journal for Infectious Diseases* 190.9 (2004): 1677–84; R. H. Lyles et al., "Prognostic Value of Plasma HIV RNA in the Natural History of *Pneumocystis carinii* Pneumonia, Cytomegalovirus and *Mycobacterium avium* Complex: Multicenter AIDS Cohort Study," *AIDS* 13 (1999): 341–49; C. E. Bush et al., "A Study of RNA Viral Load in AIDS Patients with Bacterial Pneumonia," *Journal of Acquired Immune Deficiency Syndrome Human Retrovirology* 13 (1996): 23–26; R. M. Donovan et al., "Changes in Virus Load Markers During AIDS-Associated Opportunistic Diseases in Human Immunodeficiency Virus-Infected Persons," *Journal of Infectious Diseases* 174 (1996): 401–3; M. S. Sulkowski et al., "The Effect of Acute Infectious Illnesses on Plasma Human Immunodeficiency Virus (HIV) Type 1 Load and the Expression of Serologic Markers of Immune Activation Among HIV-Infected Adults," *Journal of Infectious Diseases* 178 (1998): 1642–48; D. Goletti et al., "Effect of Mycobacterium Tuberculosis on HIV Replication: Role of Immune Activation," Journal of Immunology 157.3 (1996): 1271–78; M. S. Cohen et al., "Reduction of Concentration of HIV-1 in Semen After Treatment of Urethritis: Implications for Prevention of Sexual Transmission of HIV-1. AIDSCAP Malawi Research Group," *The Lancet* 349 (1997): 1868–73.

318. A. Kotwal, "Innovation, Diffusion and Safety of a Medical Technology: A Review of the Literature on Injection Practices," *Social Science and Medicine* 60.5 (2005): 1133–47.

319. J. C. Petithory et al., "Prévention de la transmission par les seringues et aiguilles du V.I.H. en France et en Afrique," *Bulletin de l'Académie Nationale de Médecine* 173.4 (1989): 415–20; M. Dicko et al., "Safety of Immunization Injections in Africa: Not Simply a Problem of Logistics," *Bulletin of the World Health Organization* 78.2 (2000): 163–69.
320. E. Hooper, *The River: A Journey to the Source of HIV and AIDS* (Back Bay, 2000).
321. S. A. Plotkin, A. Lebrun, and H. Koprowski, "Vaccination with the CHAT Strain of Type 1 Attenuated Poliomyelitis in Leopoldville, Belgian Congo," *Bulletin of the World Health Organization* 22.3–4 (1960): 215–34.
322. S. A. Plotkin and H. Koprowski, "No Evidence to Link Polio Vaccine with HIV (Letter)," *Nature* 407 (2000): 941–47.
323. P. Blancou et al., "Polio Vaccine Samples Not Linked to AIDS," *Nature* 410 (2001): 1045–46.
324. Personal email communication between Hooper and myself.
325. Report of an International Commission, "Ebola Haemorrhagic Vever in Zaire, 1976," *Bulletin of the World Health Organization* 56.2 (1978): 271–93.
326. M. Hayami, E. Ido, and T. Miura, "Survey of Simian Immunodeficiency Virus Among Nonhuman Primate Populations," *Current Topics in Microbiology and Immunology* 188 (1994): 1–20.
327. C. Patience, Y. Takeuchi, and R. Weiss, "Infection of Human Cells by an Endogenous Retrovirus of Pigs," *Nature Medicine* 3 (1997): 282–86.
328. R. W. Shafer and J. M. Schapiro, "HIV-1 Drug Resistance Mutations: An Updated Framework for the Second Decade of HAART," *AIDS Reviews* 10.2 (2008): 67–84.
329. E. K. Hanners, J. Benitez-Burke, and M. E. Badowski, "HIV: How to Manage Low-Level Viraemia in People Living with HIV," *Drugs in Context* 11 (2022): 2021-8-13.
330. S. Broder, "The Development of Antiretroviral Therapy and Its Impact on the HIV-1/AIDS Pandemic," *Antiviral Research* 85.1 (2010): 1–18;

E. J. Arts and D. J. Hazuda, "HIV-1 Antiretroviral Drug Therapy," *Cold Spring Harbor Perspectives in Medicine* 2.4 (2012): a007161.

331. Arts and Hazuda, "HIV-1 Antiretroviral Drug Therapy."
332. D. Y. Lu et al., "HAART in HIV/AIDS Treatments: Future Trends," *Infectious Disorders Drug Targets* 18.1 (2018): 15–22. R. W. Shafer and D. A. Vuitton, "Highly Active Antiretroviral Therapy (HAART) for the Treatment of Infection with Human Immunodeficiency Virus Type 1," *Biomedicine and Pharmacotherapy* 53.2 (1999): 73–86.
333. T. C. Quinn et al., "Viral Load and Heterosexual Transmission of Human Immunodeficiency Virus Type 1. Rakai Project Study Group," *New England Journal of Medicine* 342.13 (2000): 921–29.
334. J. M. Lange and J. Ananworanich, "The Discovery and Development of Antiretroviral Agents," *Antiviral Therapy* 19.3 (2014): 5–14.
335. M. Angell, "Investigators' Responsibilities for Human Subjects in Developing Countries," *New England Journal of Medicine* 342.13 (2000): 967–69.
336. R. H. Gray et al., "Letter to the Editor: The Ethics of Research in Developing Countries," *New England Journal of Medicine* 343.5 (2000): 361–64.
337. S. M. Baker, O. W. Brawley, and L. S. Marks, "Effects of Untreated Syphilis in the Negro Male, 1932 to 1972: A Closure Comes to the Tuskegee Study, 2004," *Urology* 65.6 (2005): 1259–62.
338. J. Katz, "The Nuremberg Code and the Nuremberg Trial: A Reappraisal," *JAMA* 276.20 (1996): 1662–66.
339. G. J. Annas, "Beyond Nazi War Crimes Experiments: The Voluntary Consent Requirement of the Nuremberg Code at 70," *American Journal of Public Health* 108.1 (2018): 42–46.

Chapter 11

340. D. Singh et al., "Global Estimates of Incidence and Mortality of Cervical Cancer in 2020: A Baseline Analysis of the WHO Global Cervical Cancer Elimination Initiative," *Lancet Global Health* 11.2 (2023): e197–e206.

341. P. Tsikouras et al., "Cervical Cancer: Screening, Diagnosis and Staging," *Journal of BUON* 21.2 (2016): 320–25.

342. S. Zhou and F. Peng, "Patterns of Metastases in Cervical Cancer: A Population-Based Study," *International Journal of Clinical and Experimental Pathology* 13 (2020): 1615–23.

343. D. W. Thaldar, "Who Would Own the HeLa Cell Line If the Henrietta Lacks Case Happened in Present-Day South Africa?," *Journal of Law and the Biosciences* 10.1 (2023): 203–13.

344. T. Pultarova, "HeLa Cells: Immortal Space Travellers," *Space Safety* Magazine, Spring 2013, http://www.spacesafetymagazine.com/wp-content/uploads/2015/05/Focus%20-%20HeLa%20Cells,%20Immortal%20Space%20Travelellers.pdf.

345. R. Lacks, *Henrietta Lack: The Untold Story* (BookBaby, 2020).

346. L. Waelsch, "Übertragungsversuche mit spitzem Kondylom," *Archives of Dermatological Research* 124 (1917): 625–46.

347. M. J. Strauss et al., "Crystalline Virus-Like Particles from Skin Papillomas Characterized by Intranuclear Inclusion Bodies," *Proceedings for the Society for Experimental Biology and Medicine* 72 (1949): 46–50.

348. L. V. Crawford and E. M. Crawford, "A Comparative Study of Polyoma and Papilloma Viruses," *Virology* 21 (1963): 258–63.

349. P. Rous and J. W. Beard, "Progression to Carcinoma of Virus-Induced Rabbit Papillomas," *Journal for Experimental Medicine* 62 (1935): 523–45; P. Rous, J. G. Kidd, and J. W. Beard, "Observations on the Relation of the Virus Causing Rabbit Papilloma to the Cancers Deriving There From," *Journal for Experimental Medicine* 64 (1936): 385–400.

350. H. zur Hausen, "Cancers in Humans: A Lifelong Search for Contributions of Infectious Agents, Autobiographic Notes," *Annual Review of Virology* 6.1 (2019): 1–28.

351. M. Dürst et al., "A Papillomavirus DNA from a Cervical Carcinoma and Its Prevalence in Cancer Biopsy Samples from Different Geographic Regions," *PNAS* 80 (1983): 3812–15; M. Boshart et al., "A New Type of Papillomavirus DNA, Its Presence in Genital Cancer Biopsies and in Cell Lines Derived from Genital Cancer," *EMBO Journal* 3 (1984): 1151–57.

352. The Rockefeller University, "1966 Nobel Prize in Physiology or Medicine," https://www.rockefeller.edu/our-scientists/peyton-rous/2493-nobel-prize/#:~:text=Rous's%20fearless%20approach%20as%20head,Prize%20in%20Physiology%20or%20Medicine.
353. J. T. Schiller and D. R. Lowy, "An Introduction to Virus Infections and Human Cancer. Recent Results," *Cancer Research* 217 (2021): 1–11.
354. P. Farinha and R. D. Gascoyne, "Helicobacter Pylori and MALT Lymphoma," *Gastroenterology* 128 (2005): 1579–1605.
355. J. B. Park and J. S. Koo, "Helicobacter Pylori Infection in Gastric Mucosa-Associated Lymphoid Tissue Lymphoma," *World Journal of Gastroenterology* 2 (2014): 2751–59.
356. W. Yangyanqiu and H. Shuwen, "Bacterial DNA Involvement in Carcinogenesis," *Frontiers in Cellular and Infection Microbiology* 12 (2022): 996778.
357. P. Brianti, E. De Flammineis, and S. R. Mercuri, "Review of HPV-Related Diseases and Cancers," *New Microbiologica* 40.2 (2017): 80–85.
358. N. M. Reusser et al., "HPV Carcinomas in Immunocompromised Patients," *Journal of Clinical Medicine* 4.2 (2015): 260–81.
359. K. Münger et al., "Mechanisms of Human Papillomavirus-Induced Oncogenesis," *Journal of Virology* 78.21 (2004): 11451–60.
360. Q. Peng et al., "HPV E6/E7: Insights into Their Regulatory Role and Mechanism in Signaling Pathways in HPV-Associated Tumor," *Cancer Gene Therapy* 31.1 (2024): 9–17; E. K. Yim and J. S. Park, "The Role of HPV E6 and E7 Oncoproteins in HPV-Associated Cervical Carcinogenesis," *Cancer Research and Treatment* 37.6 (2005): 319–24.
361. L. Zhu, Z. Lu, and H. Zhao, "Antitumor Mechanisms When pRb and p53 Are Genetically Inactivated," *Oncogene* 34.35 (2015): 4547–57.
362. A. G. Ostör, "Natural History of Cervical Intraepithelial Neoplasia: A Critical Review," *International Journal of Gynecological Pathology* 12.2 (1993): 186–92.
363. L. S. Massad et al., "2012 ASCCP Consensus Guidelines Conference: 2012 Updated Consensus Guidelines for the Management of

Abnormal Cervical Cancer Screening Tests and Cancer Precursors," *Journal of Lower Genital Tract Disease* 17.5 (2013): S1–S27.

364. G. N. Papanicolaou, "A New Procedure for Staining Vaginal Smears," *Science* 95 (1942): 438–39.
365. M. O. Mohsen and M. F, Bachmann, "Virus-Like Particle Vaccinology, from Bench to Bedside," *Cellular and Molecular Immunology* 19.9 (2022): 993–1011.
366. M. E. Hagensee et al., "Three Dimensional Structure of Vaccinia Virus-Produced Human Papillomavirus Type 1 Capsids," *Journal of Virology* 68 (1994): 4503–5.
367. J. Zepeda-Cervantes, J. O. Ramírez-Jarquín, and L. Vaca, "Interaction Between Virus-Like Particles (VLPs) and Pattern Recognition Receptors (PRRs) from Dendritic Cells (DCs): Toward Better Engineering of VLPs," *Frontiers in Immunology* 11 (2020): 1100.
368. V. Srivastava et al., "Yeast-Based Virus-Like Particles as an Emerging Platform for Vaccine Development and Delivery," *Vaccines* 11.2 (2023): 479.
369. A. L. V. Coradini et al., "Building Synthetic Chromosomes from Natural DNA," *Nature Communications* 14 (2023): 8337.
370. J. Asami et al., "Bacterial Artificial Chromosomes as Analytical Basis for Gene Transcriptional Machineries," *Transgenic Research* 20.4 (2011): 913–24.
371. S. V. Ponomartsev, S. A. Sinenko, and A. N. Tomilin, "Human Artificial Chromosomes and Their Transfer to Target Cells," *Acta Naturae* 14.3 (2022): 35–45.
372. D. T. Burke, G. F. Carle, and M. V. Olson, "Cloning of Large Segments of Exogenous DNA into Yeast by Means of Artificial Chromosome Vectors," *Science* 236 (1987): 806–12; D. Schlessinger and R. Nagaraja, "Impact and Implications of Yeast and Human Artificial Chromosomes," *Annals of Medicine* 30.2 (1998): 186–91.
373. D. T. Le and K. M. Müller, "In Vitro Assembly of Virus-Like Particles and Their Applications," *Life* 11 (2021): 334.
374. A. Zeltins, "Construction and Characterization of Virus-Like Particles: A Review," *Molecular Biotechnology* 53.1 (2013): 92–107.

375. Table modified from N. Matsumura and I. Tsunoda, "Scientific Evaluation of Alleged Findings in HPV Vaccines: Molecular Mimicry and Mouse Models of Vaccine-Induced Disease," *Cancer Science* 113.10 (2022): 3313–20.
376. Eric Sagonowsky, "GSK Exits U.S. Market with Its HPV Vaccine Cervarix," FiercePharma, October 21, 2016, https://www.fiercepharma.com/pharma/gsk-exits-u-s-market-its-hpv-vaccine-cervarix.
377. S. M. Garland and FUTURE I Study Group, "Quadrivalent Vaccine Against Human Papillomavirus to Prevent Anogenital Diseases," *New England Journal of Medicine* 356.19 (2007): 1928–43.
378. FUTURE II Study Group, "Quadrivalent Vaccine Against Human Papillomavirus to Prevent High-Grade Cervical Lesions," *New England Journal of Medicine* 356.19 (2007): 1915–27.
379. E. A. Joura et al., "A 9-Valent HPV Vaccine Against Infection and Intraepithelial Neoplasia in Women," *New England Journal of Medicine* 372.8 (2015): 711–23.
380. J. Paavonen et al., "Efficacy of a Prophylactic Adjuvanted Bivalent L1 Virus-Like-Particle Vaccine Against Infection with Human Papillomavirus Types 16 and 18 in Young Women: An Interim Analysis of a Phase III Double-Blind, Randomised Controlled Trial," *The Lancet* 369.9580 (2007): 2161–70.
381. L. A. Laimins, "The Biology of Human Papillomaviruses: From Warts to Cancer," Infectious Agents and Diseases 2.2 (1993): 74–86; F. Stubenrauch and L. A. Laimins, "Human Papillomavirus Life Cycle: Active and Latent Phases," *Seminars in Cancer Biology* 9.6 (1999): 379–86.
382. J. Schiller and P. Davies, "Delivering on the Promise: HPV Vaccines and Cervical Cancer," *Nature Reviews Microbiology* 2 (2004): 343–47.
383. R. V. Barnabas et al., "Efficacy of Single-Dose HPV Vaccination Among Young African Women," *New England Journal of Medicine Evidence* 1.5 (2022): EVIDoa2100056.
384. A. I. Khalil et al., "Efficacy and Safety of Therapeutic HPV Vaccines to Treat CIN2/CIN3 Lesions: A Systemic Review and Meta-Analysis of Phase II/III Clinical Trials," *BMJ Open* 13.10 (2023): e069616.

385. From personal email communication.
386. M. Songane and V. Grossmann, "The Patent Buyout Price for Human Papilloma Virus (HPV) Vaccine and the Ratio of R&D Costs to the Patent Value," *PLoS One* 16.1 (2021) :e0244722.
387. S. Padmanabhan et al., "Intellectual Property, Technology Transfer and Manufacture of Low-Cost HPV Vaccines in India," *Nature Biotechnology* 28 (2010): 671–78.
388. A. Darby, "Frazer vs Schlegel April 8, 2021," *Embryo Project Encyclopedia*, August 4, 2021, https://embryo.asu.edu/pages/frazer-v-schlegel-2007.
389. Heather Tomlinson, "Glaxo and Merck Agree Deal on Cervical Cancer Vaccine," *The Guardian*, February 4, 2005, http://amp.theguardian.com/society/2005/feb/04/medicineandhealth.cancercare.
390. Elizabeth Walker, "HPV Vaccine Deal Gives GSK Royalties From Merck's Product," CiteLine, February 3, 2005, https://pink.citeline.com/PS061653/HPV-Vaccine-Deal-Gives-GSK-Royalties-From-Mercks-Product#:~:text=Executive%20Summary,receive%20payments%20from%20both%20companies.
391. L. Farrow, "Seven Added to National Living Treasure List," *Canberra Times*, March 5, 2012.
392. J. H. Tanne, "Texas Governor Is Criticised for Decision to Vaccinate All Girls Against HPV," *BMJ* 334.7589 (2007): 332–33.
393. R. Lizza, "HPV, Perry, and Bachman," *The New Yorker*, September 13, 2011, https://www.newyorker.com/news/news-desk/hpv-perry-and-bachmann.
394. European Medicines Agency, "Funding," https://www.ema.europa.eu/en/about-us/how-we-work/governance-reporting/funding.
395. D. F. Thompson, "Understanding Financial Conflicts of Interest," *New England Journal of Medicine* 329.8 (1993): 573–76.
396. K. Sonawane et al., "Trends in Papilloma Vaccine Safety Concerns and Adverse Event Reporting in United States," *JAMA Network Open* 4.9 (2021): e2124502.
397. D. Ward et al., "A Cluster Analysis of Serious Adverse Event Reports After Human Papillomavirus (HPV) Vaccination in Danish Girls and

Young Women, September 2009 to August 2017," *Euro Surveillance* 24.19 (2019): 1800380.

398. M. Holland, K. M. Rosenberg, and E. Iorio, *The HPD Vaccine on Trial: Seeking Justice for a Generation Betrayed* (Simon & Schuster, 2018); C. England, *Shattered Dreams: The HPV Vaccine Exposed* (CreateSpace, 2019).
399. Verbal communication with Ron Miller from Miller & Zois Attorneys at Law.
400. K. Stratton et al., eds., *Adverse Effects of Vaccines: Evidence and Causality* (National Academies Press, 2011).
401. Verbal communication with Ron Miller from Miller & Zois Attorneys at Law.
402. A. Di Pasquale et al., "Vaccine Adjuvants: From 1920 to 2015 and Beyond," *Vaccines* 3.2 (2015): 320–43.
403. M. Lehtinen and J. Dillner, "Clinical Trials of Human Papillomavirus Vaccines and Beyond," *Nature Reviews Clinical Oncology* 10 (2013): 400–410; P. E. Gravitt and R. L. Winer, "Natural History of HPV Infection Across the Lifespan: Role of Viral Latency," *Viruses* 9 (2017): 266–76.
404. C. D. Harro et al., "Safety and Immunogenicity Trial in Adult Volunteers of a Human Papillomavirus 16 L1 Virus-Like Particle Vaccine," *Journal of the National Cancer Institute* 93.4 (2001): 284–92.
405. L. Montagnier in Holland, Rosenberg, and Iorio, *HPV Vaccine on Trial*, xv–xvi.
406. L. Montagnier in Holland, Rosenberg, and Iorio, *HPV Vaccine on Trial*, xv–xvi.
407. V. Indla and M. S. Radhika, "Hippocratic Oath: Losing Relevance in Today's World?," *Indian Journal of Psychiatry* 61.4 (2019): S773–S775.
408. J. E. Balog, "The Moral Justification for a Compulsory Human Papillomavirus Vaccination Program," *American Journal of Public Health* 99.4 (2009): 616–22.

Chapter 12

409. M. Zhao, Y. Li, and Z. Wang, "Mercury and Mercury-Containing Preparations: History of Use, Clinical Applications, Pharmacology,

Toxicology, and Pharmacokinetics in Traditional Chinese Medicine," *Frontiers in Pharmacology* 13 (2022): 807807.

410. J. Martín-Gil et al., "The First Known Use of Vermillion," *Experientia* 51.8 (1995): 759–61.
411. E. Gliozzo, "Pigments: Mercury-Based Red (Cinnabar-Vermilion) and White (Calomel) and Their Degradation Products," *Archaeological and Anthropological Sciences* 13 (2021): 210.
412. M. G. Antony, "On the Spot: Seeking Acceptance and Expressing Resistance Through the Bindi," *Journal of International and Intercultural Communication* 3.4 (2010): 346–68.
413. S. Bucklow, *The Alchemy of Paint: Art, Science and Secrets from the Middle Ages* (Equinox, 2009).
414. J. Liu et al., "Mercury in Traditional Medicines: Is Cinnabar Toxicologically Similar to Common Mercurials?," *Experimental Biology and Medicine* 233.7 (2008): 810–17.
415. J. Bostock, trans., *Pliny The Elder: Natural History. An Illustrated Selection* (Antiqua Sapientia, 2022).
416. J. Wisniak. "The History of Mercury: From Discovery to Incommodity," *Revista CENIC Ciencias Quimicas* 39.3 (2008): 147–56.
417. L. K. Herrera et al., "Studies of Deteriorated Tin-Mercury Alloy with Ancient Spanish Mirrors," *Journal of Cultural Heritage* 9.3 (2008): e41–e46.
418. B. Watson, trans., *Sima Qian* (Columbia University Press, 1995), see chapter 6.
419. M. Sheer, "A Secret Tunnel Found in Mexico May Finally Solve the Mysteries of Teotihuacán," *Smithsonian Magazine*, June 2016, https://www.smithsonianmag.com/history/discovery-secret-tunnel-mexico-solve-mysteries-teotihuacan-180959070/.
420. M. García Gómez et al., "Exposure to Mercury in the Mine of Almaden," *Occupational and Environmental Medicine* 64.6 (2007): 389–95.
421. UNESCO World Heritage Convention, "Heritage of Mercury. Almadén and Idrija," https://whc.unesco.org/en/list/1313.
422. K. W. Brown, "The Spanish Imperial Mercury Trade and the American Mining Expansion Under the Bourbon Monarchy," in *The Political*

Economy of Spanish America in the Age of Revolution, ed. K. J. Andrien and L. L. Johnson (University of New Mexico Press, 1994), 137–68.

423. Indiana University Center for Underwater Study, "Guadalupe Underwater Archaeological Preserve," https://underwaterscience.indiana.edu/research/dominican-republic/guadalupe-underwater-archaeological-preserve.html.
424. See E. A. Barber, "Maiolica Tiles of Mexico," *Bulletin of the Pennsylvania Museum* 6.23 (1908): 37–41.
425. A. Seaton and C. M. Bishop, "Acute Mercury Pneumonitis," *British Journal of Industrial Medicine* 35.3 (1978): 258–61.
426. M. T. Slois et al., "Family Poisoned by Mercury Vapor Inhalation," *American Journal of Emergency Medicine* 18 (2000): 599–602.
427. J. D. Park and W. Zheng, "Human Exposure and Health Effects of Inorganic and Elemental Mercury," *Journal of Preventive Medicine and Public Health* 45.6 (2012): 344–52; T. W. Clarkson and L. Magos, "The Toxicology of Mercury and Its Chemical Compounds," *Critical Reviews in Toxicology* 36 (2006): 609–62.
428. F. L. Lorscheider, M. J. Vimy, and A. O. Summers, "Mercury Exposure from 'Silver' Tooth Fillings: Emerging Evidence Questions a Traditional Dental Paradigm," *FASEB Journal* 9.7 (1995): 504–8; J. F. Risher et al., "Elemental and Inorganic Mercury Compounds Human Health Aspects," World Health Organization, September 10, 2003, https://www.who.int/publications/i/item/elemental-mercury-and-inorganic-mercury-compounds-human-health-aspects; L. Björkman et al., "Mercury in Human Brain, Blood, Muscle, and Toenails in Relation to Exposure: An Autopsy Study," *Environmental Health* 6 (2007): 30.
429. H. V. Worthington et al., "Direct Composite Resin Fillings Versus Amalgam Fillings for Permanent Posterior Teeth," *Cochrane Database Systematic Reviews* 8.8 (2021): CD005620.
430. A. M. Mark, "Amalgam Fillings: Safe, Strong, and Affordable," *JADA* 150.10 (2019): P894.
431. K. G. Homme et al., "New Science Challenges Old Notion That Mercury Dental Amalgam Is Safe," *BioMetals* 27 (2014): 19–24.

432. D. C. Evers et al., *Phasing Out/Phasing Down Mercury-Added Products: What to Know About Consumer and Commercial Products Outlined in the Minamata Convention* (Biodiversity Research Institute, 2018).

433. British Dental Association, "The Amalgam Ban: What You Need to Know," BDA Website, January 17, 2024, https://www.bda.org/news-and-opinion/news/the-amalgam-ban-what-you-need-to-know/.

434. T. J. Svensen. "Chess Player Suspended After Allegedly Poisoning Her Rival," Chess.com, August 17, 2024, https://www.chess.com/news/view/russian-chess-player-suspended-after-allegedly-poisoning-her-rival.

435. T. S. Putnam et al., "Severe Mercury Toxicity from Gunshot Wounds: 28-Year Case Review and Current Management Guideline," *Critical Care Medicine* 49.1 (2021): 661.

436. Documentary Central, "The Shocking JFK Confession from Prison: Files on JFK," YouTube, posted August 11, 2024, https://www.youtube.com/watch?v=44x5I-kP48o&t=735s.

437. B. J. Baker et al., "Advancing the Understanding of Treponemal Disease in the Past and Present," *American Journal of Physical Anthropology* 171 (2020): 5–41.

438. G. Bjørklund, "Mercury and Acrodynia," *Journal of Orthomolecular Medicine* 10.3–4 (1995): 145–46.

439. J. Warkany and D. M. Hubbard, "Mercury in the Urine of Children with Acrodynia," *American Journal of Diseases of Children* 79 (1950): 388.

440. S. Cappelletti et al., "Mercuric Chloride Poisoning: Symptoms, Analysis, Therapies, and Autoptic Findings. A Review of the Literature," *Critical Reviews in Toxicology* 49.4 (2019): 329–41.

441. B. Desoize, "Metals and Metal Compounds in Cancer Treatment," *Anticancer Research* 24 (2004): 1529–44.

442. J. G. O'Shea, "Two Minutes with Venus, Two Years with Mercury as an Antisyphilitic Treatment," *Journal of the Royal Society of Medicine* 83 (1990): 392–95.

443. T. Gjestland, "The Oslo Study of Untreated Syphilis: An Epidemiologic Investigation of the Natural Course of the Syphilitic Infection Based upon a Re-Study of the Boeck-Bruusgaard Material," *Acta Dermo-Venereologica. Supplementum* 35 (1955): 3–368.

444. M. J. Tobin, "Fiftieth Anniversary of Uncovering the Tuskegee Syphilis Study: The Story and Timeless Lessons," *American Journal of Respiratory and Critical Care Medicine* 205.10 (2020): 1145–58.

445. K. Swain, "Extraordinarily Arduous and Fraught with Danger: Syphilis, Salvarsan and General Paralysis of the Insane," *The Lancet* 5 (2018): 702–3.

446. W. Russell, "The Diagnosis of General Paralysis of the Insane," *Buffalo Medical Journal* 42.10 (1903): 723–30.

447. J. H. Gao, "Clinical Manifestations, Fluid Changes and Neuroimaging Alterations in Patients with General Paresis of the Insane," *Neuropsychiatric Disease and Treatment* 17 (2021): 69–78.

448. A. S. Weissfeld, "Infectious Diseases and Famous People Who Succumbed to Them," *Clinical Microbiology Newsletter* 31 (2009): 169–72.

449. H. Noguchi and J. W. Moore, "A Demonstration of *Treponema pallidum* in the Brain in Cases of General Paralysis," *Journal of Experimental Medicine* 17 (1913): 232–38.

450. S. Y. Tan and J. Furubayashi, "Hideyo Noguchi (1876–1928): Distinguished Bacteriologist," *Singapore Medical Journal* 55.10 (2014): 550–51.

451. S. Y. Tan and Y. Tatsumura, "Alexander Fleming (1881–1955): Discoverer of Penicillin," *Singapore Medical Journal* 56.7 (2015): 366–67.

452. P. Heiberg, "Is General Paresis Dependent upon Previous Treatment with Mercury?," *Journal of Hygiene* 38.4 (1938): 500–506.

453. C. C. Leong, N. I. Syed, and F. L. Lorscheider, "Retrograde Degeneration of Neurite Membrane Structural Integrity of Nerve Growth Cones Following *in vitro* Exposure to Mercury," *Neuroreport* 12.4 (2001): 733–37.

454. M. K. Zuckerman, "More Harm than Healing? Investigating the Iatrogenic Effects of Mercury Treatment on Acquired Syphilis in Post-Medieval London," *Open Archaeology* 2.1 (2016): 42–55.

455. T. Dover, *Encomium argenti vivi: A Treatise upon the Use and Properties of Quicksilver* (Austen, 1733).

456. "Good Results of Donovan's Solution in Psoriasis," *The Lancet* 70.1770 (1770): 116.

457. J. B. Vander Veer, et al., "The Prolonged Use of an Oral Mercurial Diuretic in Ambulatory Patients with Congestive Heart Failure," *American Heart Association Journal* 1.4 (1950): 516–22.
458. R. E. O'Carroll et al., "The Neuropsychiatric Sequelae of Mercury Poisoning: The Mad Hatter's Disease Revisited," *British Journal of Psychiatry* 167.1 (1995): 95–98.
459. A. R. Barron, "The Myth, Reality, and History of Mercury Toxicity," Chemistry LibreTexts Chemistry, https://chem.libretexts.org/Bookshelves/Inorganic_Chemistry/Chemistry_of_the_Main_Group_Elements_(Barron)/05%3A_Group_12/5.05%3A_The_Myth_Reality_and_History_of_Mercury_Toxicity.
460. F. Bakir et al., "Methylmercury Poisoning in Iraq," *Science* 181 (1973): 230–41.
461. S. Lemonick, "25 Years After Karen Wetterhahn Died of Dimethylmercury Poisoning, Her Influence Persists," *ACS Chemical Health and Safety* 29.4 (2022): 327–32.
462. T. I. Alekseeva, G. P. Mishin, and V. G. Turkova, "Organization of Aid to Patients with Granosan Poisoning," *Sovetskaia Meditsina* 34.5 (1971): 137–38 (in Russian).
463. J. Zhang, "Clinical Observations in Ethyl Mercury Chloride Poisoning," *American Journal of Industrial Medicine* 5.3 (1984): 251–58.
464. I. Cinca et al., "Accidental Ethyl Mercury Poisoning with Nervous System, Skeletal Muscle, and Myocardium Injury," *Journal of Neurology, Neurosurgery and Psychiatry* 43.2 (1980): 143–49.
465. J. P. Baker, "Mercury, Vaccines, and Autism: One Controversy, Three Histories," *American Journal of Public Health* 98.2 (2008): 244–53.
466. M. Tan M and J. E. Parkin, "Route of Decomposition of Thiomersal (Thimerosal)," *International Journal of Pharmokinetics* 208.1–2 (2000): 23–34.
467. D. A. Geier, L. K. Sykes, and M. R. Geier, "A Review of Thimerosal (Merthiolate) and Its Ethylmercury Breakdown Product: Specific Historical Considerations Regarding Safety and Effectiveness," *Journal of Toxicology and Environmental Health B* 10 (2007): 575–96.

468. S. Basu and R. Rustagi, "Multi-Dose Vials Versus Single-Dose Vials for Vaccination: Perspectives from Lower-Middle Income Countries," *Human Vaccines and Immunotherapies* 18.6 (2022): 2059310.
469. D. G. Fagan et al., "Organ Mercury Levels in Infants with Omphaloceles Treated with Organic Mercurial Antiseptic," *Archives of Disease in Childhood* 52.12 (1977): 962–64.
470. Geier, Sykes, and Geier, "Review of Thimerosal."
471. L. O. Nascimento, G. Lorenzi Filho, and S. Rocha Ados, "Intoxicação letal por mercúrio através da ingestão de 'merthiolate,'" *Revista do hospital das clínicas* 45.5 (1990): 216–18.
472. G. Gillett et al., "The Prevalence of Autism Spectrum Disorder Traits and Diagnosis in Adults and Young People with Personality Disorders: A Systematic Review," *Australian and New Zealand Journal of Psychiatry* 57.2 (2023): 181–96.
473. A. J. Wakefield et al., "Ileal-Lymphoid-Nodular Hyperplasia, Non-Specific Colitis, and Pervasive Developmental Disorder in Children," *The Lancet*, 351.9103 (1998): 637–41. This article has since been retracted by the journal.
474. K. M. Madsen et al., "A Population-Based Study of Measles, Mumps, and Rubella Vaccination and Autism," *New England Journal of Medicine* 347.19 (2002): 1477–82.
475. J. Guy et al., "Reversal of Neurological Defects in a Mouse Model of Rett Syndrome," *Science* 315 (2007): 1143–47.
476. D. Kirby, *Evidence of Harm: Mercury in Vaccines and the Autism Epidemic. A Medical Controversy* (Saint Martin's, 2006), see esp. chapter 1: "Mothers on a Mission."
477. D. Quade et al., "Effects of Misclassifications on Statistical Inferences in Epidemiology," *American Journal of Epidemiology* 111.5 (1980): 503–15.
478. R. E. Frye et al., "Emerging Biomarkers in Autism Spectrum Disorder: A Systematic Review," *Annals of Translational Medicine* 23 (2019): 792.
479. A. Stojsavljević, N. Lakićević, and S. Pavlović, "Mercury and Autism Spectrum Disorder: Exploring the Link through Comprehensive Review and Meta-Analysis," *Biomedicines* 11.12 (2023): 3344.

480. S. Sun and L. B. Barreiro, "The Epigenetically-Encoded Memory of the Innate Immune System," *Current Opinion in Immunology* 65 (2020): 7–13.
481. A. R. Isles, "The Contribution of Imprinted Genes to Neurodevelopmental and Neuropsychiatric Disorders," *Translational Psychiatry* 12.1 (2022): 210.
482. E. P. Susser and S. P. Lin, "Schizophrenia After Prenatal Exposure to the Dutch Hunger Winter of 1944–1945," *Archives in General Psychiatry* 49.12 (1992): 983–88; S. Song, W. Wang, and P. Hu, "Famine, Death, and Madness: Schizophrenia in Early Adulthood After Prenatal Exposure to the Chinese Great Leap Forward Famine," *Social Science and Medicine* 68.7 (2009): 1315–21.
483. F. A. Azevedo et al., "Equal Numbers of Neuronal and Nonneuronal Cells Make the Human Brain an Isometrically Scaled-Up Primate Brain," *Journal of Comparative Neurology* 513.5 (2009): 532–41.
484. D. A. Drachman, "Do We Have Brain to Spare?," *Neurology* 64.12 (2005): 2004–5.
485. "Joint Statement of the American Academy of Pediatrics (AAP) and the United States Public Health Service (USPHS)," *Pediatrics* 104.3 (1999): 568–69; Centers for Disease Control, "Notice to Readers: Thimerosal in Vaccines: A Joint Statement of the American Academy of Pediatrics and the Public Health Service," *Morbidity and Mortality Weekly Report* 48.26 (1999): 563–65.
486. R. F. Kennedy, *Thimerosal: Let the Science Speak. The Evidence Supporting the Immediate Removal of Mercury* (Skyhorse, 2014).
487. J. S. Reif, A. M. Schaefer, and G. D. Bossart, "Atlantic Bottlenose Dolphins (*Tursiops truncatus*) as a Sentinel for Exposure to Mercury in Humans: Closing the Loop," *Veterinary Science* 2.4 (2015): 407–22.
488. L. T. Kurland, S. N. Faro, and H. Siedler, "Minamata Disease: The Outbreak of a Neurologic Disorder in Minamata, Japan, and Its Relationship to the Ingestion of Seafood Contaminated by Mercuric Compounds," *World Neurology* 1 (1960): 370–95.
489. S. Ekino et al., "Minamata Disease Revisited: An Update on the Acute and Chronic Manifestations of Methyl Mercury Poisoning," *Journal of the Neurological Sciences* 262.1–2 (2007): 131–44.

490. H. Lin et al., "Mercury Methylation by Metabolically Versatile and Cosmopolitan Marine Bacteria," *ISME Journal* 15.6 (2021): 1810–25.

491. A. T. Schartup et al., "A Model for Methylmercury Uptake and Trophic Transfer by Marine Plankton," *Environmental Science and Technology* 52.2 (2018): 654–62

492. K. Kondo, "Congenital Minamata Disease: Warnings from Japan's Experience," *Journal of Child Neurology* 15.7 (2000): 458–64.

493. T. D. Solan and S. W. Lindow, "Mercury Exposure in Pregnancy: A Review," *Journal of Perinatal Medicine* 42.6 (2014): 725–29.

494. S. Mohammadi et al., "Contamination of Breast Milk with Lead, Mercury, Arsenic, and Cadmium in Iran: A Systematic Review and Meta-Analysis," *BioMetals* 35.4 (2022): 711–28.

495. T. M. Burbacher et al., "Comparison of Blood and Brain Mercury Levels in Infant Monkeys Exposed to Methylmercury or Vaccines Containing Thimerosal," *Environmental Health Perspectives* 113.8 (2005): 1015–21.

496. L. K. Ball, R. Ball, and R. D. Pratt, "An Assessment of Thimerosal Use in Childhood Vaccines," *Pediatrics* 107.5 (2001): 1147–54.

497. J. G. Dórea, M. Farina M, and J. B. Rocha, "Toxicity of Ethylmercury (and Thimerosal): A Comparison with Methylmercury," Journal of Applied Toxicology 33.8 (2013): 700–711; M. Bigham and R. Copes, "Thimerosal in Vaccines: Balancing the Risk of Adverse Effects with the Risk of Vaccine-Preventable Disease," *Drug Safety* 28.2 (2005): 89–101; A. M. Hurley, M. Tadrous, and E. S. Miller, "Thimerosal-Containing Vaccines and Autism: A Review of Recent Epidemiologic Studies," *Journal of Pediatric Pharmacology and Therapeutics* 15.3 (2010): 173–81.

498. C. Lamborg et al., "A Global Ocean Inventory of Anthropogenic Mercury Based on Water Column Measurements," *Nature* 512 (2014): 65–68.

499. See United States Food and Drug Administration 21CFR610.15, "Constitutent Materials" (https://www.ecfr.gov/current/title-21/chapter-I/subchapter-F/part-610/subpart-B/section-610.15).

Chapter 13

500. Quote from book 1, chapter 5 of *Sartor Resartus* (Munroe, 1834).

501. W. M. Haynes, ed., *CRC Handbook of Chemistry and Physics*, 97th ed. (CRC Press. 2017), 14–17.

502. R. W. Hughes, *Ruby and Sapphire* (RWH Publishing, 1997).

503. T. Geller, "Aluminum: Common Metal, Uncommon Past," *Chemical Heritage Magazine* 27.4 (2007).

504. K. Grjotheim et al., *Aluminium Electrolysis: Fundamentals of the Hall-Héroult Process*, 2nd ed. (International Publishers Service, 1982).

505. C. Butler, "Why Aluminium Smelters Are a Critical Component in Australian Decarbonisation," Institute for Energy Economics and Financial Analysis, June 2020, https://ieefa.org/wp-content/uploads/2020/06/IEEFA_Why-Aluminium-Smelters-are-a-Critical-Component-in-Australian-Decarbonisation_June-2020.pdf

506. H. Kvande, "The Aluminum Smelting Process," Journal of Occupational and Environmental Medicine 56.5 (2014): S2–S4.

507. P. Hoffman. *Wings of Madness: Alberto Santos-Dumont and the Invention of Flight* (Grand Central, 2003).

508. National Air and Space Museum, "The Wright Engine Aluminum Crankcase," https://airandspace.si.edu/multimedia-gallery/5817hjpg.

509. R. Byers, *Flying Man: Hugo Junkers and the Dream of Aviation* (Texas A&M University Press, 2016).

510. W. J. Troff and M. E. Thomas, "Aluminum Oxynitride (ALON) Spinel," in *Handbook of Optical Constant of Solids*, ed. E. D. Palik, 2 vols. (Academic Press, 1998), 2:777–87.

511. M. Viikinkoski et al., "16 Psyche: A Mesosiderite-Like Asteroid? *Astronomy and Astrophysics* 619 (2018): L3.

512. I. Whitcomb, "There's an Asteroid Out There Worth $100,000 Quadrillion. Why Haven't We Mined It?," *Live Science,* February 16, 2024, https://www.livescience.com/space/asteroids/theres-an-asteroid-out-there-worth-dollar100000-quadrillion-why-havent-we-mined-it.

513. A. Drozdov, *Aluminum: The Thirteenth Element* (RUSAL Library, 2007).

514. J. Waldman, "The Secret Life of the Aluminum Can, a Feat of Engineering," *Wired*, March 9, 2015, https://www.wired.com/2015/03/secret-life-aluminum-can-true-modern-marvel/.

515. N. Chuchu et al., "The Aluminum Content of Infant Formulas Remains Too High," *BMC Pediatrics* 13 (2013): 162.

516. J. Dórea, and R. Marques, "Infants' Exposure to Aluminum from Vaccines and Breast Milk During the First 6 Months," *Journal of Exposure Science and Environmental Epidemiology* 20 (2010): 598–601.

517. J. Windisch, B. K. Keppler, and F. Jirsa, "Aluminum in Coffee," *ACS Omega*, June 15, 2020, https://pubs.acs.org/doi/10.1021/acsomega.0c01410.

518. S. Sanajou, G. Şahin, and T. Baydar, "Aluminium in Cosmetics and Personal Care Products," *Journal of Applied Toxicology* 41.11 (2021): 1704–18.

519. R. L. Poole et al., "Aluminum in Pediatric Parenteral Nutrition Products: Measured Versus Labeled Content," *Journal of Pediatric Pharmacology and Therapeutics* 16.2 (2011): 92–97.

520. P. Edde et al., "The First Reported Mortality from Aluminum Phosphide Poisoning in Lebanon: A Case Report," *International Journal of Emergency Medicine* 17 (2024): 18.

521. L. V. Kochian, "Cellular Mechanisms of Aluminum Toxicity and Resistance in Plants," *Annual Review of Plant Molecular Biology* 46(1995): 237–60.

522. C. A. C. Crusciol et al., "Methods and Extractants to Evaluate Silicon Availability for Sugarcane," *Scientific Reports* 8 (2018): 916.

523. H. R. von Uexküll and E. Mutert, "Global Extent, Development and Economic Impact of Acid Soils," *Plant and Soil* 171 (1995): 1–15.

524. L. V. Kochian et al., "Plant Adaptation to Acid Soils: The Molecular Basis for Crop Aluminum Resistance," *Annual Review of Plant Biology* 66 (2015): 571–98.

525. E. Delhaize and P. Ryan, "Aluminum Toxicity and Tolerance in Plants," *Plant Physiology* 107 (1995): 315–21.

526. T. B. Kinraide et al., "Interactive Effects of Al+3, H+, and Other Cations on Root Elongation Considered in Terms of Cell Surface Electrical Potential," *Plant Physiology* 99 (1992): 1451–68.

527. C.-K. Au et al., "Effects of Heavy Metal Co-Exposure on the formation of DNA Adducts from Aristolochic Acid I: Implications for Balkan Endemic Nephropathy Development," *Chemical Research in Toxicology* 37.4 (2024): 545–48.

528. C. M. Reinke, J. Breitkreutz, and H. Leuenberger, "Aluminium in Over-the-Counter Drugs: Risks Outweigh Benefits?," *Drug Safety* 26.14 (2003): 1011–25.

529. A. C. Alfrey, G. R. LeGendre, and W. D. Kaehny, "The Dialysis Encephalopathy Syndrome: Possible Aluminum Intoxication," *New England Journal of Medicine* 294.4 (1976): 184–88.

530. M. Perazella and E. Brown, "Acute Aluminum Toxicity and Alum Bladder Irrigation in Patients with Renal Failure," *American Journal of Kidney Diseases* 21.1 (1993): 44–46.

531. N. J. Bishop et al., "Aluminum Neurotoxicity in Preterm Infants Receiving Intravenous-Feeding Solutions," *New England Journal of Medicine* 336.22 (1997): 1557–61.

532. B. F. Boyce et al., "Hypercalcaemic Osteomalacia Due to Aluminum Toxicity," *The Lancet* 2.8306 (1982): 1009–13; T. W. Bauer et al., "Osteomalacia Associated with Aluminum Intoxication in a Patient with Chronic Renal Failure," *Cleveland Clinic Quarterly* 52 (1985): 271–78.

533. O. Guillard et al., "Hyperaluminemia in a Woman Using an Aluminum-Containing Antiperspirant for 4 Years," *American Journal of Medicine* 117.12 (2004): 956–59.

534. A. Di Pasquale et al., "Vaccine Adjuvants: from 1920 to 2015 and Beyond," *Vaccines* 3.2 (2015): 320–43.

535. G. Ramon, "Sur la toxine et l'anatoxine diphtérique. Pouvoir floculant et propriétés immunisantes," *Annales de l'Institut Pasteur* 38 (1924): 1–10; J. P. Chippaux, "Gaston Ramon's Big Four," *Toxins* 16.1 (2024): 33.

536. T. Zhao et al., "Vaccine Adjuvants: Mechanisms and Platforms," *Signal Transduction and Targeted Therapy* 8 (2023): 283; J. de S. Apostólico, "Adjuvants: Classification, Modus Operandi, and Licensing," *Journal of Immunology Research* 2016 (2016): 1459394.

537. J. C. C. Chang et al., "Adjuvant Activity of Incomplete Freund's Adjuvant," *Advanced Drug Delivery Reviews* 32.3 (1998): 173–86.
538. C. S. Constantinescu et al., "Experimental Autoimmune Encephalomyelitis (EAE) as a Model for Multiple Sclerosis (MS)," *British Journal of Pharmacology* 164.4 (2011): 1079–106.
539. Y. Adachi et al., "Animal Models of Bone Marrow Transplantation for Autoimmune Diseases," in *Hematopoietic Stem Cell Transplantation and Cellular Therapy for Autoimmune Diseases*, ed. R, Burt et al. (CRC Press, 2022), 189–203.
540. A. Matsiko, "Alum Adjuvant Discovery and Potency," *Nature Portfolio*, September 28, 2020, https://www.nature.com/articles/d42859-020-00011-w; A. T. Glenny et al., "Immunological Notes. XVI1.–XXIV," *Journal of Pathology and Bacteriology* 29 (1926): 31–40.
541. J. Yao et al., "The Role of Inflammasomes in Human Diseases and Their Potential as Therapeutic Targets," *Signal Transduction and Targeted Therapy* 9.1 (2024): 10; F. A. Sharp et al., "Uptake of Particulate Vaccine Adjuvants by Dendritic Cells Activates the NALP3 Inflammasome," *Proceedings of the National Academy of the Sciences of the United States of America* 106 (2009): 870–75.
542. T. Marichal et al., "DNA Released from Dying Host Cells Mediates Aluminum Adjuvant Activity," *Nature Medicine* 17 (2011): 996–1002.
543. S. M. Lee et al., "Role of Damage-Associated Molecular Pattern/Cell Death Pathways in Vaccine-Induced Immunity," *Viruses* 13.12 (2021): 2340; A. S. McKee et al., "Host DNA Released in Response to Aluminum Adjuvant Enhances MHC Class II-Mediated Antigen Presentation and Prolongs CD4 T-Cell Interactions with Dendritic Cells," *Proceedings of the National Academy of the Sciences of the United States of America* 110 (2013): E1122–E1131.
544. D. Laera et al., "Aluminum Adjuvants—'Back to the Future,'" *Pharmaceutics* 15.7 (2023): 1884.
545. N. Gruber and Y. Shoenfeld, "A Link Between Human Papilloma Virus Vaccination and Primary Ovarian Insufficiency: Current Analysis," Current Opinion in Obstetrics and Gynecology 27.4 (2015): 265–70.

546. L. E. Guimarães et al., "Vaccines, Adjuvants and Autoimmunity," *Pharmacological Research* 100 (2015): 190–209.
547. R. K. Gherardi et al., "Macrophagic Myofasciitis Lesions Assess Long-Term Persistence of Vaccine-Derived Aluminium Hydroxide in Muscle," *Brain* 124.9 (2001): 1821–31.
548. R. Ostuni et al., "Latent Enhancers Activated by Stimulation in Differentiated Cells," *Cell* 152.1–2 (2013): 157–71.
549. Modified from two sources: H. HogenEsch et al, "Optimizing the Utilization of Aluminum Adjuvants in Vaccines: You Might Just Get What You Want," *npj Vaccines* 3 (2018): 51; Laera et al., "Aluminum Adjuvants."
550. Zhao et al., "Vaccine Adjuvants."

Chapter 14

551. From the introduction of the film on the Ebola virus called *Outbreak* (1995).
552. K. M. Johnson et al., "Isolation and Partial Characterization of a New Virus Causing Acute Haemorrhagic Fever in Zaire," *The Lancet* 1 (1977): 569–71.
553. J. H. Kuhn et al., "Reidentification of Ebola Virus E718 and ME as Ebola Virus/H.sapiens-tc/COD/1976/Yambuku-Ecran," *Genome Announcements* 2.6 (2014): e01178-14.
554. Report of an International Commission, "Ebola Haemorrhagic Fever in Zaire, 1976," *Bulletin of the World Health Organization* 56.2 (1978): 271–93.
555. S. T. Jacob et al., "Ebola Virus Disease," *Nature Reviews Disease Primers* 6 (2020): 13.
556. Report of a WHO/International Study Team, "Ebola Haemorrhagic Fever in Sudan, 1976. Report of a WHO/International Study Team," *Bulletin of the World Health Organization* 56.2 (1978): 247–70.
557. H. Feldmann and T. W. Geisbert, "Ebola Haemorrhagic Fever," *The Lancet* 377.9768 (2011): 849–62.

558. D. Yosban, F. Walkite, and Y. Nesradin, "Ebola Virus and Its Public Health Significance: A Review," *Journal of Veterinary Science and Research* 3.3 (2018): 000165.

559. B. N. Fields and K. Hawkins, "Human Infection with the Virus of Vesicular Stomatitis During an Epizootic," *New England Journal of Medicine* 277.19 (1967): 989–94.

560. E. Quiroz et al., "A Human Case of Encephalitis Associated with Vesicular Stomatitis Virus (Indiana Serotype) Infection," *American Journal of Tropical Medicine and Hygiene* 39.3 (1988): 312–14.

561. A. Roberts et al., "Attenuated Vesicular Stomatitis Viruses as Vaccine Vectors," *Journal of Virology* 73.5 (1999): 3723–32.

562. S. Jones et al., "Live Attenuated Recombinant Vaccine Protects Nonhuman Primates Against Ebola and Marburg Viruses," *Nature Medicine* 11 (2005): 786–90.

563. J. A. Regules et al., "rVSVΔG-ZEBOV-GP Study Group. A Recombinant Vesicular Stomatitis Virus Ebola Vaccine," *New England Journal of Medicine* 376.4 (2017): 330–41.

564. A. M. Henao-Restrepo· et al., "Efficacy and Effectiveness of an rVSV-Vectored Vaccine Expressing Ebola Surface Glycoprotein: Interim Results from the Guinea Ring Vaccination Cluster-Randomised Trial," *The Lancet* 386 (2015): 857–66.

565. N. E. Dean et al., "Transmissibility and Pathogenicity of Ebola Virus: A Systematic Review and Meta-Analysis of Household Secondary Attack Rate and Asymptomatic Infection," *Clinical Infectious Diseases* 62.10 (2016): 1277–86.

566. J. L. Vernon, "Understanding the Butterfly Effect," *American Scientist,* May/June 2017, https://www.americanscientist.org/article/understanding-the-butterfly-effect.

Chapter 15

567. V. M. Corman et al., "Hosts and Sources of Endemic Human Coronaviruses," *Advances in Virus Research* 100 (2018): 163–88.

568. D. S. Hui and P. K. Chan, "Severe Acute Respiratory Syndrome and Coronavirus," *Infectious Disease Clinics of North America* 24.3 (2010): 619–38.

569. J. Watts, "China Culls Wild Animals to Prevent New SARS Threat," *The Lancet* 363.9403 (2004): 134.

570. Y. C. Wu, C. S. Chen, and Y. J. Chan, "The Outbreak of COVID-19: An Overview," *Journal of the Chinese Medical Association* 83.3 (2020): 217–20.

571. D. Klepper, F.Amiri, and B. Dupuy, "The Superspreaders Behind Top COVID-19 Conspiracy Theories," *AP News*, February 14, 2021, https://apnews.com/article/conspiracy-theories-iran-only-on-ap-media-misinformation-bfca6d5b236a29d61c4dd38702495ffe.

572. J. Kaiser, "House Panel Concludes That COVID-19 Pandemic Came from a Lab Leak," Science Insider, December 3, 2024, https://www.science.org/content/article/house-panel-concludes-covid-19-pandemic-came-lab-leak.

573. K. Subbarao et al., "Characterization of an Avian Influenza A (H5N1) Virus Isolated from a Child with a Fatal Respiratory Illness," *Science* 279 (1998): 393–96.

574. M. Ozawa and Y. Kawaoka, "Crosstalk Between Animal and Human Influenza Viruses," *Annual Review of Animal Biosciences* 1 (2013): 21–42.

575. D. B. Resnik, "H5N1 Avian Flu Research and the Ethics of Knowledge," *Hastings Center Report* 43.2 (2013): 22–33.

576. S. Herfst et al., "Airborne Transmission of Influenza A/H5N1 Virus Between Ferrets," *Science* 336 (2012): 1534–41; C. A. Russell et al., "The Potential for Respiratory Droplet-Transmissible A/H5N1 Influenza Virus to Evolve in a Mammalian Host," *Science* 336 (2012): 1541–47; M. Imai et al., "Experimental Adaptation of an Influenza H5 HA Confers Respiratory Droplet Transmission to a Reassortant H5 HA/H1N1 Virus in Ferrets," *Nature* 486.7403 (2012): 420–28.

577. M. W. Leigh et al., "Receptor Specificity of Influenza Virus Influences Severity of Illness in Ferrets," *Vaccine* 13 (1995): 1468–73.

578. M. Tu, "Between Publishing and Perishing? H5N1 Research Unleashes Unprecedented Dual-Use Research Controversy," Nuclear Threat Initiative, May 2, 2012, https://www.nti.org/analysis/articles/between-publishing-and-perishing-h5n1-research-unleashes-unprecedented-dual-use-research-controversy/.

579. R. A. Fouchier et al., "Pause on Avian Flu Transmission Research," *Science* 335 (2012): 400–401.

580. A. S. Fauci, "Research on Highly Pathogenic H5N1 Influenza Virus: The Way Forward," *mBio* 3.5 (2012): e00359-12.

581. C. Porterfield, "Dr. Fauci on GOP Criticism: 'Attacks on Me, Quite Frankly, Are Attacks on Science,'" *Forbes*, January 29, 2021, https://www.forbes.com/sites/carlieporterfield/2021/06/09/fauci-on-gop-criticism-attacks-on-me-quite-frankly-are-attacks-on-science/.

582. A. S. Fauci, *On Call: A Doctor's Journey in Public Service* (Viking, 2024), 455.

583. Fauci, *On Call*, 357

584. Fauci, "H5N1 Influenza Virus."

585. T. Kuiken, "Global Pandemics: Gain of Function Research Concern," November 21, 2022, *Congressional Research Service*, https://www.congress.gov/crs-product/IF12021; J. Kaiser, "Moratorium on Risky Virology Studies Leaves Work at 14 Institutions in Limbo," Science Insider, November 17, 2014, https://www.science.org/content/article/moratorium-risky-virology-studies-leaves-work-14-institutions-limbo.

586. W. Duprex et al., "Gain-of-Function Experiments: Time for a Real Debate," *Nature Reviews Microbiology* 13 (2015): 58–64.

587. F. Collins, "NIH Lifts Funding Pause on Gain of Function Research," *National Institutes of Health*, December 19, 2017, https://www.nih.gov/about-nih/who-we-are/nih-director/statements/nih-lifts-funding-pause-gain-function-research.

588. National Institutes of Health, "Research Involving Enhanced Potential Pandemic Pathogens," last update June 5, 2023. https://www.nih.gov/news-events/research-involving-potential-pandemic-pathogens.

589. V. Menachery et al., "A SARS-Like Cluster of Circulating Bat Coronaviruses Shows Potential for Human Emergence," *Nature Medicine* 21 (2015): 1508–13.

590. D. Butker, "Engineered Bat Virus Stirs Debate over Risky Research," *Nature*, November 12, 2015, https://www.nature.com/articles/nature.2015.18787#citeas.

591. National Research Council and Institute of Medicine, *Potential Risks and Benefits of Gain-of-Function Research: Summary of a Workshop* (National Academies Press, 2015).

592. Butker, "Engineered Bat Virus."

593. Butker, "Engineered Bat Virus."

594. Centers for Disease Control and Prevention and US Department of Agriculture, *2022 Annual Report of the Federal Select Agent Program*, https://selectagents.gov/resources/publications/docs/FSAP_Annual_Report_2022_508.pdf.

595. N. Balbontin et al., "Canadian Laboratory Incidents with Human Pathogens and Toxins: An Overview of Reports, 2016–2022," *Canada Communicable Disease Report* 50 (2024): 144–52.

596. Y. Zhiming, "Current Status and Future Challenges of High-Level Biosafety Laboratories in China," *Journal of Biosafety and Biosecurity* 1.2 (2019): 123–27.

597. J. Qiu, "Meet the Scientist at the Center of the Covid Lab Leak Controversy," *MIT Technology Review*, February 9, 2022, https://www.technologyreview.com/2022/02/09/1044985/shi-zhengli-covid-lab-leak-wuhan/.

598. J. Qui, "How China's 'Bat Woman' Hunted Down Viruses from SARS to the New Coronavirus," *Scientific American*, June 1, 2020, https://www.scientificamerican.com/article/how-chinas-bat-woman-hunted-down-viruses-from-sars-to-the-new-coronavirus1/?amp=true.

599. Fauci, *On Call*, 419.

600. National Institutes of Health RePORTER, "Understanding the Risk of Bat Coronavirus Emergence: 1R01AI110964-01," https://reporter.nih.gov/search/KUZIl7-gLEeHjNoHzOFChw/project-details/8674931#similar-Projects.

601. S. Payne, "Virus Evolution and Genetics," *Viruses* (2017): 81–86.

602. K. G. Andersen et al., "The Proximal Origin of SARS-CoV-2," *Nature Medicine* 26 (2020): 450–52.

603. J. Farrar and A. Ahuja, *Spike: The Virus Versus the People. The Inside Story* (Profile Books, 2021), 52.

604. Rand Paul, *Deception: The Great COVID Cover-Up* (Simon & Schuster, 2023).

605. The following account of events and emails comes from J. Gorman and C. Zimmer, "Scientist Opens Up About His Early Email to Fauci on Virus Origins," *The New York Times*, updated June 20, 2021, https://www.nytimes.com/2021/06/14/science/covid-lab-leak-fauci-kristian-andersen.html; "US Immunologist Who Had Emailed Fauci That Coronavirus 'Looks Engineered' Deletes Twitter Account After His Lies Were Exposed," *OpIndia*, June 7, 2021, https://www.opindia.com/2021/06/scripps-immunologist-deletes-twitter-account-fauci-emails-coronavirus-engineered-lab-leak-hypothesis/; J. Tobias, "Unredacted NIH E-Mails Show Efforts to Rule Out a Lab Origin of Covid," *The Intercept*, January 19, 2023, https://theintercept.com/2023/01/19/covid-origin-nih-emails/.

606. F. Collins, "Genomic Study Points to Natural Origin of COVID-19," *NIH Director's Blog*, March 26, 2020, https://directorsblog.nih.gov/2020/03/26/genomic-research-points-to-natural-origin-of-covid-19/comment-page-1/.

607. K. Holland, "Sorry, Conspiracy Theorists. Study Concludes COVID-19 'Is Not a Laboratory Construct,'" *ABC News*, March 27, 2020, https://abcnews.go.com/US/conspiracy-theorists-study-concludes-covid-19-laboratory-construct/story?id=69827832.

608. Tobias, "Unredacted NIH E-Mails."

609. B. Bernstein, "'Antithetical to Science': Ex-CDC Director Takes Fauci to Task for Suppressing Lab-Leak Theory," *National Review*, March 8, 2023, https://www.nationalreview.com/news/antithetical-to-science-ex-cdc-director-takes-fauci-to-task-for-suppressing-lab-leak-theory/.

610. J. P. Chretien and G. Cutlip, "Critical Analysis of Andersen et al on the Proximal Origin of SARS-Cov-2," May 26, 2020, https://docs.house

.gov/meetings/VC/VC00/20230711/116185/HHRG-118-VC00-20230711-SD005.pdf.

611. J. E. Barnes, "Lab Leak Most Likely Caused Pandemic. Energy Dept. Says," *The New York Times*, February 26, 2023, https://www.nytimes.com/2023/02/26/us/politics/china-lab-leak-coronavirus-pandemic.html; House Oversight Committee, "Classified State Department Documents Credibly Suggest COVID-19 Lab Leak, Wenstrup Pushes for Declassification," Committee on Oversight and Government Reform, May 7,2024 https://oversight.house.gov/release/classified-state-department-documents-credibly-suggest-covid-19-lab-leak-wenstrup-pushes-for-declassification/.
612. S. Singh, "Coronavirus Man-Made in Wuhan Lab: Nobel Laureate," *The Times of India*, April 19, 2020, https://timesofindia.indiatimes.com/india/coronavirus-man-made-in-wuhan-lab-nobel-laureate/articleshow/75227989.cms.
613. Klepper, Amiri and Dupuy, "Superspreaders."
614. B. Reed, "Leading Biologist Dampens His 'Smoking Gun' Covid Lab Leak Theory," *The Guardian*, June 9, 2021, https://www.theguardian.com/world/2021/jun/09/leading-biologist-dampens-his-smoking-gun-covid-lab-leak-theory.
615. S. Xia et al., "The Role of Furin Cleavage Site in SARS-CoV-2 Spike Protein-Mediated Membrane Fusion in the Presence or Absence of Trypsin," *Signal Transduction and Targeted Therapy* 5 (2020): 92.
616. Farrar and Ahuja, *Spike*, 60–61.
617. Ozawa and Kawaoka, "Crosstalk."
618. Tu, "Publishing and Perishing."
619. Andersen et al., "Proximal Origin."
620. A. Chan and M. Ridley, *Viral: The Search for the Origin of COVID-19* (Harper, 2021), see chapter 4.
621. Chan and Ridley, *Viral*, 82
622. Chan and Ridley, *Viral*, 82–83.
623. Farrar and Ahuja, *Spike*, 65–72.
624. J. Coopersmith, *The Lazy Universe: An Introduction to the Principle of Least Action* (Oxford University Press, 2017).

625. Farrar and Ahuja, *Spike*, 65–72.

626. J. Tobias, "At the NIH, a Scandal Grows Around an Official's Evasion of Public Records Law," *The Nation*, May 28, 2024, https://www.thenation.com/article/archive/nih-foia-covid-origins-morens-hearing/. J. Tobias, "A house subcommittee releases key documents on the pandemic origin.," *The Nation*, April 10, 2023.

627. C. Calisher et al., "Statement in Support of the Scientists, Public Health Professionals, and Medical Professionals of China Combatting COVID-19," *The Lancet* 395.10226 (2020): e42–e43.

628. C. Calisher et al., "Science, Not Speculation, Is Essential to Determine How SARS-CoV-2 Reached Humans," *The Lancet* 398.10296 (2021): 209–11.

629. World Health Organization, "Origin of the SARS-Cov-2 Virus," March 30, 2021, https://www.who.int/emergencies/diseases/novel-coronavirus-2019/origins-of-the-virus.

630. World Health Organization, "WHO-Convened Global Study of Origins of SARS-CoV-2: China Part," February 10, 2021, https://www.who.int/docs/default-source/coronaviruse/who-convened-global-study-of-origins-of-sars-cov-2-china-part-joint-report.pdf.

631. A. Lardieri, "WHO: 'Extremely Unlikely' Coronavirus Came From Lab in China," *US News and World Report*, February 9, 2021, https://www.usnews.com/news/health-news/articles/2021-02-09/who-extremely-unlikely-coronavirus-came-from-lab-in-china.

632. A. Maxmen, "WHO Report into COVID Pandemic Origins Zeroes In on Animal Markets, Not Labs," *Nature* 592 (2021): 173–74.

633. J. D. Bloom et al., "Investigate the Origins of COVID-19," *Science* 372 (2021): 694.

634. J. Zarocostas, "Calls for Transparency After SARS-CoV-2 Origins Report," *The Lancet* 397.10282 (2021): P1335.

635. US Department of State, "Joint Statement on the WHO-Convened COVID-19 Origins Study," March 30, 2021, https://2021-2025.state.gov/joint-statement-on-the-who-convened-covid-19-origins-study/#:~:text=Together%2C%20we%20support%20a%20transparent,of%20the%20COVID%2D19%20pandemic.

636. Delegation of the European Union to the UN and other International Organizations in Geneva, "EU Statement on the WHO-Led COVID-19 Origins Study," *European Union External Action*, March 30, 2021, https://eeas.europa.eu/delegations/un-geneva/95960/eu-statement-who-led-covid-19-origins-study_en.
637. "China Rejects WHO's Phase-2 COVID-19 Origins Study, Calling It 'Lack of Respect for Common Sense, Arrogant Toward Science,'" *People's Daily Online*, July 23, 2021, http://en.people.cn/n3/2021/0723/c90000-9875832.html.
638. Porterfield, "Dr. Fauci on GOP Criticism."
639. Chan and Ridley, *Viral*, 333–34.
640. J. Alwine et al., "The Harms of Promoting the Lab Leak Hypothesis for SARS-CoV-2 Origins Without Evidence," Journal of Virology 98.9 (2024): e0124024.
641. Project DEFUSE, "Defusing the Threat of Bat-Borne Coronavirus," *EcoHealth Alliance*, March 24, 2018, https://assets.ctfassets.net/syq3snmxclc9/4NFC6M83ewzKLf6DvAygb4/0cf477f75646e718afb332b7ac6c3cd1/defuse-proposal_watermark_Redacted.pdf.
642. J. D. Sachs et al., "The Lancet Commission on Lessons for the Future from the COVID-19 Pandemic," *The Lancet* 400.10359 (2022): 1224–80.
643. N. L. Harrison and J. Sachs, "A Call for an Independent Inquiry into the Origin of the SARS-CoV-2 Virus," *PNAS* 119.21 (2022): e2202769119.
644. P. Kota et al., "The N Terminus of α-ENaC Mediates ENaC Cleavage and Activation by Furin," *Journal of General Physiology* 150 (2018): 1179–87.
645. R. Garry, "SARS-CoV-2 Furin Cleavage Site Was Not Engineered," *PNAS* 119.40 (2022): e2211107119.
646. N. Robinson with J. Sachs, "Current Affairs. Why the Chair of *The Lancet*'s COVID-19 Commission Thinks the US Government Is Preventing a Real Investigation into the Pandemic," JeffSachs.org, August 2, 2022. https://www.jeffsachs.org/interviewsandmedia/64rtmykxdl56ehbjwy37m5hfahwnm5.

647. T. Opeka, "Former CDC Director Claims That COVID-19 Emanated from UNC-Chapel Hill," *The Carolina Journal*, November 19, 2024, https://www.carolinajournal.com/former-cdc-director-claims-that-covid-19-emanated-from-unc-chapel-hill/.
648. A. Schemmel, "Fauci said 'I Don't Recall' 174 Times During Deposition About Collusion with Social Media," *The National Desk*, December 6, 2022, https://mynbc15.com/news/nation-world/fauci-says-i-dont-recall-174-times-during-deposition-about-collusion-with-social-media-missouri-attorney-general-eric-schmitt-louisiana-attorney-general-jeff-landry.
649. C. Cacciatore et al., "Extracorporeal Membrane Oxygenation (ECMO) During Aplasia: A Bridge Towards Myopericarditis Recovery After Autologous Hematopoietic Stem Cell Transplant for Systemic Sclerosis and Recent Coronarovirus Disease (COVID-19) Vaccination," *Current Research in Translational Medicine* 72 (2024): 103449.
650. A. S. Fauci and G. K. Folkers, "HIV/AIDS and COVID-19: Shared Lessons from Two Pandemics," *Clinical Infectious Diseases* (2024): ciae585.

Chapter 16

651. Carl Jung with John Freeman, "Face to Face," *BBC*, aired October 22, 1959, https://www.bbc.co.uk/programmes/p04qhvyj.
652. "The Administration: Instituting a War," *Time Magazine*, September 4, 1950, https://time.com/archive/6794101/the-administration-instituting-a-war/.
653. S. Subramanian, "John von Neumann Thought He Had the Answers," *The New Republic*, March 8, 2022, https://newrepublic.com/article/165581/john-von-neumann-man-from-future-book-review.
654. S. Kuhn, "Prisoner's Dilemma," *Stanford Encyclopedia of Philosophy*, last revised April 2, 2019, https://plato.stanford.edu/entries/prisoner-dilemma/#Sym2t2PDOrdPay.
655. R. Axelrod, "More Effective Choice in the Prisoner's Dilemma," *Journal of Conflict Resolution* 24.1 (1980): 3–25.

656. B. O'Neill, "A Survey of Game Theory Models of Peace and War," in *Handbook of Game Theory with Economic Applications*, ed. R. Aumann and S. Hart, vol. 2 (Elsevier, 1994), 995–1053.
657. K. G. Andersen et al., "The Proximal Origin of SARS-CoV-2," *Nature Medicine* 26 (2020): 450–52.
658. R. Grim, "Key Scientist in COVID Origin Controversy Misled Congress," *The Intercept*, July 21, 2023, https://theintercept.com › covid-origin-nih-lab-leak.
659. E. M. Tichy et al, "National Trends in Prescription Drug Expenditures and Projections for 2022," *American Journal of Health-System Pharmacy* 79.14 (2022): 1158–72.
660. J. Hopkins Tanne, "National Institutes of Health Criticised for Not Preventing Conflicts of Interest," *BMJ* 329.7456 (2004): 10; J. Hopkins Tanne, "Royalty Payments to Staff Researchers Causes New NIH Troubles," *BMJ* 330.7484 (2005): 162.
661. A. Andrzejewski, "NIH Scientists Made $710M in Royalties from Drug Marketing—A Fact They Tried to Hide," *New York Post*, June 2, 2024, https://nypost.com/2024/06/02/opinion/nih-scientists-made-710m-in-royalties-from-drug-makers-a-fact-they-tried-to-hide/.
662. R. Lewis, "DOGE Says Funding for Anthony Fauci Museum Exhibit Scrapped," *The National Desk*, February 10, 2025, https://thenationaldesk.com/news/americas-news-now/doge-says-funding-for-anthony-fauci-museum-exhibit-scrapped-elon-musk-department-of-government-efficiency-department-of-health-and-human-services-hhs-government-spending.
663. J. Cohen, "Accusers' Bad Math: NIH Researchers Did Not Pocket $710 Million in Royalties During Pandemic," Science Insider, June 7, 2024, https://www.science.org/content/article/bad-math-nih-researchers-didn-t-pocket-710-million-royalties-during-pandemic.
664. A. S. Fauci, *On Call: A Doctor's Journey in Public Service* (Viking, 2024), 357.
665. J. Salvucci and B, O'Connell, "Who Are the Highest Paid News Anchors?," *The Street*, November 19, 2024, https://www.thestreet.com/lifestyle/highest-paid-news-anchors-15062420.

666. J. Root, "Under Scrutiny, Perry Walks Back HPV Decision," *The Texas Tribune*, August 15, 2011, https://www.texastribune.org/2011/08/15/facing-new-scrutiny-perry-walks-back-hpv-decision/.
667. UNESCO, "Afghanistan: 1.4 Million Girls Still Banned from School by *de facto* Authorities," August 15, 2024, https://www.unesco.org/en/articles/afghanistan-14-million-girls-still-banned-school-de-facto-authorities.
668. Senator Bernie Sanders, "While the Ten Largest Drug Companies Made Over $112 Billion in Profits Last Year," YouTube, November 8, 2023, https://www.youtube.com/watch?v=rvC2fB8yLEs.
669. New York Public Interest Group, "The Supreme Court Delivers Another Blow to Representative Democracy," *NYPIRG*, July 1, 2019, https://www.nypirg.org/capitolperspective/the-supreme-court-deals-another-blow-to-representative-democracy/.
670. C. Berlet. "Mussolini on the Corporate State," Political Research Associates, January 12, 2005. https://politicalresearch.org/2005/01/12/mussolini-corporate-state.
671. George Washington, "Farewell Address, 19 September, 1796," Founders Online, https://founders.archives.gov/documents/Washington/05-20-02-0440-0002.
672. D. L. Baldwin, "How Universities Exploit the Tax-Exempt Status of Campus Land," The Law and Political Economy Project, May 15, 2024, lpeproject.org https://lpeproject.org/blog/universities-exploit-tax-exemptions-campus/#:~:text=Because%20higher%20education%20institutions%20provide,holdings%20are%20exempt%20from%20taxation.

Also Available by Richart K. Burt, MD

Everyday Miracles

Curing Multiple Sclerosis, Scleroderma, and Autoimmune Diseases by Hematopoietic Stem Cell Transplant

Foreword by His Holiness the 14th Dalai Lama

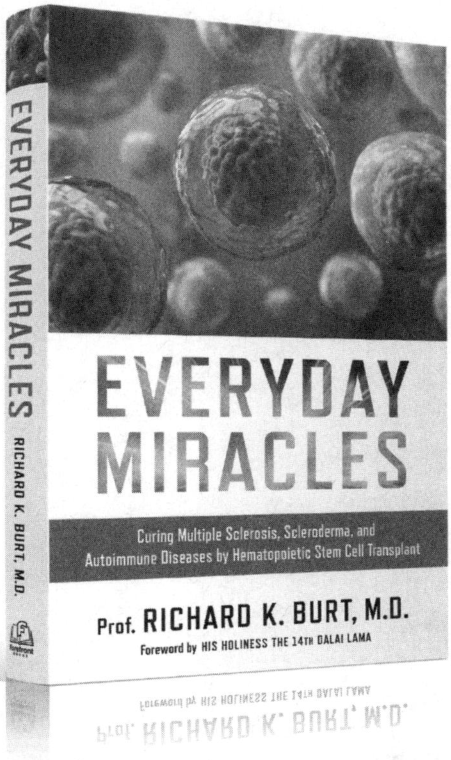

ISBN: 978-1-63763-125-6